Health Promotion for C

Maya Rom Korin

Editor

Health Promotion
for Children and Adolescents

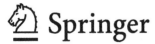 Springer

Editor
Maya Rom Korin, Ph.D., M.S.
Department of Preventive Medicine
Icahn School of Medicine at Mount Sinai
New York, NY, USA

ISBN 978-1-4939-7957-8   ISBN 978-1-4899-7711-3   (eBook)
DOI 10.1007/978-1-4899-7711-3

Printed on acid-free paper

This Springer imprint is published by Springer Nature
The registered company is Springer Science+Business Media LLC New York

Preface

Children are the most vulnerable members of society and are dependent on adults for their well-being. Communities, schools, parents, government, and various institutions strive to protect our children and provide them the environment and tools necessary to grow into healthy adults. The well-being of children determines the health of the next generation. Indeed, many of society's most severe health and social problems are caused by issues that develop during childhood and adolescence. As Healthy People 2020 points out, professionals in policy, research, and clinical practice fields are cognizant that childhood provides the physical, cognitive, and social-emotional foundation for lifelong, health, learning, and well-being, and thus health promotion strategies need to be well researched, executed, and assessed. Even from an economic perspective, investment in childhood health promotion pays off greatly.

Health promotion for children and adolescents involves a range of academic disciplines and fields in order to be successful. And thus, this book is for readers of all kinds—professionals and students in public health, public policy, education, social work, medicine and health care, and of course parents and children themselves. This book aims to bridge the gap between what is discussed in theory and academia and what health promotion programs are working on the ground.

This book presents the latest findings on the most effective methods for health promotion for children. Theory driven, the chapters highlight a multifaceted approach to health promotion, incorporating community, families, schools, and policies. Rather than using the same framework and applying it to different problems, each author presented in the book relies on different prevention and health behavior models in order to best understand the issue at hand and address the problem from a multitude of perspectives. Throughout the book, various solutions will be given using evidence-based principles to plan, implement, and evaluate community health programs that target health problems of children and adolescents. While this book was written with a US focus, the theories and approaches that are addressed are universal in nature and can easily be translated to many countries and settings.

Health Promotion for Children and Adolescents begins with an overview of health promotion theories and models in order to orient and familiarize the reader with the different theoretical approaches or tools available in conducting health promotion. The book then has two chapters that discuss the role that socioeconomics, poverty, and culture play in providing the context in which health promotion for children occurs. Part III of the book will focus on psychological wellness in children and adolescents, with Chap. 5 describing what stress and resiliency look like in children, Chap. 6 exploring recent developments in child mental health, Chap. 7 discussing youth suicide, and Chap. 8 highlighting health-related concerns among children with ADD/ADHD. Social and behavioral wellness will be the focus of Part IV. Sexual behavior, sexuality, and gender issues will be discussed in Chaps. 9 and 10, highlighting the latest research findings and debates. Chapter 11 will focus on the latest research findings in the field of alcohol, tobacco, and drug use prevention for children, while violence and aggressive behavior are covered in Chap. 12. While childhood obesity is all over news headiness these days (Chap. 13), it is unhealthy eating habits that are the root cause of both obesity and eating disorders (Chap. 14), which Chap. 15 will thoroughly address. As number of children with chronic illnesses has been increasing, Chap. 16 will cover how dealing with these illnesses is of particular challenge among children. The need for confidentiality in health services for children will appropriately follow in Chap. 17, with a look at the ethical and legal issues involved in having children be more autonomous in their health care. Chapter 18 will focus on child abuse and the foster care system.

This book was a project that could not have been completed without the hard work of so many people. Each contributing author put in time, effort, and hard work for which I am so grateful given everyone's very busy schedule and competing interests. The authors that took part in this book are some of the top scholars in the field of health promotion for children and adolescents and have been instrumental in conducting both research and programmatic efforts in their area of interest. I am appreciative of their commitment to this book and the high-quality chapters that are presented within. I would also like to thank my editors at Springer, Janet Kim and Khristine Queja, for their guidance, patience, and support throughout each step of this project. A special thanks to my family, especially my husband, Ittai, and my children, Benjamin and Gabriel, for their endless support and love.

New York, NY, USA   Maya Rom Korin, Ph.D., M.S.

Contents

Part I
The Foundation

Chapter 1
Introduction: What Is Health Promotion for Children and Adolescents?

Maya Rom Korin

1.1 What Is Health?

The concept of health has been a contested topic among public health practitioners. For many centuries, the notion of health was described as the absence of disease. With the discovery of the germ theory in the nineteenth century, the focus of public health in Western society was centered on the concept of a single cause for every disease. As chronic and noninfectious diseases started to increase in significance, it was clear that a multifactor model of disease and health was required (Blair, Stewart-Brown, Waterston, & Crowther, 2010a). The concept of human health shifted from that of a disease model to that of a health model.

The WHO historically defined health as a state of "complete physical, social, and mental well-being" and that its goal is "the attainment by all citizens of the world… of a level of health that will permit them to lead socially and economically productive lives (WHO Alma Ata 1977)." With the WHO's conceptualization of health as a human right also came the assertion that all people should have access to basic resources for health. It also emphasized that there were certain prerequisites for health, such as peace, economic resources, food, shelter, and a stable ecosystem. In addition to the WHO's definition, optimal health has also been explained as the "dynamic balance of physical, emotional, social, spiritual, and intellectual health" (ODonnell, 2009). Newer definitions of health have adopted the concept of achieving personal potential. In this context, the state of one's health is dependent upon various factors that serve as foundations for such achievement.

Perhaps a more useful metric for a given definition of health is how it is interpreted by the general public, the target of health promotion activities. Laypeople described health as the absence of illness, being physically fit, leading a "healthy"

M.R. Korin, Ph.D., M.S. (✉)
Department of Preventive Medicine, Icahn School of Medicine at Mount Sinai,
New York, NY, USA
e-mail: maya.korin@gmail.com

© Springer Science+Business Media New York 2016
M.R. Korin (ed.), *Health Promotion for Children and Adolescents*,
DOI 10.1007/978-1-4899-7711-3_1

lifestyle, having energy, having positive social relationships, being psychologically healthy, and being able to work and function in society (Lucas & Lloyd, 2005).

There has been some criticism of these definitions of health, as they are utopian in nature and unattainable, as anyone with any imperfection in their body, social, or psychological functioning is therefore not "healthy." These broad definitions are perhaps too inclusive and difficult to measure and are thought of as too vague to be practical. Additionally, health and illness are social constructs: what counts as "normal" greatly depends on cultural norms, individual interpretations, and scientific knowledge (Blaxter, 2010). Thus, while there is no clear and concise definition of health, a broad definition that includes well-being and the absence of illness is necessary for effective health promotion efforts (Institute of Medicine, 2004).

1.2   Child Health

Children have their own set of considerations for what is necessary to be healthy. While the idea of a "healthy child" seems to be factual, historically, the notion of child health was constructed through social and political considerations. It was only in the mid-eighteenth century that the concept of "childhood" even existed. The twentieth century brought a turn in ideology where the child became centered in policy and practice and children were considered in social life. Yet, childhood is more than just a social phenomenon. It has its own set of biological, physical, psychological, and environmental concerns. How we define a child matters as it determines their relation and responsibilities, their rights, and their ability to consent. This book does not define childhood by particular ages, as growth into adulthood is a process which occurs at different paces and may, in fact, never have a definitive and clear ending.

Just as the concept of childhood has changed over time, so have ideas of child health. Historically, children were seen as being part of the economic workings of a family, expected to help in household activities and contribute to the family's economic situation from a very early age. In addition to the high rate of infant and childhood mortality, there was little done to provide education, health, or other provisions specifically to children. As the shift in germ theory led to improvements in overall mortality, there was also a transformation in which children were no longer thought of as being solely the responsibility of their family but also society at large. Increased evidence of how child health was influenced by both family and social conditions led to a broadening of the definition of what was required for children to be healthy (Blair, Stewart-Brown, Waterston, & Crowther, 2010b; Kohler, 1998; Macleod, Crowther, & Stewart-Brown, 2012).

Child health has been defined as "the extent to which individual children or groups of children are able or enabled to (a) develop and realize their potential, (b) satisfy their needs, and (c) develop the capacities that allow them to interact successfully with their biological, physical, and social environments" (Institute of Medicine, 2004). This definition builds on the Ottawa Charter definition and reflects the importance of development and its multiple influences. Child health is seen as a positive resource that allows children the ability to interact with their environment and adapt to challenges and changes accordingly and acknowledges the influences of the biological, behavioral, social, and physical environments on health trajectories (Kuo, Etzel, Chilton, Watson, & Gorski, 2012). The United Nations Convention on the Rights of the Child outlines several principles that are important in child health, including the right of children to health, safety, identity, to be heard and listened to, and to participate in their health care.

While child public health shares many approaches of general public health practice, it is a distinct subspecialty that takes into account the developmental changes of children, as well as their dependence on adults for much of this period (Macleod et al., 2012). Children learn about health from a variety of sources, both formally in a school setting and through their own experiences in their family and communities, in addition to what they are exposed to through media. Children go through both sensitive and critical periods in their development, in which they are especially receptive and deterministic to influences and experiences (Institute of Medicine, 2004). Children's early experiences help shape how they will respond to challenges later on in life and how their health develops over time.

Child health and well-being is thus complicated by the fact that it encompasses both children's present lives and their future development. It is both "being" and "becoming"—life as it is experienced and life as it develops—and having the balance between those tenses. One does not want to only invest in a child's future at the expense of their current state. Thus, child health and well-being must be placed within a life course framework in which both the present and future are taken into account (Ben-Aryeh, Frønes, Casas, & Korbin, 2013).

There are numerous influences to children's health that start as early as the intrauterine environment. Children are dependent on adults for many of these influences, such that parenting, family structure, communities, and media play a large role in how children are not only perceived but also in how they perceive themselves and their well-being. As children are not able to play a part in the circumstances in which they were born and raised, they are more susceptible to social and ecological factors such as inequalities and unsafe environments. Their vulnerability makes it particularly challenging and important for public health practitioners to make sure that all the factors that play a role in child health are adequately accounted for.

1.3   Health Promotion

With all the varying definitions of health, what exactly is the definition of health promotion? Health promotion has been defined as a *process* that empowers people to change their personal behavior and lifestyle and creates and supports environments that contribute to healthy living (Nutbeam, 1986; Simons-Morton, 2013). It takes on the complicated web of health-related behavior and is often defined as a combination of health education and economic, organizational, and environmental support for healthy behaviors in individuals and communities (Green, Wilson, & Lovato, 1986). Taken out of the boundaries of health institutions, health promotion utilizes all aspects that related to the health of humans — policies, programs, science, and practices (Green, 1999). It is then any combination of educational, political, regulatory, and organizational interventions that work toward improving the health of individuals and communities (Green & Kreuter, 2005).

Health promotion has often been described as the actual practice of public health. While epidemiology is often thought of as the "science" of public health, health promotion is the actionable arm (McQueen, 2000). A newer definition has termed health promotion as the "art and science" of helping people strive for optimal health through learning experiences as well as a supportive environment (ODonnell, 2009). The WHO defines it as:

> ... the process of enabling people to increase control over, and to improve, their health. To reach a state of complete physical, mental and social well-being, an individual or group must be able to identify and to realize aspirations, to satisfy needs, and to change or cope with the environment. Health is, therefore, seen as a resource for everyday life, not the objective of living. Health is a positive concept emphasizing social and personal resources, as well as physical capacities. Therefore, health promotion is not just the responsibility of the health sector, but goes beyond healthy life-styles to well-being. (World Health Organization, 1986)

An important aspect of health promotion is that it empowers people to control and improve their health. Health promotion aims to enhance the participation of individuals to improve their living circumstances which contribute to health. While much of health promotion goes beyond the realm of the individual, the concept of empowerment is an especially significant component in children and adolescents. This notion of power and control over one's own health and the health of one's community plays out in the types of interventions health promotion utilizes (Laverack, 2007). For example, while health education strategies increase knowledge and awareness so that people can make more informed choices about their own health on an individual level, community development and capacity building allow for increased resources that can be drawn upon for the same purpose.

Thus, health promotion is a social and political process that empowers individuals through actions that strengthen skills and capabilities, as well as those that change the social, environmental, and economic conditions required to support health. It demands participation in order to sustain its efforts, with people at the center of health promotion action and decision making. Health promotion must also be comprehensive in scope, including advocacy for health to create health conditions, enabling and empowering people to reach their full potential, and mediating between competing interests in order to best enhance health (Nutbeam, 1986; World Health Organization, 1986).

1.4   Health Promotion for Children and Adolescents

There is no clear definition of health promotion for children and adolescents that is utilized throughout the field. Much of the strategies employed in health promotion for children stem from those used in adult health promotion. For the purposes of this book, we will define health promotion for children and adolescents as those strategies that promote child and young people's health, prevent disease in children and young people, and foster equity for children and young people, within a framework of sustainable development (Kohler, 1998). This involves advocating for children and enabling their voices to be heard, promoting a broad sense of health and well-being, assessing health needs, implementing a range of public health interventions, seeing children in the context of their families and communities, and cooperating between a wide network of individuals and organizations. Using the Ottawa Charter for Health Promotion, health promotion for children and adolescents needs to include five "pillars":

1. Building healthy public policy that takes into account child health concerns.
2. Creating supportive environments that allow children to make healthy choices.
3. Strengthening communities such that children feel safe and that there is a sense of equity.
4. Reorienting health services to ensure that children's health care is easily accessed and that service needs are met.
5. Developing personal knowledge and skills so that children receive appropriate health knowledge that support physical, emotional, and social development.

Health promotion for children thus operates in a variety of levels, involving a broad range of individuals and organizations, all for the goal of improving children health and wellness (Macleod et al., 2012).

One of the key tenets of health promotion is the active participation of individuals. Yet children are often left out of health promotion efforts, instead subjected to a top-down approach where they are treated as passive consumers. By not including them in the dialogue, children are given the message that they are not worth listening to and that others should make decisions for them. Children should be seen as active and competent subjects in the planning of interventions, as mastery over their health and lives is an important part of development. Many studies have shown that children's participation in their health is a crucial tool in health promotion efforts and children who learn by doing are better equipped to handle the social pressures of various detrimental health behaviors (Bandura, 2004; De Winter, Baerveldt, & Kooistra, 1999).

This book will highlight the breadth of health promotion efforts for children and adolescents. From fostering resilience, to obesity prevention, to tackling issues in confidentiality, the following chapters will demonstrate the public health challenges currently facing children and adolescents and the wide range of interventions that are utilized in health promotion. As demonstrated above, health and wellness are broad concepts that when applied to children require distinct strategies and special attention.

References

Bandura, A. (2004). Health promotion by social cognitive means. *Health Education & Behavior: The Official Publication of the Society for Public Health Education, 31*(2), 143–64. http://doi.org/10.1177/1090198104263660.

Ben-Aryeh, A., Frønes, I., Casas, F., & Korbin, J. E. (2013). *Handbook of child well-being: Theories, methods and policies in global perspective*. Dordrecht, The Netherlands, Springer. Retrieved from http://dx.doi.org/10.1007/978-90-481-9063-8.

Blair, M., Stewart-Brown, S., Waterston, T., & Crowther, R. (2010a). Key concepts and definitions. In *Child Public Health* (2nd ed.). Oxford: Oxford University Press. http://doi.org/10.1093/acprof:oso/9780199547500.003.005.

Blair, M., Stewart-Brown, S., Waterston, T., & Crowther, R. (2010b). Why child public health? In *Child Public Health* (2nd ed.). Oxford: Oxford University Press. http://doi.org/10.1093/acprof:oso/9780199547500.003.000.

Blaxter, M. (2010). How is health constructed? In M. Blaxter (Ed.), *Health* (pp. 28–47). Cambridge: Polity.

De Winter, M., Baerveldt, C., & Kooistra, J. (1999). Enabling children: participation as a new perspective on child-health promotion. *Child: Care, Health and Development*, 25(1), 15–23. http://doi.org/10.1046/j.1365-2214.1999.00073.x.

Green, L. W. (1999). Health education's contributions to public health in the twentieth century: A glimpse through health promotion's rear-view mirror. *American Review of Public Health, 20*, 67–88.

Green, L. W., & Kreuter, M. W. (2005). *Health program planning: An educational and ecological approach* (4th ed.). New York: McGraw-Hill Higher Education.

Green, L. W., Wilson, A. L., & Lovato, C. Y. (1986). What changes can health promotion achieve and how long do these changes last? The trade-offs between expediency and durability. *Preventive Medicine, 15*(5), 508–521. http://doi.org/http://dx.doi.org/10.1016/0091-7435(86)90027-7.

Health Resources and Services Administration—Maternal and Child Health Bureau. (2014). *Child Health USA 2014*. Rockville.

Institute of Medicine. (2004). *Children's health, the nation's wealth: Assessing and improving child health*. Washington, DC: National Academies Press.

Kohler, L. (1998). Child public health. *European Journal of Public Health, 8*(3), 253–255. Retrieved from http://eurpub.oxfordjournals.org/content/8/3/253.abstract.

Kuo, A. A., Etzel, R. A., Chilton, L. A., Watson, C., & Gorski, P. A. (2012). Primary care pediatrics and public health: Meeting the needs of today's children. *American Journal of Public Health, 102*. http://doi.org/10.2105/AJPH.2012.301013.

Laverack, G. (2007). *Health promotion practice: Building empowered communities*. Buckingham, GBR: Open University Press.

Lucas, K., & Lloyd, B. (2005). *Health promotion: Evidence and experience*. London: Sage.

Macleod, K. L., Crowther, R., & Stewart-Brown, S. (2012). The health of children and young people. In S. Gillam, J. Yates, & P. Badrinath (Eds.), *Essential public health* (pp. 209–226). Cambridge: Cambridge University Press.

McQueen, D. V. (2000). Perspectives on health promotion: theory, evidence, practice and the emergence of complexity. *Health Promotion International, 15*(2), 95–97. http://doi.org/10.1093/heapro/15.2.95.

Nutbeam, D. (1986). Health promotion glossary. *Health Promotion. 1* (1), 113–27. http://doi.org/10.1093/heapro/1.1.113.

ODonnell, M. P. (2009). Definition of health promotion 2.0: Embracing passion, enhancing motivation, recognizing dynamic balance, and creating opportunities. *American Journal of Health Promotion, 24*. http://doi.org/10.4278/ajhp.24.1.iv.

Simons-Morton, B. (2013). Health Behavior in Ecological Context. *Health Education & Behavior, 40*(1), 6–10. http://doi.org/10.1177/1090198112464494.

World Health Organization. (1986). *The Ottawa Charter for health promotion*. Geneva: Author.

Chapter 2
Theory and Fundamentals of Health Promotion for Children and Adolescents

Maya Rom Korin

2.1 The Importance of Theory

Health promotion, and more broadly, public health, is very much a discipline of "action." While one may not need to understand theory to promote health, for an intervention to be effective, it is helpful to understand the theories surrounding health behavior, health promotion, and public health.

What exactly is theory? In simplest terms, theories are ways in which we can explain a phenomenon. A theory is an explanatory framework in which helps us understand and predict the ways in which individuals or societies operate. And although theories are abstract and conceptual, they can be tested in a systematic fashion (Viswanath, Orleans, Glanz, & Rimer, 2008). A fully developed theory can explain (1) factors that influence the phenomenon, (2) the relationship between these factors, and (3) the circumstances in which these relationships occur (Nutbeam, Harris, & Wise, 2010). Theory helps bind a discipline as well as provide boundaries, while on a pragmatic level, it provides a guide for a discipline's practice.

In many ways, theory and practice have often been pitted as opposite concepts, with research or empirical investigation serving as a way to bridge these two ideas by testing the theory in action. Indeed, "theory, research, and practice are a continuum along which the skilled professional should move with ease. Not only are they related but they are each essential to health education and health behavior" (Viswanath et al., 2008). The relationship between theory, research, and practice is complex and perhaps can better be described as a cycle of interacting endeavors that feed off of each other. Theory provides the conceptual underpinning to research and practice, while both research and practice provide the empirical evidence to better shape concepts within theory.

M.R. Korin, Ph.D., M.S. (✉)
Department of Preventive Medicine, Icahn School of Medicine at Mount Sinai, New York, NY, USA
e-mail: maya.korin@gmail.com

© Springer Science+Business Media New York 2016
M.R. Korin (ed.), *Health Promotion for Children and Adolescents*,
DOI 10.1007/978-1-4899-7711-3_2

Theory needs to be understood and applicable in a variety of settings in order to be useful. In essence, theories are distilled representations of our reality, and while they can never be totally encompassing of all the nuances of behavior, a good theory can be a helpful guide toward effective programming. Theories can help define the problem, provide guidance on how and where to target change, and determine a benchmark to implement and evaluate the program (Nutbeam et al., 2010). Within health promotion, theories can both explain health behavior and propose ways to change behavior. Explanatory theories explain the origin of a certain health behavior, while theories of action help guide the development of interventions (Viswanath et al., 2008).

2.1.1 Two Theoretical Paradigms

Given the diversity of the field of public health and health promotion, people often draw upon varying theories depending on the focus of their work. While some argue that this diversity brings about contention and competing public health action, the multidisciplinary nature of public health must include a variety of theories, as the reasons for health behavior are complex and multilayered.

One of the main contentions in the field of health promotion is the dualism between the individualist and structuralist approaches to health. Those that promote individualist theories argue that people exercise control over their health, and thus it is their responsibility to maintain it. Structuralist proponents argue that one cannot extricate an individual's health from the social, environmental, political, and economic conditions in which it occurs, and of which individuals have little control (Bandura, 2004).

Recently, the focus of "changing health behavior through a sequential change in knowledge, attitudes, and beliefs is no longer a prevailing paradigm in health promotion research" (Crosby & Noar, 2010). Intervening at multiple levels across the ecological spectrum is accepted as the better approach. Thus, there is a disconnect between current theories in health promotion, which are centered on the individual, and the broad set of influences on health behavior. Much of medicine depends on a "single cause-single disease" model, which proves to be insufficient when addressing the complexities of health behaviors and health problems (Livingood et al., 2011). There is the need for a better understanding of "how social factors regulate behaviors, or distribute individuals into risk groups, and how these social factors come to be embodied" (Glass & McAtee, 2006). Understanding how the more "upstream" factors influence the "downstream" individual factors has been essential to producing effective health promotion programs.

This chapter will first look at both individual-based theories and models to better understand the psychological frameworks that are used within health promotion. Broader social and ecological models will then be described. Intervention and planning models will be reviewed in order to provide a structured sequence in which to guide and conduct health promotion interventions.

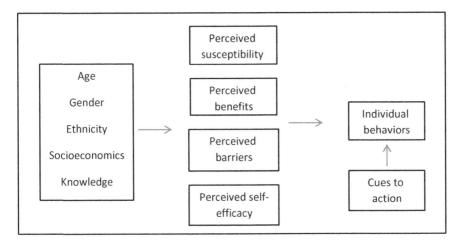

Fig. 2.1 Health belief model

2.2 Individual-Based Theories and Models

2.2.1 The Health Belief Model

The health belief model (HBM) was established in the early 1950s to understand why many people do not adhere to preventive health efforts. It has been one of the most widely used conceptual frameworks in health behavior research and interventions (Viswanath et al., 2008). This model takes into consideration psychological and behavior theories that posit the value a person places on a goal and their interpretation of how likely it is that that goal can be achieved. When put into a health context, the health behavior model attempts to predict the likelihood of person taking action for health problem using several concepts: susceptibility, severity, and the benefits and barriers to a behavior.

HBM suggests that individuals will take action if they perceive themselves to be susceptible to the illness or condition (perceived susceptibility), that this illness will have serious consequences (perceived severity), a course of action will minimize consequences (perceived benefits), and the benefits of taking action will outweigh the costs or barriers (perceived barriers) (Janz & Becker, 1984; Rosenstock, Strecher, & Becker, 1988; Rosenstock, 1974). The HBM suggests that before people change their behavior, they go through a process in which they weigh information before they reach a decision. Later iterations of the model have included modifying factors that are associated with personal characteristics and social circumstances, as well as Bandura's concept of self-efficacy (Fig. 2.1).

Critical reviews of HBM have shown empirical support for the model, through both prospective and retrospective studies (Harrison, Mullen, & Green, 1992; Janz & Becker, 1984; Rosenstock et al., 1988). In a 10-year review, Jan and Becker (1984) found that perceived barriers were the most powerful predictors across all studies and perceived susceptibility was a strong predictor of preventive health behavior. Nevertheless, HBM has been criticized as a psychosocial model; it is limited to only what can be explained by individuals' attitudes and beliefs. HBM leaves out things such as the habitual nature of many behaviors, that many people take on behaviors for non-health-related outcomes, and that people are often constrained from making rational choices because of their environment. Additionally, the model is based on the premise that most people value health and their behaviors are driven by health goals (Janz & Becker, 1984).

Despite these critiques, the Health Behavior Model is still a widely used and helpful model, particularly for traditional preventive health behaviors such as screening and immunization. It is also helpful in providing a simple way to illustrate the importance of individual's belief about health and can assist practitioners to focus on ways to personalize and facilitate individual behavior change.

2.2.2   Reasoned Action and Planned Behavior

The theory of reasoned action and its subsequent extension, the theory of planned behavior, have been highly utilized in health promotion. The theory of reasoned action assumes that human behavior is for the most part rational and controllable. It posits that people's likelihood to engage in a behavior, or behavioral intention, is predicated by their attitudes and subjective norms. One's attitude toward a behavior is determined by the sum of one's beliefs in that behavior and one's evaluations of this belief. For example, one may believe that exercise is healthy and improves appearance but is also hard and time-consuming. Each of these beliefs is then weighted (looking good may be more important to than comfort) to form an attitude. Subjective norms are the influence and expectations in one's social environment on performing the behavior in question. For example, a person may have many friends that exercise and encourage group participation, but also a significant other that is more sedentary. He or she then weighs the importance of each of those people's opinions. For any specific behavior, personal attitudes may be more or less important, depending on the weight attributed to subjective norms. Thus, in order for a health behavior intervention to be effective, it needs to take into account how the behavior is influenced by social norms and personal attitudes (Fishbein & Ajzen, 1975; Madden, Ellen, & Ajzen, 1992).

The theory of planned behavior (Ajzen, 1991) expanded the theory of reasoned action and targeted situations where individuals do not have full control over the behavior in question. While behavioral intention is still of central importance, it is not only influenced by attitude and subjective norms, but also by one's perceived control over said behavior. Perceived behavioral control refers to an individual's perception of the ease or difficulty with which they can change a particular behavior; this perceived control varies across situations and actions. It can not only have a direct effect on behavior but also an indirect effect through behavioral intentions.

Thus, when a person believes that they have little resources or ability to engage in a behavior, their behavioral intention may be low even if they have positive attitudes and subjective norms toward the behavior.

Together, these two theories are useful to think about the information that is needed from individuals in order to create a program or intervention that meets their health needs. They both underscore the importance of taking into account people's beliefs around an issue, who are the main influencers to those beliefs, and how much control they think they have around this behavior (Willis & Earle, 2007). Several meta-analyses (Armitage & Conner, 2001; Godin & Kok, 1996) found that social norms seem to be less important in predicting behavior than attitude and perceived behavioral control. While issues have been raised in the measuring of these constructs (Ajzen, 2011), the theory of planned behavior has been shown to accurately predict intentions and behavior, making it an important theory to consider in health promotion.

2.2.3   Stages of Change/Transtheoretical Model of Change

The transtheoretical model of change, also known as the stages of change model, was developed to explain the different stages individuals go through in adopting a behavior (Prochaska & DiClemente, 1986). It is based on the premise that behavior change is an ongoing process and that people have different motivations or readiness to change. Because it utilizes constructs and processes from different theories, it is dubbed "transtheoretical."

The five stages are as follows:

- Precontemplation—when an individual is not even considering changing their behavior or those that are consciously intending not to change
- Contemplation—the stage at which a person is considering making a change to a specific behavior
- Determination—the stage in which a person makes a commitment to change
- Action—the stage in which the behavior change is initiated and the individual is explicitly changing their behavior
- Maintenance—the stage of sustaining the change and achievement of health gains

A sixth stage, *termination*, has been identified as being appropriate for certain behaviors such as addiction. It is the stage in which individuals who have changed their behavior have no temptation to return to their old behavior.

The model was based on observations that people appear to move through these stages in predictable ways, although some move through them quicker than others, and others get "stuck" at a particular stage. People can also move backward and forward through the stages, and as the model is circular, people can enter or exit at any point. It applies to both people who self-initiate and those who respond to advice and encouragement to change.

The transtheoretical model is helpful in tailoring interventions to the stage at which people are in the change process. On the individual level, for example, it can provide a useful way for health-care providers to think about the advice that they give their patients, establishing whether their patient wants to change, determining what are the barriers to change, and understanding that relapse is a common problem. For planning intervention programs, the model is useful in figuring out how activities should be staged. For example, for those populations in the precontemplation stage, education and consciousness raising will be important, while for those that have already initiated the behavior, programs that provide social support are more relevant.

DiClemente (2005) emphasized a third dimension of the model, the context of change. He argues that the environment, both internal and external, in which the targeted behavior change occurs is an important contribution to the process of the change and the ability to move through the process. For example, in order for people to eat healthy and make healthy food choices, they need to be in an environment where there is easy access and availability to healthy food.

The transtheoretical model has been used as an important reference point in health interventions ranging from smoking cessation, to physical activity, to HIV prevention (DiClemente et al., 1991; Prochaska, Redding, Harlow, Rossi, & Velicer, 1994; Sarkin, Johnson, Prochaska, & Prochaska, 2001). It emphasizes the range of needs in any population and the necessity for sequencing the interventions so that interventions address all the different stages of change. A 2005 review (Bridle et al., 2005) found that there was limited evidence in the effectiveness from interventions using this model, although the methodological quality of these studies was questionable. Nevertheless, the model is useful in settings such as behavioral psychology and clinical settings.

2.3 Social/Ecological Theories of Health

2.3.1 Social Cognitive Theory

The social cognitive theory (SCT) was built on the understanding of the reciprocal interaction between an individual and their environment and addresses both what determines health behavior and how to promote change. While most behavioral and social theories emphasize individual, environmental, and social factors that influence behavior, SCT posits that there is a dynamic interplay between these factors and that the relationship between people and their environment can be both subtle and complex. This emphasis on *reciprocal determinism*, as Bandura labels it, calls for an understanding of the continuous interaction between individuals, their environment, and their behavior. Thus, while environments can influence how people behave, people can also alter and construct environments to suit their purposes (Bandura, 1986).

In addition to this interactive dynamic, Bandura also explains a range of personal cognitive factors that affect behaviors and the environment. It lays out that people's actions are not only based on an objective reality but rather their perceptions of it. First, knowledge of health risks and benefits are the precondition for change, as people need to know how their lifestyle habits affect their health in order to embark to change habits that they enjoy (Bandura, 2004). People often learn about certain behaviors by observing others (*observational learning*), marking the importance of peer influence and social norms on health behavior. Second, people place value on *expectations*, such that in order to embark on a new behavior, they need to understand what the potential outcome will be when the behavior is repeated. These expectancies are greatly influenced by the environment of the observer and highlight the importance of understanding the motivations behind different behaviors. Third, and most importantly, is the concept of *self-efficacy*. Self-efficacy is one's belief in their ability to perform a behavior. Bandura states that self-efficacy is the most important prerequisite to behavior change and will greatly affect how much effort is placed into the task. People with high self-efficacy are more likely to take on challenges and recover quickly from setbacks and disappointments, while those with low self-efficacy are less confident and thus less likely to embark on tasks deemed to be difficult. Meta-analyses have shown that self-efficacy plays an influential role across multiple domains of health functioning and indeed is the focal determinant. It affects people's goals and aspirations, how they view barriers, and shapes the outcomes people expect to produce (Bandura, 1986, 1991, 2004).

In terms of the environmental influences, social cognitive theory describes how the environment needs to support behavior modification. One such way is through *incentive motivation* which provides rewards or punishment depending on the behavior, through such things as policies or punitive laws (i.e., tobacco taxation). Another approach is *facilitation* which provides resources that allows behaviors easier to perform (i.e., free condom distribution).

Overall, the social cognitive theory provides a comprehensive base for health promotion programs. It gives a conceptual framework for understanding what influences individual human behavior, the processes in which learning occurs, and the broader environmental concerns. SCT also offers practical directions for health practitioners to modify these various influences through individual, community, and policy changes.

2.3.2 Ecological Model of Health Promotion

A broader view of health behavior takes into account an individual's lifetime exposure to the influences of family, community, and society (Glass & McAtee, 2006). The ecological model of health promotion, having its roots in the earliest iterations of public health, presents health as an "interdependence between the individual and subsystems of the ecosystem" (Green, Richard, & Potvin, 1996). It acknowledges multiple levels and dimensions of determinants of health, ranging from environmental, policy, social, and psychological. Because of this explicit consideration of multiple levels of influence, interventions stemming from this model are more comprehensive.

At its core, the ecological model of health promotion presents health "as the product of the interdependence between the individual and subsystems of the ecosystem" (Green, Richard, & Potvin, 1996). These subsystems include intrapersonal (psychological, biological), interpersonal (social, cultural, family), community, physical environment, and policy (McLeroy, Bibeau, Steckler, & Glanz, 1988). This behavior-environment interaction is reciprocal in nature, where the environment controls and influences behavior and the behavior of individuals, groups, and organizations influences and changes their environment. This comprehensive framework allows for intervention approaches to target changes at multiple levels of influence and posits that multi-level interventions are the most effective in changing behavior.

The four main principles of the ecological perspective are the following: (1) there are multiple levels of factors that influence health behavior and some concepts cut across levels such as sociocultural factors and physical environment; (2) there is interaction across levels such that variables work together; (3) multi-level interventions are most effective in changing behavior and having sustaining effects; and (4) ecological models are most useful when they are behavior specific. The ecological approach posits features of the social and built environment above and before the individual that constrain, limit, reward, and induce the behavior of the individual (Glass & McAtee, 2006).

The ecological model takes into account the importance of *contextualizing* individual behavior. People act differently in different environments, and effectiveness of any health promotion strategy depends on its fit to the specific environment in which the intervention is to be applied. Educating and providing skills to change behavior is not sufficient if the existing environment and policies stand in the way of making healthy choices. Thus, one can teach and motivate people to eat healthy foods and exercise, but if their environment does not consist of places to purchase healthy food or safe places to exercise, much of the "choice" behind the behaviors disappears.

One critique of the ecological model is that it offers limited guidance on the dynamic interactions of these factors and the unique elements of settings (Livingood et al., 2011). Because of its complexity, the model lacks specificity about what is most important and burdens the health professional with the task of figuring out what the critical factors are for each health behavior. The ecological model makes it difficult to create testable hypotheses and is challenging to manipulate experimentally. Thus, while it broadens the perspective of understanding health, it is problematic to operationalize. Additionally, the ecological perspective is that everything influences everything, leading many to throw their hands up in despair at the lack of parameters or control over these complex, intertwined systems (Green, Richard, & Potvin, 1996).

A review of 157 intervention articles over 20 years (Golden & Earp, 2012) found that the majority of interventions targeted only one or two ecological levels and most remained focused on individual beliefs and attitudes of social networks. This is perhaps because given limited funding and resources, it is unrealistic for an intervention to tackle three or more ecological levels. Given its limitations, some have argued that the ecological model may be most useful as a tool to help frame and contextualize health behavior rather than a guideline for interventions. Nevertheless, the ecological framework highlights that it is important to consider multi-level approaches to improving health behavior and to create environments and policies that make it possible to make healthy choices.

2.4 Intervention Models

2.4.1 Tiered Prevention

Much of health promotion involves prevention, which are those interventions that occur before the onset of disease or disorder. Health promotion can occur at multiple levels, but, in order to best intervene, it is important to tailor efforts according to "disease-risk cycle." This categorization can distinguish between a person's and community's current health status (Martin, Haskard-Zolnierek, & DiMatteo, 2009).

Disease prevention strategies were often defined as being either primary (before the onset of disease via risk reduction), secondary (detecting the disease and treating preclinical changes), or tertiary (to soften the impact after disease progression). There is an implied understanding of the etiology of the disease in question, such that there is a clear mechanism between cause of the disease and the occurrence and clinical manifestations. While this long-used classification was useful when diseases were pathogenic in nature, it is not as useful for those chronic disease or lifestyle health behaviors.

In response, Gordon (1983) proposed a model where interventions are broken down into three areas based on the costs and benefits of delivering the intervention to the targeted population. *Universal prevention* is defined as interventions that are offered to the general population regardless of risk. *Selective prevention* refers to interventions that are targeted to the subpopulation that are at high risk for developing the disorder or problem. *Indicated prevention* includes interventions that are targeted to individuals identified to be at high risk based on individual assessment but are currently asymptomatic (Gordon, 1983). This hierarchy recognizes the more complex interaction between risk and protective factors and the need to balance where people are in the spectrum of risk and the cost and discomfort of the preventive intervention.

Within the realm of public health and health promotion, there has been a blending of these classification systems where they are often used interchangeably. Yet Gordon believed that there was an important distinction between prevention and treatment, especially with conditions that are chronic and behavior driven (National Research Council, 1994). The tiered model of prevention has been extensively used within health promotion for children, particularly in the school setting. Using this model, a universal intervention would include all the children in a school or making a particular change school-wide. A selective intervention would target students in a smaller setting that are at-risk for a particular behavior. An indicated intervention would be for those particular students that are exhibiting some problem behaviors (Fedewa, Candelaria, Erwin, & Clark, 2013; Kratochwill, Albers, & Steele Shernoff, 2004; Lane, Oakes, Menzies, Oyer, & Jenkins, 2013; Tomb & Hunter, 2004).

2.4.2   PRECEDE-PROCEED

One attempt to create a comprehensive model for planning and evaluating a range of health issues at all levels (individual behavioral to environmental to national and policy) is the PRECEDE-PROCEED model (L.W. Green & Kreuter, 2005). The PRECEDE-PROCEED diagnostic approach to program planning is comprised of two steps: (1) PRECEDE (predisposing, reinforcing, and enabling constructs in educational/environmental diagnosis and evaluation) which is known as the diagnostic stage and (2) the development stage, PROCEED (policy, regulatory, and organizational constructs in educational and environmental development). This model provides systematic steps to both diagnose and plan interventions in a way that takes the ecological paradigm and breaks it down into manageable applications. As such, it involves all stakeholders affected by the health issue from the beginning and assumes that health is a community issue that is an integral part of a larger context. Health has a reciprocal relationship with the environment and is comprised of a constellation of factors.

The diagnostic part of the model, PRECEDE, is split into four phases:

- Phase 1 identifies and evaluates the social problems that have an impact on the population of interest. This is done by engaging the audience and finding out what it is that their community needs and then determining the desired outcome.
- Phase 2 diagnoses the epidemiological, behavioral, and environmental issues and factors that might cause or influence the desired outcome. This involves looking at epidemiological data such as vital statistics and health surveys, analyzing behavioral links to the health issue, and assessing the environmental factors that are beyond the control of the individual that influence the health outcome.
- Phase 3 isolates the predisposing, enabling, and reinforcing factors that influence the behaviors, attitudes, and environment. Predisposing factors are characteristics that motivate behavior—knowledge, beliefs, and values often fall into this category. Enabling factors are programs, services, and resources that help facilitate action to attain a behavior. Reinforcing behaviors are the attitudes and consequences that support or make it difficult to adopt a behavior.
- Phase 4 focuses on the administrative, policy, and regulatory issues that can influence the implementation of the intervention.

The PROCEED phases involve the implementation and evaluation of the intervention:

- Phase 5 implements an intervention based on the analysis conducted during the PRECEDE phases.

- Phase 6 evaluates the process of implementing the intervention and determines if the program is being implemented according to protocol with its objectives being met.
- Phase 7 measures the effectiveness of the intervention with regard to both the immediate objectives and changes in the predisposing, enabling, and reinforcing factors.
- Phase 8 evaluates the outcome in terms of both the overall objectives of the intervention and the changes in health and quality of life.

The PRECEDE-PROCEED model provides a stepwise structure or a road map within which a health intervention can be evaluated and planned. Its inclusion of community member participation allows for a feedback loop through which ideas are tested and adjusted for greater effectiveness. The model has the ability to adapt the chosen structure to fit the needs of a specific environment and community. It is a flexible, comprehensive, and scaleable model that has been used in thousands of applications in both global and national settings.

2.5 Conclusion

The theories outlined in this chapter highlight both individual and environmental approaches to health promotion. Yet it is important to highlight that these theories are not specifically geared toward children and as such are limited in their applicability. Children's health behaviors change as they develop and mature, and it is necessary to identify the changing biological, cognitive, social, and environmental factors over time. There has yet to be a health promotion theory that integrates the developmental perspectives into the existing models of understanding health behaviors. There are distinct opportunities to influence children's health behaviors across the developmental stages that need to be taken into account when designing health promotion interventions.

The field of modern health promotion is still trying to define itself, and, as such, the theories that are highlighted in this chapter are still not very well developed in their guidance of the field. Many theories have stemmed from other fields within public health, and while they have been tested, there is still no overarching theory that encompasses a comprehensive health promotion model. The challenge is to pair the appropriate theories of health behavior within a comprehensive planning process. This chapter provided an introduction to various theories and indicates their potential application within health promotion for children and adolescents. Many of the contributing authors in this book discuss the applications of these theories within their chapters.

References

Ajzen, I. (1991). The theory of planned behavior. *Organizational Behavior and Human Decision Processes, 50*(2), 179–211. http://doi.org/10.1016/0749-5978 (91)90020-T.

Ajzen, I. (2011). The theory of planned behaviour: Reactions and reflections. *Psychology and Health, 26*(9), 1113–1127. http://doi.org/http://dx.doi.org/10.1080/08870446.2011.613995.

Armitage, C., & Conner, M. (2001). Efficacy of the theory of planned behaviour: A meta-analytic review. *British Journal of Social Psychology, 40*, 471–499. http://doi.org/10.1348/014466601164939.

Bandura, A. (Ed.). (1986). *Social foundations of thought and action: A social cognitive theory* (Vol. 13). Englewood Cliffs, NJ: Prentice-Hall. 617 p.

Bandura, A. (1991). Social cognitive theory of self regulation. *Organizational Behavior and Human Decision Processes, 50*, 248–287.

Bandura, A. (2004). Health promotion by social cognitive means. *Health Education & Behavior : The Official Publication of the Society for Public Health Education, 31*(2), 143–164. http://doi.org/10.1177/1090198104263660.

Bridle, C., Riemsma, R. P., Pattenden, J., Sowden, A. J., Mather, L., Watt, I. S., & Walker, A. (2005). Systematic review of the effectiveness of health behavior interventions based on the transtheoretical model. *Psychology & Health*. http://doi.org/10.1080/08870440512331333997.

Crosby, R., & Noar, S. M. (2010). Theory development in health promotion: Are we there yet? *Journal of Behavioral Medicine, 33*(4), 259–263. http://doi.org/http://dx.doi.org/10.1007/s10865-010-9260-1.

DiClemente, C. C., Prochaska, J. O., Fairhurst, S. K., Velicer, W. F., Velasquez, M. M., & Rossi, J. S. (1991). The process of smoking cessation: an analysis of precontemplation, contemplation, and preparation stages of change. *Journal of Consulting and Clinical Psychology, 59.*

Fedewa, A. L., Candelaria, A., Erwin, H. E., & Clark, T. P. (2013). Incorporating physical activity into the schools using a 3-tiered approach. *Journal of School Health, 83*(4), 290–297. http://doi.org/10.1111/josh.12029.

Fishbein, M., & Ajzen, I. (1975). *Belief, attitude, intention, and behavior*. Reading, MA: Addison-Wesley.

Glass, T. A., & McAtee, M. J. (2006). Behavioral science at the crossroads in public health: Extending horizons, envisioning the future. *Social Science & Medicine, 62*(7), 1650–1671. http://doi.org/http://dx.doi.org/10.1016/j.socscimed.2005.08.044.

Godin, G., & Kok, G. (1996). The theory of planned behavior: a review of its applications to health-related behaviors. *American Journal of Health Promotion, 11*(2), 87–98.

Golden, S. D., & Earp, J. A. L. (2012). Social ecological approaches to individuals and their contexts: Twenty years of health education & behavior health promotion interventions. *Health Education & Behavior : The Official Publication of the Society for Public Health Education, 39*, 364–372. http://doi.org/10.1177/1090198111418634.

Gordon, R. S. (1983). An operational classification of disease prevention. *Public Health Reports, 98*(2), 107–109.

Green, L. W., & Kreuter, M. W. (2005). *Health program planning: An educational and ecological approach* (4th ed.). New York: McGraw-Hill Higher Education.

Green, L. W., Richard, L., & Potvin, L. (1996). Ecological foundations of health promotion. *American Journal of Health Promotion, 10*(4), 270–281. http://doi.org/10.4278/0890-1171-10.4.270.

Harrison, J. A., Mullen, P. D., & Green, L. W. (1992). A meta-analysis of studies of the health belief model with adults. *Health Education Research, 7*(1), 107–116. http://doi.org/10.1093/her/7.1.107.

Janz, N. K., & Becker, M. H. (1984). The health belief model: A decade later. *Health Education & Behavior, 11*, 1–47. http://doi.org/10.1177/109019818401100101.

Kratochwill, T. R., Albers, C. A., & Steele Shernoff, E. (2004). School-based interventions. *Child and Adolescent Psychiatric Clinics of North America, 13*(4), 885–903. http://doi.org/10.1016/j.chc.2004.05.003.

Lane, K. L., Oakes, W. P., Menzies, H. M., Oyer, J., & Jenkins, A. (2013). Working within the context of three-tiered models of prevention: Using schoolwide data to identify high school students for targeted supports. *Journal of Applied School Psychology, 29*(2), 203–229. http://doi.org/10.1080/15377903.2013.778773.

Livingood, W. C., Allegrante, J. P., Airhihenbuwa, C. O., Clark, N. M., Windsor, R. C., Zimmerman, M. A., & Green, L. W. (2011). Applied Social and Behavioral Science to Address Complex Health Problems. *American Journal of Preventive Medicine, 41* (5), 525–531. http://doi.org/http://dx.doi.org/10.1016/j.amepre.2011.07.021

Madden, T. J., Ellen, P. S., & Ajzen, I. (1992). A comparison of the theory of planned behavior and the theory of reasoned action. *Personality and Social Psychology Bulletin, 18*(1), 3–9. http://doi.org/10.1177/0146167292181001.

Martin, L. R., Haskard-Zolnierek, K. B., & DiMatteo, M. R. (2009). Understanding behavior change: The theory behind informing, motivating, and planning for health. In S. A. Shumaker, J. K. Ockene, & K. A. Reickert (Eds.), *Health behavior change and treatment adherence*. New York, NY: Oxford University Press.

McLeroy, K. R., Bibeau, D., Steckler, A., & Glanz, K. (1988). An ecological perspective on health promotion programs. *Health Education & Behavior, 15*(4), 351–377. http://doi.org/10.1177/109019818801500401.

National Research Council. (1994). *Reducing risks for mental disorders: Frontiers for preventive intervention research*. Washington, DC: The National Academies Press. Retrieved from http://www.nap.edu/catalog/2139/reducing-risks-for-mental-disorders-frontiers-for-preventive-intervention-research.

Nutbeam, D., Harris, E., & Wise, M. (2010). *Theory in a nutshell: A guide to health promotion theories* (3rd ed.). North Ryde NSW: McGraw-Hill Australia.

Prochaska, J. O., & DiClemente, C. C. (1986). Toward a comprehensive model of change. In *Treating addictive behaviors Processes of change* (pp. 3–27).

Prochaska, J. O., Redding, C. A., Harlow, L. L., Rossi, J. S., & Velicer, W. F. (1994). The transtheoretical model of change and HIV prevention: A review. *Health Education Quarterly, 21*, 471–486. http://doi.org/10.1177/109019819402100410.

Rosenstock, I. M. (1974). The health belief model and preventive health behavior. *Health Education Monographs, 2*, 354–386. http://doi.org/10.1177/109019818801500203.

Rosenstock, I. M., Strecher, V. J., & Becker, M. H. (1988). Social learning theory and the health belief model. *Health Education Quarterly, 15*, 175–183. http://doi.org/10.1177/109019818801500203.

Sarkin, J. A., Johnson, S. S., Prochaska, J. O., & Prochaska, J. M. (2001). Applying the transtheoretical model to regular moderate exercise in an overweight population: Validation of a stages of change measure. *Preventive Medicine, 33*, 462–469. http://doi.org/10.1006/pmed.2001.0916.

Tomb, M., & Hunter, L. (2004). Prevention of anxiety in children and adolescents in a school setting: The role of school-based practitioners. *Children Schools, 26*, 87–101.

Viswanath, K., Orleans, C. T., Glanz, K., & Rimer, B. K. (2008). *Health behavior and health education: Theory, research, and practice*. San Francisco, CA: Jossey-Bass. Retrieved from http://search.ebscohost.com/login.aspx?direct=true&db=nlebk&AN=238450&site=ehost-live.

Willis, J., & Earle, S. (2007). Theoretical perspectives on promoting public health. In S. Earle, C. Lloyd, & M. Sidell (Eds.), *Theory and research in promoting public health*. London: Sage.

Part II
Socioecological Approach to Child and Adolescent Health

Chapter 3
Poverty and Child Health

Renée Wilson-Simmons

3.1 Introduction

Poverty is one of the most consistent and influential risk factors for poor health and development across the life span. Even after taking into account factors such as medical care, diet and nutrition, social support, and health behavior, studies of health outcomes still generally find a large effect attributable to socioeconomic status. Therefore, it is imperative that we answer the question, "What is it about socioeconomic status, in and of itself, that affects health, both during childhood and in adulthood?"

Fifteen percent of the US population—47 million people—is living at or below the poverty line (U.S. Census Bureau, 2013). However, 22 % of the nation's 74 million children are living in poverty, making them the poorest residents of our nation (U.S. Census Bureau, 2012). In addition, poor populations in 96 of the 100 largest metro areas remain above levels recorded prior to the recession (Kneebone & Williams, 2013), and the US economic and housing crises have accelerated a longer-term trend toward the suburbanization of American poverty (Kneebone & Berube, 2013).

Unfortunately, what these data tell us about many poor children in cities and towns across America is that their chances of succeeding in school, having good mental and physical health, and realizing their full potential as adults are greatly compromised. They start out early on a path that puts them far behind more advantaged children, and many never catch up.

R. Wilson-Simmons, Dr.P.H. (✉)
Health Policy and Management, National Center for Children in Poverty, Columbia University Mailman School of Public Health, 215 W. 125th Street, New York, NY 10027, USA
e-mail: rw2502@columbia.edu

© Springer Science+Business Media New York 2016
M.R. Korin (ed.), *Health Promotion for Children and Adolescents*,
DOI 10.1007/978-1-4899-7711-3_3

Equally unfortunate—and distressing—is that efforts to address child poverty have been handicapped, in part, by inaccurate and damaging beliefs about poor adults. Chief among them is that although poor children are poor through no fault of their own and so deserve support, poor adults—their parents—are to blame for their indigent situation and so must deal with it as best they can.

However, such negative beliefs about many poor adults have put the healthy development of their children at risk, as research has clearly established that children do better when their families do better (Duncan & Brooks-Gunn, 1997; McLoyd, 1998; Mistry, Vandewater, Huston, & McLoyd, 2002). Low family income can impede children's cognitive development and their ability to learn (Aber, Bennett, Conley, & Li, 1997; Engle & Black, 2008); contribute to behavioral, social, and emotional problems (Yoshikawa, Aber, & Beardslee, 2012); and cause or exacerbate poor child health (Case, Lubotsky, & Paxson, 2002; Wood, 2003). To prevent and reduce child poverty and promote healthy growth and development, it is essential to examine child poverty in the context of family poverty to understand who is poor and why, associations between child poverty and health, and best options for prevention and intervention. This chapter attempts to cover these topics and more.

The chapter will begin by defining poverty and exploring the nature and extent of poverty in the USA, continue by describing the impact of family economic hardship on child health, then review research on the social determinants of health, and examine the effects of US antipoverty policies as well as early child development programs on poor children. This chapter concludes with recommendations for advancing poverty reduction efforts that promote child health. Because an examination of poverty and child health is inherently multidisciplinary, data are drawn from the fields of economics, maternal and child health, developmental psychology, public policy, sociology, and social welfare.

3.2   Defining and Measuring Poverty

The current federal poverty measure has two components: the **poverty threshold** and the **income measure**. Each year, the U.S. Census Bureau calculates poverty thresholds—the level of poverty in the previous year—and identifies trends in the level and composition of the poor from year to year (U.S. Census Bureau, 2014a, 2014b). These calculations are used to develop the nation's annual income measure, which is based on data from several major household surveys and programs (DeNavas-Walt & Proctor, 2013). Official national poverty estimates are derived from the *Annual Social and Economic Supplement* (*ASEC*) to the *Current Population Survey* (*CPS*); single- and multiyear estimates for smaller areas are calculated using the *American Community Survey* (*ACS*); longitudinal estimates are made using the *Survey of Income and Program Participation* (*SIPP*); and model-based poverty estimates for counties and school districts are developed with data from the *Small Area Income and Poverty Estimates* (*SAIPE*) program (Cauthen & Fass, 2008). **The poverty guidelines**, issued each year by the Department of Health and Human Services (HHS) and published in the Federal Register, are a

Table 3.1 Federal poverty guidelines, 2015

Persons in family/household	48 contiguous states and DC ($)	Alaska ($)	Hawaii ($)
1	11,770	14,720	13,550
2	15,930	19,920	18,330
3	20,090	25,120	23,110
4	24,250	30,320	27,890
5	28,410	35,520	32,670
6	32,570	40,720	37,450
7	36,730	45,920	42,230
8	40,890	51,120	47,010
For each additional person, add	4160	5200	4780

Source: Federal Register, Vol. 80, No. 14, January 22, 2015, pp. 3236–3237

simplification of the poverty thresholds and are used for administrative purposes, such as determining financial eligibility for certain federal programs (Fass, 2009). See Table 3.1 for 2014 poverty guidelines.

Devised to define and quantify poverty in America and provide a benchmark for progress or relapse, the official poverty measure was developed in the mid-1960s as part of President Lyndon Johnson's War on Poverty (Fisher, 1992). The measure is used to calculate the official poverty rate, which is determined by comparing a family's pretax cash income to an income poverty threshold. The threshold set the poverty line at three times the cost of a basic food basket because, at that time, food accounted for one-third of the cost of living. Despite the fact that food now accounts for only one-seventh of the cost of living, the threshold has only been adjusted to account for inflation. The pretax cash family income includes earnings, dividends, interest, Social Security payments, and pensions, as well as any public assistance, Supplemental Security Income (SSI), alimony, and child support payments a family receives. If a family's income falls below the threshold, it is considered to be poor (Johnson & Smeeding, 2012).

The poverty threshold has been assailed by many as an inaccurate assessment of **family needs** and **family resources** (Citro & Michael, 1995; Engelhardt & Skinner, 2013). On the needs side, it does not consider such nondiscretionary expenses as housing, child care, out-of-pocket medical expenses, and transportation, among others, or account for geographic variations in the cost of living. On the resources side, it excludes post-tax cash benefits such as the Earned Income Tax Credit (EITC), the refundable portion of the child tax credit, and in-kind government benefits such as the Supplemental Nutrition Assistance Program (SNAP), Medicaid, housing subsidies, and school lunch assistance.[1]

Although the Census Bureau continues to use its poverty measure, it also developed the Supplemental Poverty Measure, released in November 2011. In addition, the Census Bureau and many state and local entities have devised their own, place-specific measures in an attempt to better understand the level and trend of poverty in their region and to gauge the effectiveness of antipoverty efforts.

---

[1] Most of these "safety net" benefits are described later in this chapter.

3.3   International Comparisons

Despite its overall wealth, the USA has one of the highest child poverty rates among
the world's richest countries. According to a recent report published by the United
Nations Children's Fund (2012), there are 30 million children living in poverty in 35
"economically advanced countries" whose data were analyzed in Fig. 3.1. Two indi-
ces were used to conduct the calculations—the *Child Deprivation Index*, which
includes European countries only and defines children as deprived if they lack 2 or

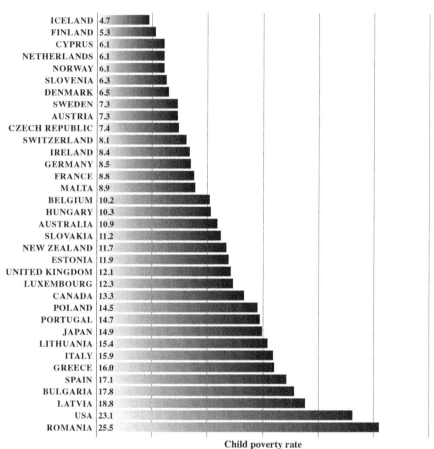

Child poverty rate
(% of children living in households with equivalent income lower than 50% of national median)

Note: Data refers to children 0-17 years old
Sources: Calculations based on European Union-Statistics on Living and Income Conditions 2009, Household, Income and Labour Dynamics
in Australia 2009, Survey of Labour and Income Dynamics 2009, Swiss Household Panel 2009, Panel Study of Income Dynamics 2007,
Household Incomes in New Zealand 2011. Results for Japan are from the Cabinet Office, Gender Equality Bureau, 2011.

Fig. 3.1 Relative child poverty in 35 economically advanced countries. Adapted from United Nations
Children's Fund. 2012. Measuring Child Poverty: New League Tables of Child Poverty in the World's
Rich Countries. Innocenti Report Card 10. Florence, Italy: UNICEF Innocenti Research Centre

more of 14 basic needs (e.g., three meals per day, a quiet place to study, educational books, an Internet connection), and the *Relative Poverty Index*, which is the percentage of children living below each country's national poverty line. The deprivation index found the highest rates of deprivation in Romania (72.6%), Bulgaria (56.6%), and Hungary (31.9%), with the least deprived children living in Norway, Sweden, and Iceland (all less than 2%). The nations with the highest relative child poverty are Romania (25.5%), the USA (23.1%), and Latvia (18.8%).

Clearly, many children do not have their basic needs met in countries that have the means to provide them, and the extremely weak US standing on child poverty is a clear sign that the nation's economy is one of the most unequal in the developed world. Thus, although Americans are, on average, six times richer than Bulgarians and Romanians, US child poverty is ranked between Bulgaria and Romania (Davies, Sandström, Shorrocks, & Wolff, 2011).

3.4 Trends in US Poverty Rates

In this section, definitions of economic hardship are provided, followed by data on poverty by age group, regional trends, and race, ethnicity, and immigrant status.

3.4.1 Economic Hardship Defined

The following definitions of economic hardship are used in this examination of child poverty:

Low income: Less than 200% of the federal poverty level
Poverty: Less than 100% of the federal poverty level
Extreme poverty: Less than 50% of the federal poverty level

The percentage of children living in low-income families, both poor and near poor, has been on the rise, increasing from 39% in 2007 to 44% in 2013 (Jiang, Ekono, & Skinner, 2015). During this time period, the overall number of children of all ages increased by less than 1%, while the numbers who were low income and poor increased by 13% and 23%, respectively (Table 3.2). Among this latter group are 7.4 million children—almost 10% of all children—who are living in extreme poverty, which is defined as an annual income of less than half the official poverty line (Institute for Research on Poverty, 2011).

Income level is the most basic measure of poverty. However, what must also be considered in any examination of child poverty are the types of hardships that the lack of household cash produces. These range from overcrowding and difficulty affording food to having utilities cut off and being behind on rent or mortgage (Sherman, 2004).

Table 3.2 Percentage change of children living in low-income and poor families, 2007–2013

Income category	2007	2013	Percent change
Low income	28,236,002	31,820,739	13
Poor	12,867,473	15,770,127	23

Source: National Center for Children in Poverty. *Basic Facts about Low-Income Children under 18 Years, 2013*

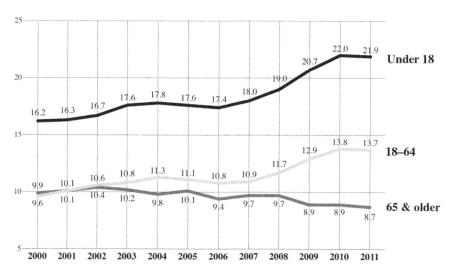

Fig. 3.2 Poverty rates of all persons by age, 2000–2011. *Source*: Poverty and income statistics: A summary of 2012 current population survey data. *ASPE Issue Brief*. Washington, DC: Department of Health and Human Services Office of the Assistant Secretary for Planning and Evaluation.

3.4.2 Poverty by Age Group

Especially notable within poverty data is the dramatic decrease in elder poverty in contrast to the consistent increase in child poverty (Fig. 3.2). Children are over twice as likely as adults 65 years and older to live in poor families. In 2013, the poverty rate for people age 65 and over was 9.1 % (Department of Health and Human Services, 2013). The benefits of Social Security have been identified as a major protector against the effects of severe economic downturns for many in this population (Hillier & Barrow, 2014).

The overall percentages of children under 18 years who live in low-income and poor families are 44 % and 22 %, respectively; however, there is variation by age group (Jiang et al., 2015):

Under 3 years: 47 % (5.3 million) live in low-income families
25 % (2.7 million) live in poor families

3–5 years: 48% (5.8 million) live in low-income families
24% (3.0 million) live in poor families

6–11 years: 45% (10.9 million) live in low-income families
22% (5.4 million) live in poor families

12–17 years: 41% (9.9 million) live in low-income families
19% (4.7 million) live in poor families

As these numbers illustrate, young children, that is, those younger than 6 years old, are more likely to live in low-income or poor families than older children.

3.4.3 Regional Trends in Poverty

The American Community Survey (ACS) is an excellent source of data on regional trends in poverty (Bishaw, 2012). The ACS collects demographic, social, economic, and housing data for the nation, states, congressional districts, counties, and other localities on an annual basis and has an annual sample size of approximately 3.3 million addresses across the USA and Puerto Rico.

According to data from the ACS, in 2013, poverty rates were highest in the South (16.1%), followed by the West (14.7%), the Midwest (12.9%), and the Northeast (12.7%). From 2012 to 2013, poverty remained statistically unchanged—measured both in terms of numbers of poor and rates—in each of the four regions (Gabe, 2014). The poorest states in the USA were almost entirely found in the South, with Mississippi being the highest (24%), followed by New Mexico (22%), Louisiana (20%), and Arkansas (20%). The lowest rates of poverty were in New Hampshire and Alaska (9%). The rate in Puerto Rico was 46% (Gabe, 2014). Puerto Rico's poverty rate hit 45% in 2013, which is nearly double that of Mississippi, the most impoverished of the 50 states (Bishaw & Fontenot, 2014).

Household incomes in rural America continue to lag behind those in suburban and urban areas, and within metropolitan areas, the incidence of poverty in central city areas (19%) is considerably higher than in suburban areas (11%) (Gabe, 2014). However, it is important to note that suburban poverty is on the rise. The trek of affluent and working-class families from urban to suburban areas during the latter half of the twentieth century, which led to increased concentrations of low-income people in the central cities, has stopped and, in some cases, reversed in recent years (Felland, Lauer, & Cunningham, 2009). By 2011, one in three poor Americans—about 16.4 million people—lived in the suburbs (Kneebone & Berube, 2013).

While these annual statistics are important, it is essential to use such data to examine the persistence of poverty over time. The Economic Research Service (ERS) of the US Department of Agriculture, which studies US counties, defines a county as being persistently poor if 20% or more of its populations have lived in poverty over the last 30 years (U.S. Department of Agriculture, 2014). ERS measured poverty via the 1980, 1990, and 2000 decennial censuses and 2007–2011

American Community Survey 5-year estimates. Using this definition, ERS identified 353 persistently poor counties in the USA, which comprise 11 % of all counties (U.S. Department of Agriculture, 2014). The large majority of the persistent, poverty counties (301 or 85.3 %) were nonmetro. As might be expected, persistent poverty also demonstrates a strong regional pattern, with 84 % of persistent poverty counties in the South.

3.4.4   Race, Ethnicity, and Immigrant Status

Poverty rates among children of color are much higher than among white children and have been so since the Census Bureau began making separate estimates by race. Although black, American Indian, and Hispanic children are disproportionately low income, whites comprise the largest group of all low-income children, and Hispanics make up the largest group of poor children under the age of 18 years (see Fig. 3.3).

Poverty is also prevalent among children of immigrants, who are significantly more likely to be economically disadvantaged than native children. Approximately one-third live in poverty—a rate close to 15 % points higher than that for native children—and nearly half receive public assistance, compared with about one-third of native children. The differences between the two groups continue into young adulthood, with the poverty and public assistance program participation

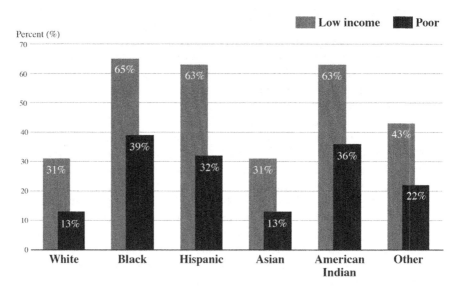

Fig. 3.3 Percentage of children in low-income and poor families in the USA, by race/ethnicity, 2013. *Source*: National Center for Children in Poverty, *Basic Facts about Low-Income Children: Children under 18 Years, 2013*

status of immigrant children in particular strongly linked to their retaining the same status as young adult (Borjas, 2011). However, there are differences among racial and ethnic groups.

Among Hispanics, low-income families are much more likely to be headed by foreign-born adults. Nearly two-thirds of low-income Hispanic families are headed by an immigrant, compared with half of middle- and high-income Hispanic families. For black and other race families, the opposite is true: Middle- and high-income families are more likely than low-income families to be headed by an immigrant. The proportion of white households that is low income is similar among the foreign born and native born (Simms, Fortuny, & Henderson, 2009a, 2009b).

3.5   Poverty and Child Health and Development

Brain, cognitive, and behavioral development early in life are strongly linked to an array of important health outcomes later in life, including cardiovascular disease and stroke, hypertension, diabetes, obesity, smoking, drug use, and depression.

—Robert Wood Johnson Foundation Commission to Build a
Healthier America (2011, p. 3)

Poverty, in and of itself, does not determine life course. However, early childhood is a time of rapid brain, nervous, endocrine, and immune system development—all of which are critical to healthy growth (Center on the Developing Child, 2010). Many infants born into poverty not only have a higher likelihood of prematurity and morbidity than those in higher-income families but also experience subsequent developmental delays (Currie, 2006; Schlee, 2009; Yeung et al., 2002). As poor children, they are more likely than their better-off peers to have cognitive and behavioral difficulties (McLoyd, 1998); complete fewer years of education (Reardon, 2011); and, as they transition to adulthood, experience more years of unemployment, underemployment, and low adult earnings (Duncan & Brooks-Gunn, 1997; Wagmiller, 2006). Those who experience economic hardship when they are very young or who experience extreme and prolonged hardship are at greatest risk for poor outcomes (Cauthen & Fass, 2009).

There are many ways in which the disadvantage of poverty affects child health and development. For example, prenatal substance exposure, the result of maternal use of tobacco, alcohol, and other drugs, is disproportionately experienced by the poor and has been associated with low birth weight, adverse cognitive outcomes, and some long-term behavioral outcomes extending from early childhood into adulthood (Brook, Brook, & Whiteman, 2000; Chasnoff, 1998; Richardson, Goldschmidt, Larkby, & Day, 2013; Weissman, 1999).

Children in many lower-income neighborhoods have higher levels of exposure to lead-based paint, a neurotoxin that accumulates in the body, putting them at risk for irreversible neurologic damage (Farah, Noble, & Hurt, 2006; Needleman, 1990). A meta-analysis of low-level lead exposure on IQ estimated that every 10 μg/dL increase in lead is associated with a 2.6-point decrease in IQ (Schwartz, 1994).

Inadequate nutrition, due in part to food insecurity, defined as limited or uncertain availability of nutritionally adequate and safe foods for all household members, is associated with childhood obesity and is a strong predictor of adult obesity and risks of morbidity and premature mortality (Drewnowski, 2004; Ogden, Lamb, Carroll, & Flegal, 2010). Infants and toddlers in food-insecure homes are 30 % more likely to have a history of hospitalization, 90 % more likely to be reported in fair or poor health by a parent, and two-thirds more likely to be at risk for developmental delays than young children in food-secure households (Rose-Jacobs, 2008).

Iron-deficiency anemia, the most common nutritional deficiency in children, is highest among those living at or below the poverty level (Cusick, Mei, & Cogswell, 2007). It has been associated with lowered scores on tests of mental and motor development in infancy (Lozoff et al., 1987), decreased attention span, reduced alertness, and deficits in cognitive achievement among infants, children, and adolescents (Halterman, 2001; Lukowski, 2010).

3.5.1   Cognitive Development

The risks to cognitive development are particularly striking and warrant further examination. In terms of language development, the effects of family socioeconomic status on children's language development can be seen as early as 18 months (Center on the Developing Child at Harvard University, 2007). Compared to their peers in higher-income families, children in low-income families have shown lags in cognitive and behavioral development as early as 24 months (Halle et al., 2009). By age 3, a child's vocabulary can predict third-grade reading achievement (O'Donnell, 2008). These findings are a warning sign of low-income children's lack of school readiness, which is comprised of five dimensions: (1) physical well-being and motor development, (2) social and emotional development, (3) approaches to learning, (4) language development (including early literacy), and (5) cognition and general knowledge (National Education Goals Panel, 1995).

As poor children move into the early elementary grades, cognitive lags affect their mastery of reading and writing, which are literacy skills essential to full participation in American society. Proficiency in reading by the end of third grade enables children to shift from learning to read to reading to learn and to mastering the more complex subject matter they will encounter in the fourth grade and beyond. Most students who fail to reach this critical milestone falter in the later grades, with many dropping out before earning a high school diploma, making the link between reading deficiencies and broader social consequences clear (Fiester, 2013). Unfortunately, four out of every five low-income students miss this critical reading proficiency milestone (Hernandez, 2011).

Weak cognitive functioning and literacy deficiencies in poor children have been associated with less home-based cognitive stimulation (McLoyd, 1998), including a lack of children's books in homes, as well as inadequate lighting and places to do homework, and the limited opportunities poor and low-income children have to learn their alphabet, a hallmark of early literacy (Piasta & Wagner, 2010; Bank, 2012). These children are also challenged by limited access to literacy opportunities in low-income communities, where there are few public places, such as well-stock libraries, where reading is a focus and other literacy-promoting resources are in short supply, making it difficult for them to test their skills by reading signs, labels, and logos (Neuman, 2001).

Parents will always be a child's first teacher and, more often than not, a child's most important teacher. They hold one of the master keys that unlocks their child's potential for positive cognitive, social, emotional, and behavioral health. As such, they are expected to serve as gatekeepers, protecting their child from harm and identifying and addressing health and developmental problems before they result in serious harm. However, many parents, especially those living in poverty, are pulled in multiple directions and cannot always make their child's development a top priority. They must address a range of competing priorities while dealing with the stress of living in poverty.

3.5.2   The Stress of Living in Poverty

While income directly influences the availability of such basic needs as food, clothing, housing, and health care, financial strain also hinders child development via a range of other mechanisms. Placed in the context of the family, many of the negative child outcomes described above have been associated with the social determinants of a mother's health, such as prepregnancy health behaviors and health status before, during, and after birth (Kahn, Wilson, & Wise, 2005; Larson & Halfon, 2010; Nagahawatte, 2008). Of course, mothers are not the only parent affected by the stresses of poverty. A range of poverty-related environmental and psychosocial factors negatively affect many poor and low-income mothers **and** fathers. The stress of dealing with limited access to health care, food insecurity, inferior housing, energy insecurity, and lack of community safety, with limited social supports to buffer their effects, is harmful to all members of the family and detrimental to young children's development (Knitzer & Lefkowitz, 2006).

Developmental psychologist Urie Bronfenbrenner's model of human ecology, which combines aspects of sociology and developmental psychology and describes the mutually shaping relationships between individuals and their environments, is relevant to the discussion of the stress of poverty (Bronfenbrenner, 1977). His ecological systems theory, which focuses on the social contexts in which children live and the people who influence their development, consists of complex systems in which evolving interactions among factors in a child's maturing biology, family, and community environments, as well as society as a whole, stimulate and guide development (Bronfenbrenner, 1986; Bronfenbrenner & Morris, 1998).

Bronfenbrenner identified five systems of interaction: (1) the **microsystem**, within which a child experiences immediate interactions with other people, which begin at the family level and become more complex as the child ages and involves more people (e.g., peers, neighbors, teachers); (2) the **mesosystem**, which makes interrelationships among settings (e.g., home, day care, schools) possible—and more powerful influences on development, based on the strength of the relationship; (3) the **exosystem**, which involves the contexts in which the child does not have an active role but affect his or her experiences in various settings that are important to development (e.g., social service agencies, workplaces); (4) the **macrosystem**, which consists of ideological and organizational patterns (e.g., culture's laws, values, customs, and resources), which have implications for child development and the allocation of resources for children; and (5) the **chronosystem**, the sociohistorical conditions of human development and the ways in which social trends are patterned over an individual's lifetime (e.g., child care outside the home) (Bronfenbrenner, 1979).

By looking at poverty through this model of human ecology, it is possible to identify many of the ways in which the stress of living in poverty affects child development. Poor and low-income parents tend to be more focused on such major priorities as providing for basic family needs, protecting their children from dangerous neighborhood conditions, and finding and/or keeping a job, despite the fact that their employment seldom offers opportunity for advancement.

The increased spatial concentration of poverty within high-poverty areas combined with increasing levels of residential segregation by race, business disinvestment, limited economic opportunities, joblessness, scarce social services, and violence have produced high levels of social isolation, depression, family conflict, and, in turn, unstable home environments, all of which exert a negative impact on child and adolescent development (McLoyd, Jayaratne, Ceballo, & Borquez, 1994; McLeod & Shanahan, 1993; Sampson, 2001; Sampson & Laub, 1994; Wilson, 2009). And while financial limitations can impede the ability of poor parents to supply their children with the intellectual stimulation provided by toys and books as well as high-quality early care and education, the stress of poverty that produces maternal depression can also have equally damaging effects on child development.

Maternal depression, alone or in combination with other risks (e.g., substance abuse, domestic violence, prior trauma), can pose serious but typically unrecognized barriers to healthy early development and school readiness, particularly for low-income young children (Knitzer, Theberge, & Johnson, 2008). The negative effects of maternal depression on children's health and development can start before birth (Bonari et al., 2004), impair parental safety and health management (e.g., breastfeeding, safety practices, preventive health measures) (Chung, McCollum, Elo, Lee, & Culhane, 2004), damage early bonding between parent and child (Essex, Klein, Cho, & Kalin, 2002), and negatively affect school readiness (Riley et al., 2009).

Although approximately 12% of all women experience depression in a given year (Isaacs, 2004), the estimated prevalence doubles to at least 25% among low-income women (Lanzi, Pascoe, Keltner, & Ramey, 1999; Siefert, Bowman, Heflin, Danziger, & Williams, 2000). Among low-income mothers of young children as well as low-income pregnant and parenting teens, reports of depressive symptoms have been in the 40–60% range, which is significantly higher than the 5–25% of pregnant, postpartum, and parenting women in the general population who have reported depressive symptoms (Knitzer et al., 2008).

Single-mother families are about five times more likely to be poor than married-couple families with children (Cancian & Reed, 2009), and nearly three out of four single parents with long-term unemployment were poor in 2011 (Nichols, 2013). Based on these data, it is not surprising that maternal depression is more prevalent among low-income mothers than among those with higher incomes (Petterson, 2001).

While research has not found a direct relationship between the chronic stress of poverty and infant mortality (Aber et al., 1997), studies have shown associations among family poverty, poor parenting behavior (e.g., punitive actions such as shouting and slapping children), and child social, emotional, and behavioral problems (Aber et al., 1997; Elder, Van Nguyen, & Caspi, 1995; McLeod & Shanahan, 1993), especially among poor parents who report receiving little to no social support (Hashima & Amato, 1994). One of the most vulnerable groups is comprised of homeless poor children, whom research has shown exhibit internalizing problem behaviors (e.g., anxiety, depression, withdrawn behavior, somatic complaints) and externalizing problem behaviors (e.g., attention difficulty, aggression, disruptive behavior) at an even greater rates than housed poor children (Buckner, Bassuk, Weinreb, & Brooks, 1999; Buckner, 2008).

3.6 Efforts to Reduce Poverty and Promote Child Health and Development

3.6.1 Safety Net Programs and Their Effects on Child Health and Development

Although there is much more to be done to reduce the poverty rate and associated trends, the situation for poor children and their families would be much worse, were it not for the nation's safety net programs. While cash welfare accounts for a small and continually smaller share of federal expenditures on poor families with children, safety net programs are a lifeline for many poor families. Those programs most relevant to poor children and families are the following:

- *Child Nutrition*: School lunch, breakfast, and after-school food programs
- *Child Care and Development Block Grant (CCDBG)*: Assists working families with the cost of providing child care
- *Earned Income Tax Credit*: Provides an income tax refund to workers in low-wage jobs
- *Child Care Tax Credit*: Provides a tax credit to working parents to help offset the cost of raising a child
- *Head Start*: Preschool program
- *Housing Assistance*: Housing and Urban Development housing programs that include rent vouchers, public housing, and community development programs
- *Lifeline*: Phone (landline and cell phone) subsidy, also known as Obama Phone

- *Low-Income Home Energy Assistance Program (LIHEAP)*: Aid for heating or cooling a residential dwelling
- *Medicaid*: Health care for low-income people
- *Supplemental Nutritional Assistance Program (SNAP)*: Debit cards for the purchase of food
- *Temporary Assistance for Needy Families (TANF)*: Cash payments to support low-income families and move them from welfare to work
- *Women, Infants, and Children (WIC)*: High-protein food for pregnant women and children up to 5 years old

Among these programs are several that deserve closer examination because of their significant role in poverty reduction. They are described below, with information drawn from the National Center for Children in Poverty website: www.nccp.org.

3.7 Earned Income Tax Credit

As the largest poverty reduction program in the USA, this tax credit alone lifts more children out of poverty than any other program. It is designed to "make work pay" by providing an income tax refund to workers in low-wage jobs. Eligibility is based on income, and the refund amount is based on income and family size. The EITC is refundable, which means that if the amount of the credit exceeds the amount of personal income tax one would otherwise owe, the taxpayer actually gets money back. Refundability is an important feature and hallmark of a truly effective low-income credit, because for most fixed-income families, sales and property taxes take a much bigger bite out of their wallets than does the personal income tax. This refundable credit on income tax forms is the most cost-effective mechanism for partially offsetting the effects of other regressive taxes on low-income families (Institute on Taxation and Economic Policy, 2013).

In 2013, over 27 million working families received the EITC, with 6.2 million brought out of poverty by the credit, including more than three million children (Center on Budget and Policy Priorities, 2015a). In addition, two-thirds of EITC recipients spend most of their refund immediately and close to home (Berube, 2007), and every increased dollar received by low- and moderate-income families has a multiplier effect of between 1.5 and 2 times the original amounts, in terms of its impact on the local economy (Rodriguez, 2013).

3.8 Child Tax Credit

According to the White House Task Force on the Middle Class (2010), since 2000, the cost of child care has increased twice as fast as the median income of families with children. The average increase among all states in the cost of care for a 4-year-old in a center also exceeds the rate of inflation; in 24 states, center-based child care fees for an infant exceeded annual rent payments; and in 40 states, the average annual cost for center-based care for an infant is higher than a year's tuition and related fees at a 4-year public college (Child Care Aware® of America, 2012; Child Care Aware® of America, 2013). Also, in every region of the USA, the average center-based child care fee for an infant exceeded the average annual amount that families spent on food (Lino, 2013).

Designed to offset some of the expense of raising a child, the Child Tax Credit (CTC) is the largest tax provision benefitting families with children, providing a per-CTC of up to $1000. A minimum annual income of $3000 is required to claim the credit, and a household income of at least $9667 is required to receive the full $1000 as a tax refund (Falk, Gabe, & Bradley, 2014). The CTC is a partially refundable credit, which means that the taxpayer does not simply get the difference between the credit and taxes owed, like the EITC. In 2013, the CTC prevented 3.1 million people from entering poverty, including 1.7 million children; it also reduced the severity of poverty for another 13.7 million people, including 6.8 million children (Center on Budget and Policy Priorities, 2014)

3.9   Child Care and Development Block Grant

This is the primary federal grant program that provides child care assistance for families and funds child care quality initiatives. Congress annually appropriates a discretionary amount that is administered to states in formula block grants, and states use the grants to subsidize child care for low-income working families. Most of this assistance is administered through vouchers or certificates, which can be used by parents for the provider or program of their choice. No less than 4 % of CCDBG funding in each state is used for activities to improve the overall quality of child care for all children within a community. The CCDBG also funds Child Care Resource and Referral services and quality projects for infants and toddlers. States may choose to use part of their federal welfare block grant for CCDBG. However, the amount varies from year to year and has decreased dramatically because of the fiscal crises that many states continue to experience, which means that not all families that qualify for child care assistance can access subsidies (Center for Law and Social Policy, 2014). According to the National Women's Law Center, in 2013, 19 states had waiting lists or had frozen intake for child care assistance (Schulman & Blank, 2013).

3.10   Supplemental Nutrition Assistance Program

Also known as food stamps, SNAP is the nation's most important anti-hunger program, providing nutritional support for low-wage working families as well as low-income seniors, people with disabilities, and those on fixed incomes. Nearly 75 % of SNAP participants are families with children. The federal government pays the full cost of SNAP benefits and splits the cost of administering the program with the states, which operate the program (Center on Budget and Policy Priorities, 2015b).

SNAP is an effective poverty-reducing program when it is counted in comprehensive poverty measures. In fiscal year 2013, more than 47 million low-income Americans participated in the program, at a cost to the federal government of approximately $82.3 billion (Center on Budget and Policy Priorities, 2015b). According to the Council of Economic Advisors (2014), in 2012, the program reduced the poverty rate by 1.6 % points among all individuals and by 3.0 % points among children.

Free school meals are also part of SNAP, and in the 2012–2013 school year, 10.8 million low-income children participated in the School Breakfast Program on an average day, and, for every 52 low-income children who participated in the breakfast program, 100 participated in the National School Lunch Program (Food Research and Action Center, 2014).

Research has shown that students who participate in school breakfast show improved attendance, behavior, and punctuality as well as improved performance on standardized achievement test scores (Murphy, 2007; Basch, 2011). In addition, children who increased their school breakfast participation as a result of a School Breakfast Program offered free to all students showed greater improvements in math scores, attendance, punctuality, depression, anxiety, and hyperactivity than children whose participation remained unchanged or decreased (Murphy et al., 1998).

3.11   State Participation in Safety Net Programs

While all of the programs described above are federally based, it is important to highlight the fact that state policy choices matter. How a state chooses to allocate federal and state funds, promote quality, and establish eligibility criteria influence who has access to essential supports and who does not. Given the state of the US economy and reductions in funds available to support federal safety net programs, it is important to look at how states are supporting low-income families via the safety net as well as other policies. The National Center for Children in Poverty's 50-State Policy Tracker is an online tool for comparing work supports that are critical to the economic security of working families (http://www.nccp.org/tools/policy/). The tool reveals striking variation among states, showing that state of residence has a major impact on whether low-income working parents succeed in making ends meet. The policy tracker enables users to compare state policies across ten programs: (1) Child Care and Development Fund subsidies, (2) State Child and Dependent Care Tax Credit, (3) State Earned Income Tax Credit, (4) minimum wage, (5) income tax liability, (6) unemployment insurance, (7) family and medical leave, (8) public health insurance, (9) Supplemental Nutrition Assistance Program, and (10) Temporary Assistance for Needy Families.

3.12   Effective Child Development Interventions

More than 20 years of longitudinal data on small- and large-scale high-quality child development programs have demonstrated their cost-effectiveness. Poor and low-income children who participate in these programs are more likely to stay in school, attend college, and become productive adults; they are less likely to need remediation, be arrested, or commit violent crimes (Campbell, Ramey, Pungello, Sparling, & Miller-Johnson, 2002; Reynolds, Temple, White, Ou, & Robertson, 2011; Schweinhart et al., 2005). High-quality programs can not only directly affect health and health care but also indirectly affect health by having an impact on social outcomes that have well-established health consequences (Anderson et al., 2003).

As discussed earlier in an examination of Bronfenbrenner's model of human ecology, child's evolving interactions with the peer group, family, community, and society stimulate and guide early childhood development. It follows that comprehensive programs are those designed to support positive interactions in all of these spheres. However, to determine which child development interventions, among the multitude that exist, are effective—and effective with low-income children—it is helpful to turn to the range of searchable online databases that catalog evidence-based interventions.

Chief among such information sources are the **National Registry of Evidence-based Programs and Practices** (http://nrepp.samhsa.gov/Index.aspx); **Social Programs that Work, Coalition for Evidence-Based Policy** (www.evidence-basedprograms.org/); **the Collaborative for Academic, Social, and Emotional Learning** (www.casel.org/guide); **Promising Practices Network on Children, Families and Communities** (www.promisingpractices.net/programs.asp); and **Blueprints for Healthy Youth Development** (www.blueprintsprograms.com/). Each database has specific criteria for program inclusion, and many criteria are similar across databases. However, for the purposes of brevity, only one database will be described here—Blueprints for Healthy Youth Development—but those interested in the range of databases currently in operation and the criteria for inclusion of those that promote healthy child development should review others.

All programs in the Blueprints database have been reviewed by an independent panel of evaluation experts and labeled *promising* or *model*, based on a set of scientific standards.

Programs deemed *promising* have met the following standards:

- *Intervention specificity*: Program description clearly identifies the outcome the program is designed to change, the population for which it is intended, the specific risk and/or protective factors targeted to produce the change, and how the components of the intervention work to produce the change.
- *Evaluation quality*: The evaluation trials produce valid and reliable findings via a minimum of one high-quality randomized control trial, or two high-quality quasi-experimental evaluations have been conducted.

- *Intervention impact*: The preponderance of evidence from the high-quality evaluations indicates significant positive change in intended outcomes that can be attributed to the program—and there is no evidence of harmful effects.
- *Dissemination readiness*: The program is currently available for dissemination and has the necessary organizational capability, manuals, training, technical assistance, and other support required for implementation with fidelity in communities and public service systems.

Programs identified as *model* have met the following additional standards:

- *Evaluation quality*: A minimum of two high-quality randomized control trials or one high-quality randomized control trial plus one high-quality quasi-experimental evaluation has been conducted.
- *Positive intervention impact*: Sustained for a minimum of 12 months after the program intervention ends.

One promising program and one model program relevant to this examination of child poverty and child development are described briefly below.

3.12.1   Promising

The **Early Literacy and Learning Model (ELLM)** was designed to help meet the challenge of improving the emergent literacy skills of young children in urban schools. It was developed by the University of North Florida, the College of Education and Human Services, and the UNF-based Florida Institute of Education, in partnership with several governmental and private organizations, Head Start Centers, public and private child care centers, and public school districts committed to improving reading among children, particularly those children who come to school underprepared. The program is designed to enhance existing classroom curricula by specifically focusing on children's early literacy skills and knowledge. Designed to be implemented year round or during the academic year, it supplements the daily activities of the classroom and includes regular teacher support and family involvement opportunities throughout the year (Cosgrove, Fountain, Wehry, Wood, & Kasten, 2006; Cosgrove, Fountain, Kasten, Wehry, & K, 2007).

Although one study found that children who received ELLM showed greater recognition of letters and better emerging literacy skills than children who did not (Cosgrove et al., 2006), the intervention is in the Blueprints promising category because a national study found no evidence of (1) impact at intervention year posttest; (2) an effect on children's mathematic understanding, early reading, phonological awareness, or behavior; or (3) an effect on teachers' overall classroom management, teacher-child relationships, or classroom instruction at any time period (Preschool Curriculum Evaluation Research Consortium, 2008). However, there was a delayed effect on vocabulary that showed up at the end of kindergarten (i.e., 1-year post-intervention).

3.12.2 Model

Nurse-Family Partnership is designed to improve the outcomes of pregnancy, improve infant health and development, and enhance the mother's personal development by helping her plan future pregnancies, continue her education, and find work. The intervention provides nurse home visits to pregnant women with no previous live births, most of whom are low income, unmarried, and teenagers. Participation in the program begins as early as possible during pregnancy, and the nurses visit the women approximately once per month during their pregnancy and the first 2 years of their children's lives, providing guidance regarding positive health-related behaviors, competent care of children, and maternal personal development, including family planning, educational achievement, and participation in the workforce. The frequency of home visits changes with the stages of pregnancy and infancy and is adapted to the mother's needs, with a maximum of 13 visits occurring during pregnancy and 47 occurring after the child's birth (Olds et al., 2002; Olds et al., 2004).

The program was developed by David Olds, a professor of pediatrics, psychiatry, and preventive medicine at the University of Colorado Denver who, while working in an inner-city day care center in the early 1970s, witnessed the developmental difficulties experienced by low-income children and realized that they and their mothers needed help even before they were born. He developed Nurse-Family Partnership, which in 2010 dollars costs approximately $12,500 per woman over the 3 years of visits. Individual programs serve a minimum of 100–200 families, supported by 4–8 trained registered nurse home visitors (each carrying a caseload of 25 families), a nurse supervisor, and administrative support.

Three program trials, each carried out in a different population and setting, all found the program to produce sizable, sustained effects on mother and child outcomes, although the types of effects often differed across the three studies. Significant program effects on risk and protective factors were in prenatal health, such as hypertension and use of cigarettes; maternal employment and use of welfare and food stamps; responsive interactions with child; child abuse and neglect and behavioral problems caused by the use of alcohol or drugs; and psychological aggression, physical assault, sexual coercion, injury, and combined forms of intimate partner violence (Olds, Henderson, Tatelbaum, & Chamberlin, 1986a; Olds, Henderson, Tatelbaum, & Chamberlin, 1986b; Olds, Henderson, & Kitzman, 1994; Olds et al., 1997).

3.13 Harlem Children's Zone

Although both the Early Literacy and Learning Model and Nurse-Family Partnership are included in several of the databases previously cited, it is important to mention one community-based program that addresses many of the risk and protective factors related to child development via the social contexts in which children live and the people who influence their development: Harlem Children's Zone (HCZ). Information about the initiative is primarily drawn from the website: http://hcz.org.

Begun in the 1990s as a pilot project that brought a range of support services to a single neighborhood block, by 2010, HCZ was a 100-block initiative that served more than 10,000 children and more than 7400 adults with a $75 million budget. HCZ is working to achieve its mission of breaking the cycle of generational poverty by developing, implementing, and evaluating a range of innovative strategies. Among them are The Baby College® parenting workshops established in 2000; the Harlem Gems® preschool program launched in 2001; and the Promise Academy public charter school, including The Renaissance University for Community Education (TRUCE), launched in 2004, and HCZ's Project Pipeline, which has two tracks—one for children who attend the Promise Academy Charter School and a second to support children who attend area public schools or who live in the area and go to school elsewhere. HCZ also developed the HCZ Asthma Initiative, which teaches families to better manage the disease, and an obesity program to help children stay healthy. There is also a Family Development Program that helps families gain access to mental health professionals who collaborate with caseworkers to support therapeutic interventions and a Family Support Center that provides crisis intervention services, referrals, advocacy, and parenting and anger management training.

According to HCZ, it tracks over 600 goals each year and its programs have produced impressive results: 100 % of the Harlem Gems pre-kindergarteners have been assessed as "school ready"; 95 % of its high school seniors have been accepted into college; more than 4000 parents have graduated from The Baby College parenting workshop series. In 2013, 12,316 children and 12,436 adults were served by HCZ, and 954 students were attending college.

In a community where 63 % of children are born into poverty, 48 % of households receive food assistance, and 59 % of children are born to single mothers, an organization such as HCZ deserves examination for its goal of becoming a national model for breaking the cycle of poverty by providing residents with what its founders believe is the right set of supports for enabling large numbers of poor children to achieve self-sufficiency. HCZ programs and processes, which focus on a birth-to-college pipeline, have received increasing attention from a range of researchers, practitioners, advocates, and policymakers who are seeking to determine cost-effectiveness, sustainability, and replicability (Grossman and Curran (2004; Dobbie & Fryer, 2011; Levin, 2013)

3.14   Recommendations

Socioeconomic factors that affect poor families represent the strongest and most consistent predictors of child health. The inequalities these families face—from disinvested communities and deficient home, work, and leisure lives to poor-quality schools to inaccessible or inadequate health care—all have a bearing on their ability to successfully achieve and maintain good health and to promote the health and development of their children. (World Health Organization Commission on Social Determinants of Health, 2008)

A 2000 Institute of Medicine report rightly states that the question is not whether early childhood programs can make a difference, because that question has been asked and answered in the affirmation many times. Instead, investigation must determine the most effective and efficient early childhood interventions, especially those for vulnerable children and families (National Research Council and Institute of Medicine, 2000).

Considering what we know about the influence of early childhood experiences on long-term outcomes, improvements in early care and education for poor children should be a priority, especially those that focus on the health and mental health of poor children and mothers. These include improving the capacity of early care and education programs to prevent and address mental health problems in young children in poverty (Azzi-Lessing, 2010) and providing screening and treatment to low-income women for postpartum depression, a serious and common psychiatric disorder that can have negative effects on women, their children, and families (Howell, Golden, & Beardslee, 2013). It has been suggested that the former could be achieved via a range of strategies that involve expanding use of early childhood mental health consultants and building effective partnerships with mental health and other community-based systems as well as providing support and training for teachers and establishing family-based supports such as those provided by Head Start and Early Head Start (Azzi-Lessing, 2010). The latter will be possible because of provisions in the Affordable Care Act that take effect in 2014 and would enable women to access screening and treatment for depression via Medicaid coverage (U.S. Department of Labor, 2014).

It should be of concern to all Americans that even the stereotypical "ideal family"—two parents with two children—will live in poverty on a full-time, minimum-wage salary. At the current federal minimum wage of $7.25, such a family cannot move above the poverty line without EITC as well as SNAP (Falk et al., 2014). It is, therefore, impossible for many families to achieve financial security, even with full-time employment.

Because children do better when families do better, what is needed to improve outcomes for low-income and poor children are policies and programs that address the needs of both parents and their children. Many recommendations have been made for moving families out of poverty. Among those that hold promise is adoption of the Supplemental Poverty Measure in order to produce a more realistic measure, one that incorporates the types of expenses families typically face (e.g., work-related expenses, shelter, and out-of-pocket medical expenses), includes some degree of geographic adjustment to account for differences in the cost of living, and enables policy analysts to determine whether federal tax and safety net programs are having an effect on income poverty (Engelhardt & Skinner, 2013).

Also needed are education and training programs, combined with language integration programs for limited English speakers, many of whom have relatively high labor force commitment but low educational attainment and so are under-employed (Simms et al., 2009a, 2009b). Unfortunately, although increasing public funding to improve job readiness and occupational skills of poor parents would improve the economic security of parents and promote the development of their children and the health of the nation (Plotnick, 1997), the federal government is funding fewer and fewer public workforce development programs (Holzer, 2008). And because higher education continues to be one of the most promising pathways out of poverty, creating a clear path to higher education is also needed. However, it is difficult for low-income parents to take that path because of welfare reform and student financial aid policies that require work before higher education and reserve Pell grants for students enrolled at least six credit hours (Jacobs & Winslow, 2003). Clearly a two-generation approach to poverty prevention is needed.

3.14.1   Two-Generation Approaches

In 2012, 66% of American households were family households (Vespa, Lewis, & Kreider, 2013). Two-generation approaches that help both parents and children can be applied to policy, practice, program, and research (Chase-Lansdale & Brooks-Gunn, 2014). Such approaches focus (1) equally on all members of a family, (2) first or primarily on the child but also offer services and opportunities for the parent, or (3) first or primarily on the parent but also provide services and opportunities for the child, with education from early childhood to postsecondary; economic supports that include care subsidies and student financial aid; and social capital components that draw on faith-based organizations and career coaches, among others (Mosle & Patel, 2012; Princeton-Brookings, 2014; Smith, 1995; St. Pierre, Layzer, & Barnes, 1995).

Several organizations are actively promoting a two-generation approach, most notably the Aspen Institute, through its Ascend initiative (www.aspeninstitute.org/policy-work/ascend), the Foundation for Child Development (http://fcd-us.org), and the Annie E. Casey Foundation (www.aecf.org). Ascend is promoting two-generation approaches by convening national forums and roundtable discussions where leaders in policy development, research, program design, evaluation, and community engagement share lessons learned; identifying and publicizing emerging and promising programs with the potential to multiply the returns on investments; and developing tools to advance its efforts. The Institute has also launched an 18-month fellows program that brings together leaders from diverse sectors and communities to tackle intergenerational poverty (Ascend Family Economic Security Program, 2012).

The three programs presented briefly below describe different ways in which services are being provided to parents and education and stimulation to children via two-generation approaches: Chicago Child-Parent Center, College Access and Success Program, and Career*Advance*.

3.15   Chicago Child-Parent Center

This program provides educational support and family support to economically disadvantaged children and their parents via a school-based, stable learning environment during preschool that involves parents as active and consistent participants in their child's education. The program requires parental participation and emphasizes a child-centered, individualized approach to social and cognitive development (Reynolds, 2000). A cost-benefit analysis of the Child-Parent Centers (CPCs) is the first for a sustained publicly funded early intervention. Using data collected up to age 26, the Chicago Longitudinal Study of over 1400 program and comparison group participants indicated that the CPCs had economic benefits in 2007 dollars that exceeded costs in terms of increased earnings and tax revenues, and averted criminal justice system costs (Reynolds et al., 2011).

3.16   College Access and Success Program

Developed in partnership with New York University and City University of New York, NY, the program ensures that children of low-income parents are enrolled in high-quality Early Head Start and Head Start and their parents are enrolled in adult education that leads to higher education opportunities and enhanced financial security. Adult education services vary based on parents' needs and can include English for Speakers of Other Languages (ESOL) courses, high school equivalency classes, and assistance with college enrollment through graduation. Also provided is a range of support services designed to strengthen family functioning, enhance family financial stability, help parents overcome obstacles to furthering their education, and inform parents about education options as their children progress in school. Evaluation of the program is currently underway ((Dropkin & Jauregui, 2015).

3.16.1   *Career*Advance

Begun in 2009 in Tulsa, Oklahoma, with a focus on nursing careers, the program provides cohort-based workforce development to parents, primarily single mothers, of Head Start and Early Head Start children. It is designed to enhance family economic success in order to protect and enhance gains made through high-quality early childhood programs even after children transition into the public school system. Over time, the program has evolved and has a sector-based focus on growing industries with high-demand occupations, good pay, and opportunities for advancement; skill training and certification geared to industry needs; conditional cash transfers that promote high performance; and peer mentoring and support (Glover, Smith, King, & Coffey, 2010). A 5-year, mixed method evaluation is currently being evaluated to better understand whether and how participating in career training may influence (1) family economic well-being; (2) parent self-confidence, self-efficacy, stress, and career success; and (3) child outcomes, including social, emotional, and cognitive development (King & Yoshikawa, 2014).

3.17 Conclusions

As adults, we have a special responsibility to support the healthy development of our most precious asset—our children—especially those whose futures are in jeopardy because of economic hardship. If we, as a nation, are truly committed to social justice, we must contribute to creating an America where all families are economically secure, strong, and nurturing and all children are supported so they thrive and grow into healthy adults. And there's a truth that should always be at the heart of our efforts, and that is: *Children do better when their families do better.*

However, negative sentiments about poor families must be changed before public policy can be more supportive. If sustainable poverty reduction is to be achieved in the USA, the public must have a more accurate understanding of who is poor and why, believe in the effectiveness of poverty reduction policies and their power to elevate the nation, and support such policies. This can only be achieved if child poverty is elevated in the public consciousness. It must be placed at the top of the country's policy agenda, and stakeholders must facilitate action on known solutions to reducing poverty and improving the health, well-being, and life outcomes of our nation's poor children and their families.

References

Aber, J. L., Bennett, N. G., Conley, D. C., & Li, J. (1997). The effects of poverty on child health and development. *Annual Review of Public Health, 18*, 463–483.

Anderson, L. M., Fullilove, M. T., Fielding, J. E., Shinn, C., Scrimshaw, S. C., Normand, J., Carande-Kulis, V. G. (2003). The effectiveness of early childhood development programs: A systematic review. *American Journal of Preventive Medicine, 24*(3), 32–46.

Ascend Family Economic Security Program. (2012). *Two generations, one future: Moving parents and children beyond poverty together.* Washington, DC: Aspen Institute.

Azzi-Lessing, L. (2010). Meeting the mental health needs of poor and vulnerable children in early care and education programs. *Early Childhood Research & Practice, 12*(1), n.p.

Bank, C. T. D. (2012). *Early school readiness: Indicators on children and youth.* Washington, DC: Child Trends.

Basch, C. E. (2011). Breakfast and the achievement gap among urban minority youth. *Journal of School Health, 81*(10), 635–640.

Berube, A. (2007). *The importance of the EITC to urban communities.* Washington, DC: Brookings Institution, Metropolitan Policy Program.

Bishaw, A. (2012). *Poverty: 2010 and 2011.* Washington, DC: American Community Survey Briefs.

Bishaw, A., & Fontenot, K. (2014). *Poverty: 2012 and 2013. American Community Survey Briefs. ACSBR/13-01.* Washington, DC: U.S. Census Bureau. Retrieved January 24, 2015, from http://www.census.gov/content/dam/Census/library/publications/2014/acs/acsbr13-01.pdf.

Bonari, L., Pinto, N., Ahn, E., Einarson, A., Steiner, M., & Koren, G. (2004). Perinatal risks of untreated depression during pregnancy. *Canadian Journal of Psychiatry, 49*(11), 726–735.

Borjas, G. J. (2011). Poverty and program participation among immigrant children. *The Future of Children, 21*(1), 247–266.

Bronfenbrenner, U. (1977). Toward an experimental ecology of human development. *American Psychologist, 32*(7), 513–531.

Bronfenbrenner, U. (1979). *The ecology of human development.* Cambridge, MA: Harvard University Press.

Bronfenbrenner, U. (1986). Ecology of the family as a context for human development: Research perspectives. *Developmental Psychology, 22,* 723–742.

Bronfenbrenner, U., Morris, P. (1998). The ecology of developmental process. In W. Damon (Series Ed.) & R.M. Lerner (Volume Ed.), *Handbook of child psychology: Vol. 1. theoretical models of human development* (pp. 993-1029). New York, NY: Wiley.

Brook, J. S., Brook, D. W., & Whiteman, M. (2000). The influence of maternal smoking during pregnancy on the toddler's negativity. *Archives of Pediatrics and Adolescent Medicine, 154*(4), 381–385.

Buckner, J. C. (2008). Understanding the impact of homelessness on children: Challenges and future directions. *American Behavioral Scientist, 51*(6), 721–736.

Buckner, J. C., Bassuk, E. L., Weinreb, L. F., & Brooks, M. G. (1999). Homelessness and its relation to the mental health and behavior of low-income school-age children. *Developmental Psychology, 35*(1), 246–257.

Campbell, F., Ramey, C., Pungello, E., Sparling, J., & Miller-Johnson, S. (2002). Early childhood education: Young adult outcomes from the Abecedarian Project. *Applied Developmental Science, 6*(1), 42–57.

Cancian, M., & Reed, D. (2009). Family structure, childbearing, and parental employment: Implications for the level and trend in poverty. *Focus, 26*(2), 21–26.

Case, A., Lubotsky, D., & Paxson, C. (2002). Economic status and health in childhood: The origins of the gradient. *American Economic Review, 92,* 1308–1334.

Cauthen, N., & Fass, S. (2009). *Ten important questions about children and economic hardship.* New York, NY: National Center for Children in Poverty, Columbia University.

Cauthen, N., & Fass, S. (2008). *Measuring poverty in the United States.* New York, NY: National Center for Children in Poverty, Columbia University. Retrieved 27, 2015, from http://www.nccp.org/publications/pub_825.html.

Center on Budget and Policy Priorities. (2015a). *Policy basics: The earned income Tax credit.* Washington, DC: Center on Budget and Policy Priorities. Retrieved January 23, 2015, from http://www.cbpp.org/files/policybasics-eitc.pdf.

Center on Budget and Policy Priorities. (2015b). *Policy basics: Introduction to the supplemental nutrition assistance program (SNAP).* Washington, DC: Center on Budget and Policy Priorities. Retrieved 23, 2015, from http://www.cbpp.org/files/policybasics-foodstamps.pdf.

Center on Budget and Policy Priorities. (2014). *The child Tax credit.* Washington, DC: Center on Budget and Policy Priorities. Retrieved January 27, 2015, from http://www.cbpp.org/files/policybasics-ctc.pdf.

Center on the Developing Child at Harvard University. (2010). *The foundations of lifelong health are built in early childhood.* Cambridge, MA: Harvard University. Retrieved June 30, 2014, from http://developingchild.harvard.edu/resources/reports_and_working_papers/foundations-of-lifelong-health/.

Center on the Developing Child at Harvard University. (2007). *A Science-Based Framework for Early Childhood Policy: Using Evidence to Improve Outcomes in Learning, Behavior, and Health for Vulnerable Children.* Retrieved July 26, 2014, from http://developingchild.harvard.edu/index.php/resources/reports_and_working_papers/policy_framework/.

Chase-Lansdale, P. L., & Brooks-Gunn, J. (2014). Two-generation programs in the twenty-first century. *The Future of Children, 24*(1), 13–39.

Chasnoff, I. J. (1998). Prenatal exposure to cocaine and other drugs: Outcome at four to six years. *Annals of the New York Academy of Sciences, 846,* 314–328.

Child Care Aware of America. (2012). *Parents and the high cost of child care: 2012 Report.* Arlington, VA: Child Care Aware of America. Retrieved June 27, 2014, from http://www.nac-crra.org/sites/default/files/default_site_pages/2012/cost_report_2012_final_081012_0.pdf.

Child Care Aware of America. (2013). *Parents and the high cost of child care: 2013 Report.* Arlington, VA: Child Care Aware of America. Retrieved June 27, 2014, from http://usa.child-careaware.org/sites/default/files/cost_of_care_2013_103113_0.pdf.

Chung, E. K., McCollum, K. F., Elo, I. T., Lee, H. J., & Culhane, J. F. (2004). Maternal depressive symptoms and infant health practices among low-income women. *Pediatrics, 113*(6), 523–529.

Citro, C. F., & Michael, R. T. (1995). *Measuring poverty: A New approach.* Washington, DC: National Academy Press.

Cosgrove, M., Fountain, C., Wehry, S., Wood, J., Kasten, K. (2006, April). *Randomized field trial of an early literacy curriculum and instructional support system.* Paper presented at the annual meeting of the American Educational Research Association, San Francisco.

Cosgrove, M., Fountain, C., Kasten, K., & Wehry, S., K (2007, April). *Examining the sustained effects of an early literacy curriculum and instructional support system using a randomized field trial.* Paper presented at the annual meeting of the American Educational Research Association, Chicago.

Council of Economic Advisors. (2014). The war on poverty 50 years later: A progress report. Washington, DC: Executive Office of the President of the United States. Retrieved July 27, 2014, from http://www.whitehouse.gov/sites/default/files/docs/50th_anniversary_cea_report_-_final_post_embargo.pdf.

Currie, J. M. (2006). *The invisible safety net: Protecting the nation's poor children and families.* Princeton, NJ: Princeton University Press.

Cusick, S., Mei, Z., & Cogswell, M. E. (2007). Continuing anemia prevention strategies are needed throughout early childhood in low-income preschool children. *Journal of Pediatrics, 150*(4), 422.

Davies, J. B., Sandström, S., Shorrocks, A., & Wolff, E. N. (2011). The level and distribution of global household wealth. *Economic Journal, Royal Economic Society, 121*(551), 223–254.

DeNavas-Walt, C., & Proctor, B. D. (2013). *Income and poverty in the United States: 2013. Current population reports* (pp. 60–249). Washington, DC: U.S. Census Bureau.

Department of Health and Human Services. (2013, September 13). *Information on poverty and income statistics: A summary of 2013 current population survey income data. ASPE Issue Brief.* Washington, DC: Office of the Assistant Secretary for Planning and Evaluation.

DeSilver, D. (2014, January 7). 5 Facts about economic inequality. *Fact Tank.* Washington, DC: Pew Research Center.

Dobbie, W., & Fryer, R. G. (2011). Are high-quality schools enough to increase achievement among the poor? Evidence from the Harlem Children's Zone. *American Economic Journal: Applied Economics, 3*(3), 158–187.

Drewnowski, A. (2004). Poverty and obesity: The role of energy density and energy costs. *The American Journal of Clinical Nutrition, 79*(1), 6.

Dropkin, E., & Jauregui, S. (2015). *Two generations together: Case studies from head start.* Washington, DC: National Head Start.

Duncan, G., & Brooks-Gunn, J. (1997). *Consequences of growing up poor.* New York, NY: Russell Sage Press.

Elder, G. H., Van Nguyen, T., & Caspi, A. (1995). Linking family hardship to children's lives. *Child Development, 56*(2), 361–375.

Engelhardt, W., & Skinner, C. (2013). *Knowing what works: States and cities build smarter social policy with new and improved poverty measurement.* New York, NY: National Center for Children in Poverty, Columbia University.

Engle, P. I., & Black, M. M. (2008). The effect of poverty on child development and educational outcomes. *Annals of the New York Academy of Sciences, 1136*, 243–256.

Essex, M. J., Klein, M. H., Cho, E., & Kalin, N. H. (2002). Maternal stress beginning in infancy may sensitize children to later stress exposure: Effects on cortisol and behavior. *Biological Psychiatry, 52*(8), 776–784.

Falk, G., Gabe, T., & Bradley, D. H. (2014). *Federal minimum wage, tax-transfer earnings supplements, and poverty.* Washington, DC: Congressional Research Service. Retrieved January 27, 2015, from http://fas.org/sgp/crs/misc/R43409.pdf.

Farah, M., Noble, K., & Hurt, H. (2006). Poverty, privilege, and brain development: Empirical findings and ethical implications. In J. Illes (Ed.), *Neuroethics* (pp. 277–289). Oxford: Oxford University Press.

Fass, S. (2009). *Measuring poverty in the United States.* New York, NY: National Center for Children in Poverty, Columbia University.

Felland, L. E., Lauer, J. R., & Cunningham, P. J. (2009). *Suburban poverty and the health care safety net. Research Brief No. 13..* Washington, DC: Center for Studying Health Care System Change.

Fiester, L. (2013). *Early warning confirmed: A research update on third grade reading.* Baltimore, MD: Annie E. Casey Foundation.

Fisher, G. M. (1992). The development and history of the poverty thresholds. *Social Security Bulletin, 55*(4), 3–14.

Food Research and Action Center. (2014). *School breakfast scorecard: 2012-2013 school year.* Washington, DC: Food Research and Action Center.

Gabe, T. (2014). *Poverty in the United States: 2013. Congressional research service report to Congress.* Washington, DC: Congressional Research Service, 7-5700, RL33069. Retrieved January 24, 2015, from https://www.fas.org/sgp/crs/misc/RL33069.pdf.

Glover, R. W., Smith, T. C., King, C. T., & Coffey, R. (2010). *CareerAdvance: A dual-generation antipoverty strategy: An implementation study of the initial pilot cohort July 2009 through June 2010.* Austin, TX: Ray Marshall Center for the Study of Human Resources, University of Texas.

Grossman, A. S., Curran, D. F. (2004, March). The Harlem Children's Zone: Driving performance with measurement and evaluation. *Harvard Business School Case 303–109.* Retrieved July 28, 2014, from http://www.hbs.edu/faculty/Pages/item.aspx?num=29945.

Halle, T., Forry, N., Hair, E., Perper, K., Wandner, L., Wessel, J., Vick, J. (2009). *Disparities in early learning and development: Lessons from the early childhood longitudinal study—birth cohort (ECLS-B).* Washington, DC: Child Trends.

Halterman, J. S. (2001). Iron deficiency and cognitive achievement among school-aged children and adolescents in the United States. *Pediatrics, 107*(6), 1381–1386.

Hashima, P. Y., & Amato, P. R. (1994). Poverty, social support and parental behavior. *Child Development, 65*(2), 394–403.

Hernandez, D. J. (2011). *Double jeopardy: How third grade reading scores and poverty influence high school graduation.* Baltimore, MD: Annie E. Casey Foundation.

Hillier, S. M., & Barrow, G. M. (2014). *Aging, the individual, and society.* Belmont, CA: Wadsworth.

Holzer, H. J. (2008). *Workforce development as an antipoverty strategy: What do we know? What should we do?* Washington, DC: Institute for the Study of Labor. Discussion Paper No. 3776.

Howell, E., Golden, O., & Beardslee, W. (2013). *Emerging opportunities for addressing maternal depression under Medicaid.* Washington, DC: Urban Institute.

Institute for Research on Poverty. (2011). *How many children are poor?* Madison, WI: University of Wisconsin-Madison. Retrieved January 24, 2015, from http://www.irp.wisc.edu/faqs/faq6.htm.

Institute on Taxation and Economic Policy. (2013). *State Tax codes as poverty fighting tools: 2013 Update on four key policies in all 50 states.* Washington, DC: ITEP.

Isaacs, M. (2004). *Community care networks for depression in low-income communities and communities of color: A review of the literature.* Submitted to Annie E. Casey Foundation.

Washington, DC: Howard University School of Social Work and the National Alliance of Multiethnic Behavioral Health Associations.

Jacobs, J. A., & Winslow, S. (2003). Welfare reform and enrollment in postsecondary education. *Annals of the American Academy of Political and Social Science, 586*(1), 194–217.

Jiang, Y., Ekono, M., & Skinner, C. (2015). *Basic facts about low-income children: Children under 18 years, 2013*. New York, NY: National Center for Children in Poverty, Columbia University. Retrieved January 23, 2015, from http://www.nccp.org/publications/pdf/text_1100.pdf.

Johnson, D. S., & Smeeding, T. M. (2012). A consumer's guide for interpreting various U.S. poverty measures. *Fast Focus, 14*, 1–7.

Kahn, R. S., Wilson, K., & Wise, P. H. (2005). Intergenerational health disparities: Socioeconomic status, women's health conditions, and child behavior problems. *Public Health Reports, 120*(4), 399–408.

King, C., & Yoshikawa, H. (2014). *Measuring two-generation results: The CareerAdvance® evaluation*. Austin, TX: TX. Retrieved January 27, 2015, from http://www.aspeninstitute.org/sites/default/files/content/docs/ascend/2-Gen_Measures_072412.pdf.

Kneebone, E., & Berube, A. (2013). *Confronting suburban poverty in America*. Washington, DC: Brookings Institution Press.

Kneebone, E., & Williams, J. (2013). New census data show metro poverty's persistence in 2012. In E. Kneebone & A. BerubeConfronting (Eds.), *Suburban poverty in America*. Washington, DC: The Brookings Institution. Retrieved March 28, 2014, from http://www.brookings.edu/~/media/research/files/reports/2013/09/19%20census%20data%20poverty/poverty2012update.pdf.

Knitzer, J., & Lefkowitz, J. (2006). *Helping the most vulnerable infants, toddlers, and their families*. New York, NY: National Center for Children in Poverty, Columbia University.

Knitzer, J., Theberge, S., & Johnson, K. (2008). *Reducing maternal depression and its impact on young children toward a responsive early childhood policy framework*. New York, NY: National Center for Children in Poverty, Columbia University.

Lanzi, R., Pascoe, J. M., Keltner, B., & Ramey, S. (1999). Correlates of maternal depressive symptoms in a national Head Start program sample. *Archives of Pediatric and Adolescent Medicine, 153*(8), 801–807.

Larson, K., & Halfon, N. (2010). Family income gradients in the health and health care access of U.S. children. *Maternal and Child Health Journal, 14*(3), 332–342.

Levin, B. (2013). *What does It take to scale up innovations? An examination of teach for America, the Harlem Children's zone, and the knowledge is power program*. Boulder, CO: National Education Policy Center. Retrieved July 28, 2014, from http://nepc.colorado.edu/publication/scaling-up-innovations.

Lino, M. (2013). *Expenditures on children by families, 2012* (pp. 1528–2012). Washington, DC: U.S. Department of Agriculture, Center for Nutrition Policy and Promotion. Miscellaneous Publication No.

Lozoff, B., Brittenham, G. M., Wolf, A. W., McClish, D. K., Kuhnert, P. M., Jimenez, E., … Krauskoph, D. (1987). Iron deficiency anemia and iron therapy effects on infant developmental test performance. *Pediatrics, 79*(6), 981–995.

Lukowski, A. F. (2010). Iron deficiency in infancy and neurocognitive functioning at 19 years: Evidence of long-term deficits in executive function and recognition memory. *Nutritional Neuroscience, 13*(2), 54–70.

McLeod, J. D., & Shanahan, M. J. (1993). Poverty, parenting and children's mental health. *American Sociological Review, 58*(3), 351–366.

McLoyd, V. C. (1998). Socioeconomic disadvantage and child development. *American Psychologist, 53*(2), 185–204.

McLoyd, V. C., Jayaratne, T. E., Ceballo, R., & Borquez, J. (1994). Unemployment and work interruption among African American single mothers: Effects on parenting and adolescent socioemotional functioning. *Child Development, 65*(2), 562–589.

Mistry, R. S., Vandewater, E. A., Huston, A., & McLoyd, V. C. (2002). Economic well-being and children's social adjustment: The role of family process in an ethnically diverse low-income sample. *Child Development, 73*(3), 935–951.

Mosle, A., & Patel, N. (2012). *Two generations, one future: Moving parents and children beyond poverty together*. Washington, DC: The Aspen Institute. Retrieved July 28, 2014, from ascend. aspeninstitute.org/resources/two-generations-one-future.

Murphy, J. M. (2007). Breakfast and learning: An updated review. *Journal of Current Nutrition and Food Science, 3*(1), 3–36.

Murphy, J. M., Pagano, M., Nachmani, J., Sperling, P., Kane, S., & Kleinman, R. (1998). The relationship of school breakfast to psychosocial and academic functioning: Cross-sectional and longitudinal observations in an inner-city sample. *Archives of Pediatric and Adolescent Medicine, 152*, 899–907.

Nagahawatte, N. T. (2008). Poverty, maternal health, and adverse pregnancy outcomes. *Annals of the New York Academy of Sciences, 1136*(1), 80–85.

National Education Goals Panel. (1995). *Reconsidering children's early development and learning: Toward common views and vocabulary*. Washington, DC: National Education Goals Panel.

National Research Council and Institute of Medicine. (2000). *From neurons to neighborhoods: The science of early childhood development*. Committee on Integrating the Science of Early Childhood Development. In J. Shonkoff & D. Phillips (Eds.). Board on Children, Youth, and Families, Commission on Behavioral and Social Sciences and Education. Washington, DC: National Academy Press.

Needleman, H. L. (1990). Low-level lead exposure and the IQ of children: A meta-analysis of modern studies. *Journal of the American Medical Association, 263*(5), 673.

Neuman, S. B. (2001). Access to print in low-income and middle-income communities: An ecological study of fur neighborhoods. *Reading Research Quarterly, 36*(1), 8–26.

Nichols, A. (2013). *Poverty and unemployment. Urban institute unemployment and recovery project*. Washington, DC: Urban Institute.

O'Donnell, K. (2008). *Parents' reports of the school readiness of young children from the national household education surveys program of 2007 (NCES 2008-051)*. Washington, DC: National Center for Education Statistics, Institute of Education Sciences, U.S. Department of Education.

Ogden, C. L., Lamb, M. M., Carroll, M. D., & Flegal, K. M. (2010). Obesity and socioeconomic status in children and adolescents: United States, 2005-2008. *National Center for Health Statistics Data Brief, 51*, 1–7.

Olds, D. L., Eckenrode, J., Henderson, C. R., Kitzman, H., Powers, J., Cole, R… Luckey, D. (1997). Long-term effects of home visitation on maternal life course and child abuse and neglect: Fifteen-year follow-up of a randomized trial. *Journal of the American Medical Association, 278*(8), 637-643.

Olds, D. L., Henderson, H. R., & Kitzman, H. (1994). Does prenatal and infancy nurse home visitation have enduring effects on qualities of parental caregiving and child health at 25 to 50 months of life? *Pediatrics, 93*(1), 89–98.

Olds, D. L., Henderson, H. R., Tatelbaum, R., & Chamberlin, R. (1986a). Improving the delivery of prenatal care and outcomes of pregnancy: A randomized trial of nurse home visitation. *Pediatrics, 77*, 16–28.

Olds, D. L., Henderson, H. R., Tatelbaum, R., & Chamberlin, R. (1986b). Preventing child abuse and neglect: A randomized trial of nurse home visitation. *Pediatrics, 78*, 65–78.

Olds, D. L., Robinson, J., O'Brien, R., Luckey, D. W., Pettitt, L. M., Henderson, C. R., … Talmi, A. (2002). Home visiting by paraprofessionals and by nurses: A randomized, controlled trial. *Pediatrics, 110*, 486–496.

Olds, D. L., Robinson, J., Pettitt, L., Luckey, D. W., Holmberg, J., Ng, R. K… Henderson, C. R. (2004). Effects of home visits by paraprofessionals and by nurses: Age 4 follow-up results of a randomized trial. *Pediatrics, 114*, 1560–1568.

Piasta, S. B., & Wagner, R. K. (2010). Developing early literacy skills: A meta-analysis of alphabet learning and instruction. *Reading Research Quarterly, 45*(1), 8–38.

Petterson, S. M. (2001). Effects of poverty and maternal depression on early child development. *Child Development, 72*(6), 1794–1813.

Plotnick, R. D. (1997). Child poverty can be reduced. *The Future of Children: Children and Poverty, 7*(2), 72–87.

Preschool Curriculum Evaluation Research Consortium (PCERC) (2008). *Effects of preschool curriculum programs on school readiness* (NCER 2008-2009, pp. 99-108, C-17, C-18, D-17, D-18). National Center for Education Research, Institute of Education Sciences, U.S. Department of Education. Washington, DC: Government Printing Office.

Princeton-Brookings. (2014). Helping parents, helping children: Two generation mechanisms. *The Future of Children, 24*(1).

Reardon, S. F. (2011). The widening academic achievement gap between the rich and the poor: New evidence and possible explanations. In R. Murnane & G. Duncan (Eds.), *Whither opportunity? Rising inequality and the uncertain life chances of Low-income children.* New York, NY: Russell Sage.

Reynolds, A. J. (2000). *Success in early intervention: The Chicago child-parent centers.* Lincoln, NE: University of Nebraska Press.

Reynolds, A. J., Temple, J. A., White, B. A. B., Ou, S., & Robertson, D. L. (2011). Age 26 cost–benefit analysis of the child-parent center early education program. *Child Development, 82*(1), 379–404.

Richardson, G. A., Goldschmidt, L., Larkby, C., & Day, N. L. (2013). Effects of prenatal cocaine exposure on child behavior and growth at 10 years of age. *Neurotoxicology and Teratology, 40*(1), 1–8.

Riley, A. W., Coiro, M .J., Broitman, M., Colantuoni, E., Hurley, K. M., Bandeen-Roche, K., Miranda, J. (2009). Mental health of children of low-income depressed mothers: influences of parenting, family environment, and raters. *Psychiatric Services, 60*(3), 329–336.

Robert Wood Johnson Foundation Commission to Build a Healthier America. (2011). *Early childhood experiences and health.* Princeton, NJ: Robert Wood Johnson Foundation. Issue Brief 2.

Rodriguez, E. (2013). *Federal policies to reward and support work in a difficult economy.* Washington, DC: National Council of La Raza. Submitted to Subcommittee on Human Resources of the Committee on Ways and Means. Retrieved January 27, 2015, from http://docs.house.gov/meetings/WM/WM03/20130618/101003/HHRG-113-WM03-Wstate-RodriguezE-20130618.pdf.

Rose-Jacobs, R. (2008). Household food insecurity: Associations with at-risk infant and toddler development. *Pediatrics (Evanston), 121*(1), 65–72.

Sampson, R. J. (2001). How do communities undergird or undermine human development? Relevant contexts and social mechanisms. In A. Booth & A. C. Crouter (Eds.), *Does It take a village? Community effects on children, adolescents, and families* (pp. 3–30). Mahwah, NJ: L Erlbaum.

Sampson, R., & Laub, J. H. (1994). Urban poverty and the family context of delinquency: A new look at structure and process in a classic study. *Child Development, 65*(2), 523–540.

Schlee, B. M. (2009). Parents social and resource capital: Predictors of academic achievement during early childhood. *Children and Youth Services Review, 31*(2), 227–234.

Schwartz, J. (1994). Low-level lead exposure and children's IQ: A meta-analysis and search for a threshold. *Environmental Research, 65*(1), 42–55.

Schweinhart, L. J., Montie, J., Xiang, Z., Barnett, W. S., Belfield, C. R., & Nores, M. (2005). *Lifetime Effects: The High/Scope Perry Preschool Study through Age 40.* Ypsilanti, MI: HighScope Press.

Sherman, A. (2004). *Hardships are widespread among families in poverty.* Washington, DC: Center for Budget and Policy Priorities. Retrieved July 11, 2014, from http://www.cbpp.org/files/12-20-04pov.pdf.

Siefert, K., Bowman, P. J., Heflin, C. M., Danziger, S., & Williams, D. R. (2000). Social and environmental predictors of maternal depression in current and recent welfare recipients. *American Journal of Orthopsychiatry, 70*(4), 510–522.

Simms, M. C., Fortuny, K., & Henderson, E. (2009a). *Children of immigrants: National and state characteristics.* Washington, DC: The Urban Institute.

Simms, M. C., Fortuny, K., & Henderson, E. (2009b). *Racial and ethnic disparities among low-income families.* Washington, DC: Low-Income Working Families Project Fact Sheet.

St. Pierre, R. G., Layzer, J. I., & Barnes, H. V. (1995). Two-generation programs: Design, cost, and short-term effectiveness. *The Future of Children, 5*(3).

Smith, S. (Ed.). (1995). *Two generation programs for families in poverty: A new intervention strategy. Advances in developmental psychology.* Norwood, NJ: Alex.

United Nations Children's Fund. (2012). *Measuring child poverty: New league tables of child poverty in the World's rich countries. Innocenti report card 10.* Florence, Italy: UNICEF Innocenti Research Centre.

Census Bureau, U. S. (2014a). How the census bureau measures poverty. *Social, Economic, and Housing Statistics Division: Poverty.* Last revised September 16, 2014. Retrieved January 22, 2015, from https://www.census.gov/hhes/www/poverty/about/overview/measure.html.

Census Bureau, U. S. (2014b). *Measuring America: How census measures poverty.* Washington, DC: U.S. Department of Commerce, Economics and Statistics Administration. Retrieved January 24, 2015, from http://www.census.gov/library/infographics/poverty_measure-how.html.

U.S. Census Bureau. (2013). *Current population survey, 2013 annual social and economic supplement.* Washington, DC: Author.

U.S. Census Bureau. (2012). Estimates of the population of the United States by single years of age, color, and sex: Data for 2013 were derived from the national population projections released in December 2012. *Current Population Reports.* Washington, DC: U.S. Census Bureau.

U.S. Department of Agriculture. (2014). *Geography of poverty.* Washington, DC: USDA, Economic Research Service. Retrieved June 30, 2014, from http://www.ers.usda.gov/topics/rural-economy-population/rural-poverty-well-being/geography-of-poverty.aspx#.U7GkvKhn7YY.

U.S. Department of Labor. (2014). *FAQs about Affordable Care Act Implementation (Part XVIII) and mental health parity implementation.* Washington, DC: DOL. Retrieved July 28, 2014, from http://www.dol.gov/ebsa/faqs/faq-aca18.html.

Vespa, J., Lewis, J. M., & Kreider, R. M. (2013, August). *America's families and living arrangements: Population characteristics.* Washington, DC: U.S. Department of Commerce, Economics and Statistics Administration, U.S. Census Bureau. Report P20-570.

Wagmiller, R. L. (2006). The dynamics of economic disadvantage and Children's life chances. *American Sociological Review, 71*(5), 847–866.

White House Task Force on the Middle Class. (2010). *Annual report of the White House Task Force on the middle class.* Washington, DC: Office of the Vice President of the United States.

Weissman, M. M. (1999). Maternal smoking during pregnancy and psychopathology in offspring followed to adulthood. *Journal of the American Academy of Child and Adolescent Psychiatry, 38*(7), 892–899.

Wilson, W. J. (2009). *More than just race: Being black and poor in the inner city.* New York, NY: Norton.

Wood, D. (2003). Effect of child and family poverty on child health in the United States. *Pediatrics, 112*(3), 707–711.

World Health Organization Commission on Social Determinants of Health. (2008). *Closing the gap in a generation: Health equity through action and the social determinants of health.* Geneva: World Health Organization.

Yeung, W. J., Linver, M. R., & Brooks–Gunn, J. (2002). How Money Matters for Young Children's Development: Parental Investment and Family Processes. Child Development, 73, 1861–1879. doi:10.1111/1467-8624.t01-1-00511.

Yoshikawa, H., Aber, J. L., & Beardslee, W. R. (2012). The effects of poverty on the mental, emotional, and behavioral health of children and youth: Implications for prevention. *American Psychologist, 67*(4), 272–284.

Chapter 4
Impact of Family Structure, Functioning, Culture, and Family-Based Interventions on Children's Health

Karol L. Kumpfer, Cátia, Magalhães, and Sheetal A. Kanse

4.1 Introduction

There are many different types of family structures worldwide that can have differing impacts on children's health and well-being. In Western and Eastern cultures, children have been raised primarily by two biological parents with large extended families and communities.

In other cultures, parents might not be the primary caretakers or advisors, and that role is assumed by a grandparent, aunt, or uncle. The head of the household or who has the most power also varies greatly—the mother, the grandmother, the father, the grandfather, or another family member.

4.1.1 History of the Breakdown in Family Support Structures

During the Industrial Revolution, many families moved from small farming and fishing villages to work in urban factories (De Vries, 2008). This trend continues today, with one or both parents moving to cities, leaving their children to be raised by grandparents or relatives in small rural towns. In rapidly developing countries such as China, India, and Brazil, there has been a massive migration of rural parents

K.L. Kumpfer, Ph.D. (✉) • S.A. Kanse, M.P.H., Ph.D.
Department of Health Promotion and Education, University of Utah,
Salt Lake City, UT 84112, USA
e-mail: kkumpfer@xmission.com; drsheetal15@yahoo.co.in

C. Magalhães, Ph.D.
Polytechnic Institute of Viseu, ESEV-Department of Psychology,
Rua Maximiano Aragão, 3504-501 Viseu, Portugal
e-mail: catiacmagalhaes@gmail.com

© Springer Science+Business Media New York 2016
M.R. Korin (ed.), *Health Promotion for Children and Adolescents*,
DOI 10.1007/978-1-4899-7711-3_4

to cities. These parents hope to pay for their children's education, welfare, and a better life (Child Trends, 2013) but are leaving their children at higher risk for academic and developmental problems because of loss of parental supervision, protection, and support (Bowlby, 2008).

In developed countries, immigrant or refugee families from developing or war-torn countries often arrive first to cities and then bring over as many relatives as possible. They live in one household or closely, so children have many "parents" and lots of siblings and cousins to play with. These families slowly become more isolated as they move up to better jobs and their own homes in the suburbs. As both parents work to pay for a house and birth control reduces family size, children are eventually left with almost no one to support and nurture them (Zhou, 2009). Because school ends long before parents return from work, children come home to an empty house (Reno & Riley, 2000). This breakdown of the family is happening worldwide.

4.1.2   Stresses on the Traditional Institutions of Marriage and Family

For most of the twentieth century, the two-parent family was the norm in the USA. Between 1880 and 1970, about 85 % of all children lived in two-parent house-holds (Kreider & Renee, 2009; Lang & Zagorsky, 2001). With the advent of the Second Demographic Transition (SDT), starting in the 1970s, the numbers of divorces and single-parent families increased rapidly, leveling off in 1995 at 67 % and continuing to today (Child Trends, 2013). These dramatic changes in family structure have resulted in ever-widening health disparities including educational, economic, and social hardships for the children born in fragile homes of the less educated parents (McLanahan, 2004; McLanahan & Jacobsen, 2015; Putmam, 2015). Increases in divorce, separation, cohabitation, out-of-wedlock births, single-parent families, and changes in gender roles and sexuality since the 1970s have reduced the percentage of traditional mother/father families (Popenoe, 2009). Single-parent American households increased from 11 % in 1970 to 29 % by 2007. About a third of the US children under 18 live in biological father-absent homes, and about a third of these children are under 9 years of age (Mather, 2010). The collapse of the traditional family structure hit the African American families even sooner in the 1960s (Moynihan, 1965). Contributing to increased poverty and health disparities, more African American children (52 %) than white children live with single mothers (Mather, 2010). Most children who live with a divorced parent live with their moth-ers and only 20 % with their fathers (United States Census Bureau, 2011a, 2011b) leaving 10 % of children who live with a grandparent, with other relatives, or with nonrelatives. Of the children who live in nonrelatives' homes, about a third live with foster parents (United States Census Bureau, 2012).

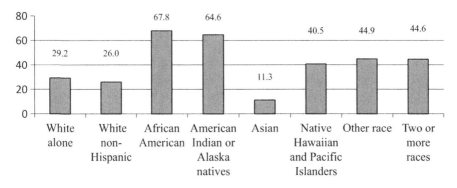

Fig. 4.1 Percentage of nonmarital births to unmarried women aged 15–50, by race and ethnicity (US Census Statistics, 2011a, 2011b)

Single mother households have increased primarily because of a sharp rise in births to unmarried women that has more than doubled in the last 30 years to 41 % by 2011. According to Putnam (2015), "the class divide is growing even as the racial gap is shrinking" as manifested in a fourfold increase in part of this decrease was due to a recent 8 % decline in the birth rate for teenagers. In 2011, the National Vital Statistics System reported that nonmarital birth rates were highest among African American women (68 %), followed by American Indians and Alaska natives (64 %) and Hispanic women (43 %) as compared to non-Hispanic whites (29 %) and Asian or Pacific Islanders (11.3 %) (Shattuck & Kreider, 2013) (Fig. 4.1).

In a new book, *Our Kids: The American Dream in Crisis*, Robert Putnam (2015) argues that class, and not race, is related most to health disparities and unwed births, leading to a bifurcation into two different family structures. The college-educated upper third of society tend to have stable "neo-traditional" two-parent marriages, in which both parents work and share household duties. Divorce rates have gone down from their peak in the 1970s and mother's age of first birth has increased. With two incomes and higher education, these parents provide more opportunities for their children. In contrast, in the only high-school educated, a much more diverse pattern of family structure emerged with sexual partnership being less durable. Sara McLanahan (2004) labeled these "fragile families" where the parents may have never been married or divorced later, resulting in more single-parent families and poverty. Age of first birth has also decreased to 10 years earlier than in the better-educated mothers.

Putnam (2015) highlights that these very different family structures are resulting in an ever-widening gap or inequality of opportunity for children in the USA. He suggests that class (education level and income), rather than race, is the major predictor of how well children do in life because of more opportunities and effective parenting in better-educated parents. The incidence of unwed mothers and single-mother households is more related to lower education levels today than race. By 2012, the percent of children aged 0–7 living in a single-parent household was lower than 10 % in parents with a bachelor's degree but over 65 % in 2012 for parents with only a high-school degree (Putnam, 2015). Fewer than 10 % of births were nonmarital for college-educated females regardless of race, whereas it was 65 % for women with just a high-school education.

Race does make a small difference as only 2 % of births were out of wedlock for white college graduates. According to Putnam (2015), "the class divide is growing even as the racial gap is shrinking" as manifest in a fourfold increase in nonmarital births to high-school-educated whites to 50 % but a decrease by a third to 25 % in college-educated African American women.

As will be discussed in detail later in this chapter, upper- and middle-class parents are richer, are more nurturing, spend more time with their children, and provide educational opportunities. Births to underage, unmarried, and low-education-level women not only restrict children's access to social and economic resources but increase their risk of poor outcomes (e.g., low birth weight, preterm birth, infant mortality, and poorer developmental outcomes) (Chandra, Martinez, Mosher, Abma, & Jones, 2005).

4.2   Impact of Different Family Structures on Children

The social and sexual revolution in the 1970s or the SDT brought new and more fluid family structures such as cohabitation, divorce, and step-, adoptive-, foster-, and single-parent families. These changing family structures increase children's stress, reduce attachment to significant others, and decrease time with pro-social fathers or male role models, which can negatively affect children's psychosocial development as well as physical and mental health (McLanahan, 2004; Lamb & Lewis, 2011).

The Impact on Children of Single-Parent Families: Most children who grow up with a single parent can have positive health and psychosocial developmental outcomes if the family has adequate resources, time for parents or other caring adults to spend with their children, and effective parenting skills. Unfortunately, children in father-absent homes are almost four times more likely to be poor (44 % compared to 12 % in married-couple families) (United States Census Bureau, 2011a, 2011b). Unless child support is paid, children in single-parent families with little extended family support typically are negatively impacted. As discussed earlier, parents' low levels of education can also negatively affect children's well-being. Single mothers are generally poorer, more highly stressed, and less well educated (McLanahan & Jacobsen, 2015).

Most research focuses on the impact of fathers' absence, but mothers' absence also puts children at risk. The differences in single-parent and two-parent families are insufficient to support the claim that parental absence is the *primary* cause of children with worse behavioral and physical health. There is evidence, however, that above the mediating factor of poverty, the absence of fathers is responsible for at least some negative child outcomes (McLanahan & Sandefur, 1994).

The Effect of Divorce on Children: Unfortunately about 50 % of US marriages end in divorce (CDC, 2011). Family conflict, separation, and litigation are stressful for the couple and the children too. Children who experienced divorce have strained family relationships, poorer academic achievement, more school dropout, delayed psychosocial development, higher levels of anxiety and depression, anger management and trust issues, and early sexual behavior. As adults, they have higher chances of divorcing, choosing cohabitation over marriage, and negative religious feelings (Carrier & Utz, 2012).

The Effects of Cohabitation on Children: Compared to only 5 % of unmarried pregnant women who choose a "shotgun" wedding, 18 % opted to move in with their boyfriends before the child was born (CDC, 2014). Of all births in the 2000s, 60 % were to married mothers, 24 % to cohabiting mothers, and 16 % to single mothers. This increase is attributed to reduced social stigma for out-of-wedlock births and cohabitation (Bramlett & Mosher, 2002). Cohabitation is more likely to lead to stable relationships and marriage as well as lower pregnancy rates in the more highly educated cohabiting couples. But in contrast for high-school-educated Americans, cohabitation is a considered way station to finding the right person and to permanent partnership (Putnam, 2015). McLanahan and associates (2005) found that 5 years after the birth of a child, about 50 % of cohabitating women, but more than 66 % of unmarried women, were no longer in any romantic relationship with the father. Some couples cohabitate to save money, learn if they are really compatible, or wait for more stable jobs and better finances. Forty percent of children are expected to spend some time in a cohabiting parent family because of being born to already cohabiting parents or one of their biological parents opting for cohabitation (Bumpass & Lu, 2000; Fields & Casper, 2000). Children of cohabiting partners or cohabitating grandparents tend to follow the same lifestyle of cohabitation (Sassler, Cunningham, & Lichter, 2009).

Cohabiting parents have slightly more negative parenting practices because they are more highly stressed by family instability and lack of financial resources (Brown, 2002; Hofferth & Anderson, 2003; Morrison, 2000). Children residing in cohabiting stepfather families experience higher rates of school suspension or expulsion, delinquency, lower grades, lack of college expectations, and increased emotional and behavioral problems than teenagers living with two married biological parents (Manning & Lamb, 2003). However, children in cohabitating families have better outcomes than those living with single parents because they have better financial security and more positive parent support and nurturing.

The Impact of Stepfamilies on Children: The number of stepfamilies in the USA has risen because of high rates of divorce and remarriage. About 40 % of US families are stepfamilies or "blended" families. Almost half of US adults have at least one step relationship (e.g., being a stepchild, a stepsibling, or a stepparent), including 15 % of men being stepfathers and about 12 % of women who are stepmothers (Deal, 2013; Parker, 2011).

Joining a stepfamily can be especially stressful for adolescents as it often also involves ending any lingering hopes of the biological parents reuniting. Research shows that younger children adjust more easily than teens (Amato, 2005). Adolescents living with a single parent tend to have more autonomy and lack of interference by parents. Parental monitoring by a stepparent can be viewed by teens as interference, and sometimes they react with aggression. Children may suffer from loyalty conflicts between their stepparent and the biological parent because of a belief that accepting their new stepparent would mean betraying their biological parent. They can also experience insecurity, abandonment, resentment, and jealousy when having to share parental time and attention with a stepparent or siblings (Hetherington & Kelly, 2002). These children often have less mother-child interaction, more mother-child disagreement, and more problem behaviors than children in two-biological-parent families (Amato, 2005; Demo & Acock, 1996; Hoffmann, 2006). Hence, remarriage of a single parent does not necessarily ensure better psychological well-being for the children. Factors that can impact children's health and well-being in new stepfamilies include ages of the children and *adults*, length of time since the divorce and remarriage, and, most importantly, the stepfamily's functioning—the type of relationship between stepparents and children and between the biological parents and children (Hoffmann, 2006).

Impact on Children of Adoption and Foster Care: Research on the impact on children of foster care is complicated because children may have been exposed to maltreatment before placement, leading to negative outcomes, feelings of being unloved, and lack of attachment and bonding (Erickson & Egeland, 2002). Children are removed from their homes primarily because of maltreatment, including neglect and abuse (physical, emotional, sexual), and also because of poverty, caretaker death, and incapacity. The impact on the children's health and psychosocial development depends primarily on the quality of the child/foster parent relationship, the length of time in foster care, and number of placements. Multiple failures or rejections by foster parents are related to increased behavioral health problems such as substance abuse and delinquency. Children from unstable foster homes are more likely than children in the general population to suffer poorer developmental outcomes (e.g., poor physical and mental health, lower academic performance and increased school dropout, teen pregnancies, attachment problems, low self-esteem, failed marriages, social isolation) (Rubin, O'Reilly, Luan, & Localio, 2007; Simms, Dubowitz, & Szilagyi, 2000). Outcomes are improved, however, if the child gets a stable long-term foster home and nurturing parents or is adopted.

Lawrence, Carlson, and Egeland (2006) suggested that adoption could better serve these children because of economic advantage, stability, and positive parenting. Adoption to long-term loving families has positive impact on children, but foster care can negatively impact children if they are moved from home to home.

One hopeful statistic is that the number of children in foster care has dropped by about a quarter since 2002 and the average number of months in foster care has declined from 31 to 22 months. More judges are requiring parents reported for child maltreatment to participate in parenting education courses in an effort to reduce the very high costs of foster care from about $25,000 to $75,000 per year and keep children with their parents. Effective parenting programs have cut days in foster care in half (Brook, McDonald, & Yan, 2012). However, this is still a long time for children to be in out-of-the-home placement and without their parents.

4.3   Impact of Family Functioning on Children

This section will highlight research on family or parental functioning that are mediating or more direct causal factors in negative health outcomes for children. In other words, the major risk factor for children is not the family structure directly but the impact of family structures on the parent–child relationship, parenting effectiveness or style, and functional relations within the family. For instance, research on the impact of having only one parent is confounded by moderating and mediating factors such as socioeconomic status, class, poverty, educational opportunities, amount of time spent with the child, and parental emotional or mental dysfunction. Many nontraditional family structures provide less security, protection, and care for children because overstressed or dysfunctional parents often lack the money or time to provide adequate parenting opportunities. Research on critical functional risks is discussed below.

4.3.1   Impact of Dysfunctional Parents

Clearly, mentally ill, depressed, highly stressed, and substance-abusing parents face more difficulties in child raising. Parents who are substance users are often unable to provide a safe and nurturing home for their children, as studies have found their family environment to be chaotic with reduced family organization and family routines and rituals and increased conflict between parents and children (Kumpfer & DeMarsh, 1986). Drug abusers spent about half as much time with their children as normal families. Authoritarian and inconsistent parenting was also a hallmark of substance-using and depressed parents (Dette-Hagenmeyer & Reichle, 2013). Researchers also found that parental depressive symptoms were a mediator of children's poorer social-emotional development. Children of parents with substance use disorders (SUDs) experience two to nine times greater risk of becoming substance abusers as adolescents or adults (Chassin, Carle, Nissim-Sabat, & Kumpfer, 2004). They are also at higher risk for child maltreatment and foster care placement.

Because of their higher risk, children of substance abusers need evidence-based family services and also extra community support services to prevent child maltreatment, poorer health and behavioral health outcomes, and placement into foster care (Kumpfer & Johnson, 2011). A 5-year multi-site federally funded study (Brook et al., 2012) found days in foster care reduced by half and improved parenting skills and children's behavioral and depression outcomes in families graduating from the *Strengthening Families Program*, an evidence-based 14-week family skills training program designed to improve the behavioral health of children of drug abusers.

4.3.2 Decreased Parent Time with Children

Worldwide, parents are spending less time parenting and supporting their children. The increased absence of parents and extended family is related to child health and educational risks. A study conducted by the Annenberg Center (2009) found that in just 3 years the amount of time parents in the USA spent caring, teaching, or social- izing with their children decreased by a third to only 4.5 h per week by 2008. Education level and two-parent households are related to the amount of time spent with children. In the 1970s, there was almost no difference by socioeconomic level in time that parents spent talking, reading, and playing with their children. However, for children 0–4 years, more educated parents increased their time in "developmen- tal care" from 30 min per day in 1975 to a high of 132 min per day for more edu- cated parents but only to 89 min per day for less educated parents. Today, the children of college-educated parents receive 50 % more of what Putnam (2015) calls "Goodnight Moon" time.

Few US parents still eat with their children every day, although two-thirds of children in other countries still have their main meal with their parents. Once again, parent's education is related to eating dinner together, which decreased in both lower- and higher-education-level parents to 70 % and 74 %, respectively, until 1990 for "usually eat dinner together." However, for the more highly educated parents, usually eating together increased slightly to 75 % by 2005, but decreased to 63 % in parents with only a high-school degree (Putnam, 2015). Even fewer children talk with their parents on a regular basis (UNICEF, 2007). Educated parents engage in constant dialogue with their children to teach values, skills, and expectations for their behavior. This takes time, and it helps to have a reliable and supportive spouse to share the job of child raising, not to mention cleaners, drivers, babysitters, and cash for educational and recreational opportunities. Overworked and less educated parents tend to demand from their children to just obey them or else be spanked. While this saves time, Putnam (2015) suggests that these poor parenting practices are a barrier to upward social mobility because the children do not learn to think for themselves.

This trend toward reduced parent–child involvement is particularly evident in immigrant or refugee families whose parents must often work more than one low- paid job. The loss of parent–child time together is even more apparent in develop- ing countries, such as China and India, where more parents are moving away from their rural children to cities to work in factories. Even in developed countries Europe and Australia/New Zealand, parents are spending less time in child rearing (IREFREA, 2010).

Behavioral health problems such as alcohol and drug use and delinquency in European youth are increasing particularly in girls as they did in the USA in the mid-1990s with the breakdown of the traditional family structure (Kumpfer, Smith, & Franklin Summerhays, 2008; Kumpfer, 2014). This increase in substance abuse in teen girls was related to increased divorce rates and separation of fathers in US families as well as more single-mother families living in poverty. High levels of parental absence are also related to substance abuse (Kumpfer & DeMarsh, 1986), divorce, separation, imprisonment, military deployment, foster care placement, and parental employment in another location.

Although generally parents are spending less time with their children, the good news is that fathers who do live with their children are much more involved and provide more child care than in previous generations (Livingston & Parker, 2011). The large fivefold increase from 1975 to 2013 in time spent by educated parents in child care of children under 4 years is likely due to fathers caring more for children. Even less educated parents increased their time with young children from 27 to 88 min per day (Putnam, 2015). This trend appears to be happening worldwide. Unfortunately, because of increases in nonmarital childbearing, fewer fathers now live with their children (Martin et al., 2013; CDC, 2014). The impact of nonmarital childbearing on the presence of fathers is moderated by more children being born into cohabiting unions (Martinez, Daniels, & Chandra, 2012).

4.3.3 Impact of Father Absence on Children's Developmental and Health Outcomes

Because more children today are raised without consistent father involvement, research on the impact of fathers' absence or presence on a child's development has increased (Booth & Crouter, 1998; Lamb, 1997; Lamb & Lewis, 2011). Lamb (2004) proposed that fathers influence children's outcomes, as do mothers, by their degree of emotional support, security, and encouragement. Conversely, father absence or disengagement is associated with negative effects on children (i.e., child abuse, depression, school failure, substance abuse, delinquency, early sexual activity, and teen pregnancy) (Jafee, Moffitt, Caspi, & Taylor, 2003). A child living with his/her divorced mother, compared to a child living with both parents, is 375 % more likely to suffer from anxiety or depression and hyperactivity and needs treatment (Ventura, Abma, Mostter, & Henslaw, 2008). Living with an involved father also decreases the risk of first substance use (Bronte-Tinkew, Kristin, Randolph, & Jonathan, 2006) and child maltreatment (Bendheim-Thomas Center, 2010). Even living in a neighborhood with fewer fathers increases the risk of teen violence (Resnick et al., 1997). Positive interaction by any father figure predicts better child health (Carr & Springer, 2010), including reduced obesity if the father is physically active (Trost, Kerr, Ward, & Pate, 2009). Paternal involvement in childhood is related to reduced police contact and crimes in teens (Flouri, 2005), and parent/teen closeness is correlated with greater adult marital satisfaction and happiness (Flouri & Buchanan, 2002).

4.3.4 Gender Differences in Children-Rearing Styles

Research suggests that fathers' and mothers' child rearing and discipline styles differ significantly (Lamb, 2010). The direct effects of fathering are especially salient when fathers' and mothers' interactions differ. Rowe, Coker, and Pan (2004) have suggested that, because fathers use more imperatives and attention-getting utterances and utter more complex sentences than mothers do, they contribute in unique, though still poorly understood, ways to linguistic development. Fathers also tend to stress justice, fairness, and duty (based on rules), while mothers stress sympathy, care, and help (based on relationships). Fathers tend to observe and enforce rules systematically and sternly, which teaches children the objectivity and consequences of right and wrong. Fathers tend to use more behavioral controls ("If you do that again, this is what will happen to you") as compared to mothers who tend to use more psychological controls ("If you loved me, you wouldn't disobey me"). Fathers tend to have a greater impact on their sons even if they do not refer to them as a role model (Fuhrmans & Fuhrer, 2013). Children with fathers tend to work harder to succeed in school and avoid getting into trouble. But if fathers control their children primarily through excessive physical punishment versus clear expectations, positive relationships, and time together, their children are more likely to experience emotional problems, psychosomatic disorders, and school difficulties and have lower levels of moral development (Lamb & Lewis, 2011).

4.4   Impact of Culture and Differential Cultural Acculturation on Health

Minorities now comprise 37% of the US population (US Census Bureau, 2012). Because of higher birth rates and immigration rates of minority families, particularly Latin and Asian families, they are predicted to become the majority (57%) by the year 2060 (CDC, 2013; US Census Bureau, 2012). Because of this demographic transition, racial and ethnic minorities will need increased attention from health educators, policy makers, and the government to identify and prevent health problems that afflict them. There is currently insufficient research on their cultures, traditions, health disparities, and culturally appropriate and effective health promotion programs and services.

4.4.1   Acculturation Among Minority Groups

Acculturation is defined as "the extent to which individuals have maintained their culture of origin or adapted to the larger society" (Phinney, 1996, p. 921). Acculturation is a complex multidimensional process, and the level of acculturation among minority populations depends on numerous factors such as age at immigration, circumstances during immigration, purpose of immigration, socioeconomic status, length of stay and location of residence in the host culture, exposure to host culture in work or community activities, and other cultural factors (Farver, Bhadha, & Narang, 2002).

Immigration imposes substantial pressures and increases stress in families. Immigrants are torn between retaining their original cultural identities while simultaneously accepting and assimilating into the host culture (Inman, Howard, Beaumont, & Walker, 2007). Previous research studies among Hispanic immigrants suggested that acculturation stress and deviation from the original cultural norms such as daily contact and social interaction with family and friends, language barriers, lower self-esteem, social isolation, boredom, and loneliness result in increased alcohol and substance abuse among immigrants (Gonzalez-Guarda, Ortega, Vasquez, & De Santis, 2010). Increased substance abuse is linked with negative health-related consequences such as cancer, cardiovascular disease, hepatitis, complications in pregnancy, mental illness, HIV infection, and intimate partner violence.

Differential Acculturation and Family Conflict: Children often assimilate more quickly to a new culture, creating increased family conflict because of differential generational acculturation (Chung, Flook, & Fuligni, 2009) leading to children's developmental problems such as delinquency, substance abuse, anxiety, depression, suicidal tendencies, violence, and prostitution (Dow, 2011; Farver et al., 2002; Feldman & Rosenthal, 1993). Role reversal can also happen in immigrant and refugee families when children learn the new language much faster and take on the parent role, creating a familial schism. Increased family conflict leads to a reduction in the family protective factors of family bonding, supervision, and communication of positive family values and influence (Rodnium, 2007).

Cultural Pride and Family Traditions: One of the protective factors against differential generational acculturation is the maintenance of ethnic pride and family traditions by individual family members leading to positive academic and psychological adjustment especially among adolescents and healthy familial environment (Berkel et al., 2010; Guilamo-Ramos, 2009; Smokowski, David-Ferdon, & Bacallao, 2009). Cuellar and Paniagua (2000) found that families and adolescents who strike a balance between maintaining their original family values and cultural traditions and acculturating to the new host culture have better emotional and behavioral health. Previous research suggests that parent–child communication and attachment and parental warmth promote ethnic pride among the children resulting in decreased risk of drug use and increased self-esteem (Umana-Taylor, Diversi, & Fine, 2002).

Multicultural Competencies: Research suggests that youth living in two or more cultures, while initially stressed, can acquire multicultural competencies that increase their resilience to behavioral health problems (Beauvais & Trimble, 2006). When facing additional stressors or in a new environment, they have a broader range of skills and appropriate responses. This increases the youth's confidence and self-esteem.

4.4.2 Professional Multicultural Competence

The American Association for Health Education defines cultural competence as "the ability of an individual to understand and respect values, attitudes, beliefs, and mores that differ across cultures, and to consider and respond appropriately to these differences in planning, implementing, and evaluating health education and promotion programs and interventions." One of the potential solutions to eliminate racial/ethnic disparities in health care is by developing a culturally competent health-care system (Betancourt, Green, Carrillo, & Ananeh-Firempong, 2003). However, chief barriers in achieving cultural competency include, but are not limited to, lack of cultural diversity among the health-care professionals, limited awareness regarding cultural differences in health-care professionals, and a dearth of culturally competent health programs leading to reduced enrollment of the ethnic population in health promotion and prevention programs (Johnson, Saha, Arbelaez, Beach, & Cooper, 2004).

Cultural competency can be achieved by recruiting ethnically diverse health-care professionals or training them to practice multicultural competencies, developing cultural appropriate and tailored health programs, increasing the participation of minority groups in national health surveillance and data systems, and increasing efforts toward research among ethnic minorities (Betancourt, Green, Carrilo, & Ananeh-Firempong, 2003). The greatest challenge that lies before the health-care system is developing culturally competent, evidence-based health programs that could address the health disparities among the ethnic minorities in the USA.

4.4.3 Lack of Culturally Tailored Programs for Ethnic Families

Previous research studies suggested that when family-based intervention programs are offered in schools and communities, it is difficult to recruit and retain ethnic families because most programs are not culturally appropriate nor taught in their primary language (Biglan & Metzler, 1999; McLean & Campbell, 2003; Watson, 2005). Participation of ethnic families can be as low as 10 % in these programs (Kumpfer, Alvarado, Smith, & Bellamy, 2002). Moreover, the majority of the health promotion and universal prevention programs are developed for the general American culture focusing mostly on white, middle-class values which might not be culturally appropriate or tailored to the specific needs of ethnic families.

Traditional ethnic families favor family systems change approach as compared to individual change approach for prevention, because of their cultural values that stress interconnection, reciprocity, and filial responsibility as contrasted with the Western value of individual achievement (Boyd-Franklin, 2001; Kumpfer, Alvarado, Smith, & Bellamy, 2002). Previous meta-analyses found that family-based interventions have effect sizes 2–9 times larger than youth-only interventions in decreasing youth behavioral health disorders in both traditional and acculturated minority families (Kumpfer et al., 2002; Tobler & Kumpfer, 2000). Hence, family interventions should be more effective for minority families.

4.5   Solutions to Strengthen Families

Because of the breakdown of the traditional family and the decrease in parental involvement in child rearing, parents have to be more effective and efficient with the little time they have with their children. Behavioral parenting programs and family therapy help to improve parents' child rearing skills. Evidence-based family interventions have proven to be the most cost-effective way to reduce negative health and social outcomes in youth.

4.5.1   Importance of the Family in Health Promotion and Prevention

While there are a number of different approaches to improved youth's health outcomes and delayed onset of alcohol and drug use among young people, evidence-based family skills training interventions appear to be the most effective (UNODC, 2009; Kumpfer & Hansen, 2014). Whereas youth-only programs work mostly for boys and not for girls, family interventions work for both girls and boys (Kumpfer, 2014). Meta-analyses have found that health promotion or prevention programs that improve ongoing family dynamics are the most effective (Foxcroft, Ireland, Lister-Sharp, Lowe, & Breen, 2003; Foxcroft & Tsertsvadze, 2012) because they promote healthy parent–child relationships including those causal factors found most important such as improved communication, bonding, parental monitoring, supervision, discipline, and family organization and rule setting (Petrie, Bunn, & Byrne, 2007).

4.5.2   Intervention Theories: Family Systems Theories

The family interventions found to be most effective are based on family systems theories proposed by Bowen (1991) and perfected in structural family therapy (Minuchin, 1974). The most effective parenting and family skills training programs are based on cognitive behavioral change theories including social learning/efficacy theory (Bandura, 2001). This theory emphasizes that learning occurs primarily in the social context of the family and friends and that behavior change occurs through role modeling, positive reinforcement, and even vicarious learning. These behavior change theories are targeted in effective parenting and family interventions to improve the most critical risk/resilience factors such as family attachment, supervision, and communication of positive expectations that are particularly important for preventing health problems for girls (Kumpfer, 2014). Our tested social ecology model (Kumpfer, Alvarado, & Whiteside, 2003) found that girls are slightly more impacted by these three family protective factors than are boys; hence, Evidence based (EB) family interventions are very useful in the prevention of behavioral health problems in girls as well as boys.

4.5.3 Types of Family Interventions and Effectiveness

A review of effective Evidence Based Program (EBP) approaches or types of family interventions determined that four family-based approaches demonstrated the highest level of evidence of effectiveness in reducing behavioral and emotional problems in children 5 years old and up. These evidence-based family intervention approaches include (1) behavioral parent training (primarily cognitive/behavioral parent training), (2) family skills training (including parent training, children's skills training, and family practice time together), (3) family therapy (structural, functional, or behavioral family therapy), and (4) in-home family support (Kumpfer & Alvarado, 2003).

Although these effective family interventions target different stages of a child's early development, they share certain critical core content. They all include interactive experiential teaching methods rather than didactic teaching methods and stressing knowledge change to achieve faster behavior changes. Additionally, they include methods for engaging and retaining hard-to-reach families and removing barriers to attendance (e.g., transportation, meals, child care, personal invitations, incentives for homework completions or attendance, a warm and welcoming staff and location).

4.5.4 Effective Evidence-Based Family Interventions

Periodic expert reviews conducted over the past 20 years have helped identify individual evidence-based family interventions. Criteria for evidence of effectiveness included large positive changes, randomized control trial studies of high quality, and independent replication. These reviews have found eight exemplary family interventions which include the following: Helping the Noncompliant Child (the basis of the FAST Track Project), the Incredible Years, the Strengthening Families Program, functional family therapy, multisystemic family therapy, Preparing for the Drug-Free Years (now called Guiding Good Choices), treatment foster care, and Triple P (UNODC, 2010). These family interventions are effective because they have sufficient dosage or length to meet the needs of the parents, involve the whole family in the behavior change, and target the most important family protective and risk factors (family bonding, supervision, and communication of positive values and norms). Other factors that impact attendance include attractive materials, adequate schedules, provision of meal and transportation, inclusion of child care, a warm and respectful staff, and good relationship skills.

Almost all evidence-based family programs tend to share common characteristics and focus on critical core elements that improve positive results. A CDC meta-analysis suggested that family skills trainings that include interactive training such as role playing, group discussion, and homework assignments and particularly parent–child practice time are more effective in preventing child maltreatment than training that uses reading and lecturing (Kaminski, Valle, Filene, & Boyle, 2008).

The most significant components predicting better outcomes were practicing with their child with a family coach, practicing consistent and positive communication, and home practice assignments to change behaviors at home. These components are important as they improve the parent–child relationship, which subsequently improves child behavior. Additionally, boosting children's social skills and emotion regulation skills has been shown to be the most important in preventing delinquency (Kumpfer et al., 2003). These skills create self-reinforcing pro-social behaviors that allow the child/adolescent to bond with positive adults, authority figures, and peers, and through these positive relationships, they can avoid delinquency and have more positive life outcomes. Other factors that increase program success are having a strength- and resilience-based focus, involving fathers, adapting the program to target the needs and cultural sensitivities of the families, having the appropriate intervention dose, and providing incentives and transportation to improve retention (Kumpfer & Alvarado, 2003).

The results from a meta-analysis suggested that family programs are on average nine times as effective in reducing conduct disorders, delinquency, substance abuse, and child abuse as youth-only focused programs (Tobler & Kumpfer, 2000, Tobler & Stratton, 1997). Another particular benefit of family programs is their cost benefit at $9–33 saved per dollar spent (Miller & Hendrie, 2008). Early elementary school parent training or family skills training programs have been found to be very effective in reducing aggression, conduct disorders, attention deficit/hyperactivity, and oppositional defiant disorders and preventing child abuse, drug abuse, and delinquency (Kumpfer & Alvarado, 2003; Kumpfer, 2014). Family skills training programs (e.g., SFP, Guiding Good Choices, Adolescent Transitions, Parents Who Care, Positive Parenting Program, or Triple P) appear to have particular promise. This category of program includes parent training, children's skills training, and a family practice session in family groups. The key to the success of these family skills training programs appears to be having the parents and children directly practice the new skills together and to have home practice assignments to bring their new modes of interaction into the home.

4.6 Use of Information Technology for Program Delivery and Dissemination of EBPs

Information technology has been increasingly used to obtain health-related information, manage and prevent diseases, and deliver behavioral change interventions (Budman, 2000; Moore, Fazzino, Garnet, Cutter, & Barry, 2011). In spite of promising results, information technology-based interventions (ITBI) have yet to attain their full potential. Though evidence-based family prevention programs have proven to be highly effective in preventing even inherited diseases in adolescents (Brody et al., 2012, 2014; Kumpfer, 2014; Loveland-Cherry, 2000), the cost of staff and staff training, multiple intervention sites, follow-up, and numerous implementation costs hinder their wide-scale dissemination and increase costs (Gordon, 2000; Miller & Hendrie, 2008). In addition, attendance barriers such as transportation and trouble with accessibility, busy family schedules and time constraints, inability to commit to multiple sessions, stigma associated with family therapy, or even parent education can reduce the program retention and engagement. Finally, using digital delivery technology could be beneficial for ethnic families because of the convenience of participation, lack of stigma, unwillingness to participate in group interventions, and the ability to review and practice the sessions for a longer period of time (Gordon, 2000; Ito, Kalyanaraman, Ford, Brown, & Miller, 2008; Haggerty, MacKenzie, Skinner, Harachi, & Catalano, 2006; 2007, Haggerty, Skinner, MacKenzie, & Catalano, 2007; Kumpfer & Brown, 2012; Kumpfer, 2014; Wingood et al., 2011). Haggerty et al., (2006, 2007) found that ethnic mothers benefited more from a CD of the program than attending family skills training group because they could review the video multiple times and could self-pace and were less likely to attend groups in person.

4.7   Effective Health Promotion Programs for Ethnic Families

As discussed above, immigrant and minority families have particular challenges that need to be addressed when creating family programs. Below are listed some critical protective factors in developing health promotion programs that are likely to be effective with minority or ethnic youth:

1. *Instill Cultural Pride and Competence.* Youth whose parents move to a new cultural community adapt better if they maintain pride in their ethnicity and culture of origin. Youth who feel culturally inferior feel more depressed and reject their family culture which leads to family conflict and rejection also.
2. *Promote Maintaining Cultural and Family Traditions.* Cultural traditions often help create order and predictability for children which reduce their stress. These cultural traditions often also connect the family to a cultural and religious community and increase support systems and participation in community celebrations.
3. *Build Multicultural Competencies.* As explained earlier, ethnic youth who understand and have multicultural skills to behave appropriately in both their culture and other cultures have been found to be less likely to become substance abusers and delinquent (Beauvais & Trimble, 2006). Hence, health educators should promote youth learning skills to be competent in both their culture and other cultures by exposing them to different cultures and peoples.
4. *Increase Family Attachment and Reduce Family Acculturation Conflict.* Youth who are bonded and attached to their parents are less likely to reject their culture or language of origin and have better adjustment (Champagne & Meaney, 2007; Champagne, 2010; Jirtle, 2010).

5. *Culturally Adapt Evidence-Based Health Promotion Programs.* Rather than develop culturally tailored health promotion program from scratch, it is usually more effective to select the best evidence-based program (EBP) that addresses the community's health risk and protective factors and needs and then culturally adapt the program following steps of gradual cultural adaptations and evaluation of effectiveness as recommended by the author and associates (Kumpfer, Pinyuchon, de Melo, & Whiteside, 2005; Kumpfer, Magalhães, & Xie, 2012). Five studies of cultural adaptation with the Strengthening Families Program for each major ethnic populations (rural and urban African Americans, Hispanics, American Indians, and Pacific Islanders) found that although outcomes were similar, recruitment and retention of participants were 40 % better when the program was culturally adapted (Kumpfer et al., 2002).

Hence, cultural adaptations of health promotion EBPs work to substantially improve engagement, acceptability, recruitment, and retention. Better outcomes will occur, however, only when adaptations reflect sensitivity to cultural values without affecting program fidelity (e.g., not reducing dosage, core interactive elements, and the focus on behavioral change). Culturally informed and responsive programs can both deliver the best science and address the practical concerns of a particular community (Castro, Barrera, & Martinez, 2004). And by implication, prevention interventions that are "culturally blind" will fail to appeal to local participants and likely erode the effectiveness of the original program (Kumpfer et al., 2002).

4.8 Policy Recommendations

Citizens and policy makers understand that the economic, cultural, and social future of a country depends on the quality of their young people in the next generation. Investing in children and families then should logically be a high priority, but often in budget decisions this is not the major factor considered compared to the needs of businesses and keeping taxes low. The USA trails many countries in policies that support families to raise productive and healthy children. There is a shared value in equality of opportunity, but class realities show a growing inequality of economic and social opportunity.

Effective policies to reduce the opportunity gap have been suggested by scholars in many different fields (Kenworthy, 2012), including emphasis on ways to keep families and children of all classes strong and effective, such as the following:

1. *Evidence-Based Parenting and Family Programs:* These should be funded and implemented widely in many settings, such as workplaces, community centers, child care centers, faith communities, and schools. Parenting and family skills classes should be acceptable for all families and not just high risk or failing families. EBP parenting programs should be mandated by judges for parents with open CPS reports and parents of youth involved in juvenile court.

2. *Provide EBP Parenting Programs Digitally*: Because of their high costs especially for family skills training groups or family therapy, these parenting programs should also be provided digitally without charge on the web, DVDs, smartphone apps, and TV. Because of their low cost, many more participants could be reached with equally effective outcomes to family group or individual delivery (Fang & Schinke, 2013; Haggerty et al., 2006, 2007; Kumpfer & Brown, 2012; Schinke, Fang, & Cole, 2011).
3. *Maternity and Paternity Leave for Both Parents in the First Year of the Child's Life*: Lack of bonding can lead to reactive attachment disorder, which is a known cause of violence against others due to lack of empathy.
4. *Child Care Quality Improvements*: There should be better standards, credentialing, and pay for child care workers. Evidence-based parenting programs should be offered or even made mandatory for parents to have their children attend child care programs.
5. *Reduce the Number of Children in Foster Care using EBP Family Skills Training*: Foster care is not a good substitute for helping biological parents learn to be better parents, which they can be done by mandating EBP parenting skills training courses. Family and drug court judges need the resources to mandate evidence-based parent and family skills training courses versus short but ineffective parent education classes.

4.9   Conclusions

The relationship between lack of positive parental involvement and negative outcomes in children and adolescents is well established. This relationship is not absolute; however, evidence-based prevention and treatment interventions should be disseminated widely to reduce health-care and social costs by helping parents or caregivers improve their parenting effectiveness, reunify children in foster care with their families, or help absent parents to reconnect with their children. Parent training opportunities in effective parent and family skills training programs should be disseminated widely at low or no cost to help mothers and fathers to feel more confident and competent in their parenting ability. In the end, it is the functioning and not the structure of the family that matters most. Children can be raised in stable two-parent families but still not receive the time and loving attention they need. However, in general, single parents who have not graduated from high school spend less time and provide fewer developmental learning opportunities for their children leading to increased educational, socioeconomic, and health disparities. This growing gap in opportunity for all children should be a high national priority. Since all children want and deserve loving and caring parents, policy makers should do all that they can to improve the ability of all parents to care for their children effectively regardless of income or educational level.

References

Amato, P. R. (2005). The impact of family formation change on the cognitive, social, and emotional well-being of the next generation. *The future of children, 15*(2), 75–96.

Annenberg Institute of School Reform. (2009). *Annual report.* Providence, RI: Annenberg Institute of School Reform, Brown University.

Bandura, A. (2001). Social cognitive theory and clinical psychology. In N. J. Smelser & P. B. Baltes (Eds.), *International encyclopedia of the social and behavioral sciences* (Vol. 21, pp. 14250–14254). Oxford: Elsevier Science.

Beauvais, F., & Trimble, J. E. (2003). The effectiveness of alcohol and drug abuse prevention among American-Indian youth. In Z. Sloboda & W. J. Bukoski (Eds.), *Handbook of drug abuse prevention: Theory, science, and practice* (pp. 393–410). New York, NY: Kluwer.

Bendheim-Thomas Center for Research on Child Wellbeing and Social Indicators Survey Center. (2010). *CPS involvement in families with social fathers.* Fragile Families Research Brief No.46. New York, NY: Author.

Berkel, C., Knight, G. P., Zeiders, K. H., Tein, J. Y., Roosa, M. W., Gonzales, N. A., et al. (2010). Discrimination and adjustment for Mexican American adolescents: A prospective examination of the benefits of culturally- related values. *Journal of Research on Adolescence, 20*, 893–915. doi:10.1111/j.1532-7795.2010.00668.x.

Betancourt, J. R., Green, A. R., Carrillo, J. E., & Ananeh-Firempong, O. (2003). Defining cultural competence: A practical framework for addressing racial/ethnic disparities in health and health care. *Public Health Rep, 118*, 293–302.

Biglan, A., & Metzler, C. (1999). A public health perspective for research on family-focused interventions. In R. Ashery, E. Robertson, & K. Kumpfer (Eds.), *Drug abuse prevention through family interventions.* Rockville, MD: National Institute on Drug Abuse (National Institute of Drug Abuse Research Monograph on family-focused' prevention research).

Booth, A., & Crouter, A. C. (1998). *Men in families: When do they get involved? WHAT difference does it make?* Mahwah, NJ: Erlbaum.

Bowen, M. (1991). *De la familia al individuo: la diferenciación del sí mismo en el sistema familiar.* Buenos Aires: Paidós.

Bowlby, J. (2008). *A secure base: Parent-child attachment and healthy human development.* New York: Basic Books.

Boyd-Franklin, N. (2001). Reaching out to larger systems. In interventions with multi-cultural families (Part 2). *The Family Psychologist, 17*(3), 1–4.

Bramlett, M. D., & Mosher, W. D. (2002). Cohabitation, marriage, divorce, and remarriage in the United States. *National Center for Health Statistics, Vital and Health Statistics Series 23* (22).

Brody, G. H., Chen, Y.-f., Kogan, S. M., Yu, T., Molgaard, V. K., DiClemente, R. J., & Wingood, G. M. (2012). Family-centered program to prevent substance use, conduct problems, and depressive symptoms in Black adolescents. *Pediatrics, 129*(1), 108–115.

Brody, G. H., Chen, Y. F., Beach, S. R., Kogan, S. M., Yu, T., Diclemente, R. J., ... Philibert, R. A. (2014). Differential sensitivity to prevention programming: A dopaminergic polymorphism-enhanced prevention effect on protective parenting and adolescent substance use. *Health Psychology, 33*(2):182–91.

Bronte-Tinkew, J., Kristin, M., Randolph, C., & Jonathan, Z. (2006). The influence of father involvement on youth risk behaviors among adolescents: A comparison of native-born and immigrant families. *Social Science Research, 35*(1), 181–209.

Brook, J., McDonald, T. P., & Yan, Y. (2012). An analysis of the impact of the strengthening families program on family reunification in child welfare. *Children and Youth Services Review, 34*, 691–695. doi:10.1016/j.childyouth.2011.12.018.

Brown, S. (2002). Child well-being in cohabiting families. In A. Booth & A. Crouter (Eds.), *Just living together: Implications of cohabitation for children, families and social policy* (pp. 173–188). Mahwah, NJ: Lawrence Erlbaum.

Budman, S. H. (2000). Behavioral health care dot-com and beyond: Computer-mediated communications in mental health and substance abuse treatment. *American Psychologist, 55,* 1290–1300.

Bumpass, L., & Lu, H.-H. (2000). Trends in cohabitation and implications for children's family contexts in the US. *Population Studies, 54*(1), 29–41.

Carr, D., & Springer, K. W. (2010). Advances in families and health research in the 21st century. *Journal of Marriage and Family, 72,* 743–761.

Carrier, H. U., & Utz, R. (2012). Parental divorce among young and adult children: A long-term quantitative analysis of mental health and family solidarity. *Journal of Divorce & Remarriage, 53*(4), 247–266. doi:10.1080/10502556.2012.663272.

Castro, F. G., Barrera, M., Jr., & Martinez, C. R. (2004). The cultural adaptation of preventive interventions: Resolving tensions between fidelity and fit. *Prevention Science, 5,* 41–45.

Centers for Disease Control and Prevention. (2011). *National marriage and divorce rate trends.* Retrieved from http://www.cdc.gov/nchs/nvss/marriage_divorce_tables.htm.

Centers for Disease Control and Prevention. (2013). *Asian American populations.* Retrieved from http://www.cdc.gov/minorityhealth/populations/REMP/asian.html.

Centers for Disease Control and Prevention. (2014). *National survey of family growth.* Retrieved from http://www.cdc.gov/nchs/nsfg.htm.

Champagne, F. (2010). Epigenetic influences of social interaction across the lifespan. *Developmental Psychobiology., 52*(4), 299–311. Online publication (www.interscience.wiley.com).

Champagne, F. A., & Meaney, M. J. (2007). Transgenerational effects of social environment on variations in maternal care and behavioral response to novelty. *Behavioral Neuroscience, 111*(6), 1353–1363.

Chandra, A., Martinez, G. M., Mosher, W. D., Abma, J. C., & Jones, J. (2005). Fertility, family planning, and reproductive health of U.S. women: Data from the 2002 national survey of family growth. National Center for Health Statistics. *Vital Health Stat 23, 25,* 1–160.

Chassin, L., Carle, A., Nissim-Sabat, D., & Kumpfer, K. L. (2004). Fostering resilience in children of alcoholic parents. In K. I. Maton (Ed.), *Investing in children, youth, families, and communities: Strengths-based research and policy.* Washington, DC: APA Books [PMID: 15645706].

Trends, C. (2013). *Mapping family change and child well-being out comes.* Retrieved from http://www.childtrends.org/wp-content/uploads/2013/02/Child_Trends-2013_01_15_FR_WorldFamilyMap.pdf.

Chung, G. H., Flook, L., & Fuligni, A. J. (2009). Daily family conflict and emotional distress among adolescents from Latin American, Asian, and European backgrounds. *Developmental Psychology, 45*(5), 1406–1415.

Cuellar, I., & Paniagua, F. A. (Eds.). (2000). *Handbook of multicultural mental health: Assessment and treatment of diverse population.* San Diego, CA: Academic Press.

Deal, R. L. (2013, March). *Marriage, family, & stepfamily statistics.* Retrieved from http://www.smartstepfamilies.com/view/statistics.

Demo, D. H., & Acock, A. C. (1996). Family structure, family process, and adolescent well-being. *Journal of Research on Adolescence, 6,* 457–488.

Dette-Hagenmeyer, D.E. & Reichle, B. (2013). Depressive symptoms, parenting, and child adjustment: Not just a mother-child issue. *Paper presented at the 16th European Conference on Development Psychology, Lausanne, Switzerland.*

De Vries, J. (2008). *The industrious revolution* (pp. 132–175). Cambridge: Cambridge University Press.

Dow, H. D. (2011). The acculturation processes: The strategies and factors affecting the degree of acculturation. *Home Health Care Management & Practice, 23*(3), 221–227.

Erickson, M. F., & Egeland, B. (2002). Child neglect. *The APSAC handbook on child maltreatment, 2,* 3–20.

Fang, L., & Schinke, S. P. (2013). Two-year outcomes of a randomized, family-based substance use prevention trial for Asian American adolescent girls. *Psychol Addict Behav., 27*(3), 788–98. doi:10.1037/a0030925.

Farver, J. A. M., Bhadha, B. R., & Narang, S. K. (2002). Acculturation and psychological functioning in Asian Indian adolescents. *Social Development, 11*(1), 11–29.

Feldman, S. S., & Rosenthal, D. A. (1993). Culture makes a difference…or does it? A comparison of adolescents in Hong Kong, Australia, and the USA. In R. Silbereisen & E. Todt (Eds.), *Adolescence in context*. New York, NY: Springer.

Fields, J., & Casper, L. (2000). *America's families and living arrangements* (Current population reports, pp. 20–537). Washington, DC: US Census Bureau.

Flouri, E. (2005). *Fathering and child outcomes*. Chichester, MA: Wiley. ISBN 9780470861677.

Flouri, E., & Buchanan, A. (2002). Father involvement in childhood and trouble with the police in adolescence: Findings from the 1958 British cohort. *Journal of Interpersonal Violence, 17*, 689–701.

Foxcroft, D. R., Ireland, D., Lister-Sharp, D. J., Lowe, G., & Breen, R. (2003). Longer-term primary prevention for alcohol misuse in young people: A systematic review. *Addiction, 98*, 397–411.

Foxcroft, D. R., & Tsertsvadze, A. (2012). Universal alcohol misuse prevention programmes for children and adolescents: Cochrane systematic reviews. *Perspectives in Public Health., 132*, 128–134.

Fuhrmans, F. & Fuhrer, U. (2013, September). *Intergenerational influences on fatherhood: How fathers matter for their sons' fatherhood*. Paper presented at the 16th European Conference on Development Psychology, Lausanne, Switzerland.

Gonzalez-Guarda, R. M., Ortega, J., Vasquez, E., & De Santis, J. (2010). La mancha negra: Substance abuse, violence and sexual risks among Hispanic males. *Western Journal of Nursing Research, 32*(1), 128–148.

Gordon, D. A. (2000). Parent training via CD-ROM: Using technology to disseminate effective prevention practices. *The Journal of Primary Prevention, 21*(2), 227–251.

Guilamo-Ramos, V. (2009). Maternal influence on adolescent self-esteem, ethnic pride and intentions to engage in risk behavior in Latino youth. *Prevention Science, 10*, 366–375. doi:10.1007/s11121-009-0138-9.

Haggerty, K. P., MacKenzie, E. P., Skinner, M. L., Harachi, T. W., & Catalano, R. F. (2006). Participation in "Parents Who Care": Predicting program initiation and exposure in two different program formats. *Journal of Primary Prevention, 27*(1), 47–65. doi:10.1007/s10935-005-0019-3.

Haggerty, K. P., Skinner, M. L., MacKenzie, E. P., & Catalano, R. F. (2007). A randomized trial of Parents Who Care: Effects on key outcomes at 24-month follow-up. *Prevention Science, 8*(4), 249–260.

Hetherington, E. M., & Kelly, J. (2002). *For better or for worse: Divorce reconsidered*. New York, NY: W.W. Norton.

Hoffmann, J. P. (2006). Family structure, community context, and adolescent behaviors. *Journal of Youth and Adolescence, 35*, 867–880.

Hofferth, S., & Anderson, K. (2003). Are all dads equal? Biology versus marriage as a basis for paternal investment. *Journal of Marriage and Family, 65*, 213–232.

Inman, A. G., Howard, E. E., Beaumont, R. L., & Walker, J. A. (2007). Cultural transmission: Influence of contextual factors in Asian Indian immigrant parents' experiences. *Journal of Counseling Psychology, 54*(1), 93.

IREFREA (2010): *EFE—European Family Empowerment: Improving family skills to prevent alcohol and drug related problems* (Grant agreement JLS/DPIP/2008-2/112). Co-financed by the Drug Prevention and Information Programme, European Commission, Directorate-General: JUSTICE.

Ito, K. E., Kalyanaraman, S., Ford, C. A., Brown, J. D., & Miller, W. C. (2008). "Let's Talk About Sex": Pilot study of an interactive CD-ROM to prevent HIV/STIS in female adolescents. *AIDS Education and Prevention, 20*, 78–89.

Jafee, R., Moffitt, E., Caspi, A., & Taylor, A. (2003). Life with (or without) father: The benefits of living with two biological parents depend on the father's antisocial behaviour. *Child Development, 74*(1), 109–126.

Jirtle, R. (2010, June 2). *Epigenetic mechanisms on gene expression.* Plenary Session I, Annual Conference of the Society for Prevention Research. Denver, CO.

Johnson, R. L., Saha, S., Arbelaez, J. J., Beach, M. C., & Cooper, L. A. (2004). Racial and ethnic differences in patient perceptions of bias and cultural competence in health care. *Journal of General Internal Medicine, 19*(2), 101–110.

Kaminski, J. W., Valle, L. A., Filene, J. H., & Boyle, C. L. (2008). A meta-analytic review of components associated with parent training program effectiveness. *J Abnorm Child Psychol, 36*(4), 567–89. doi:10.1007/s10802-007-9201-9.

Kenworthy, L. (2012). It's hard to make in America: How the United States stopped being the land of opportunity. *Foreign Affairs, 91,* 103–109.

Kreider, R. M. & Renee, E. (2009). *Living arrangements of children: 2009,* Current Population Reports, pp. 70–126. Washington, DC: US Census Bureau. Retrieved from http://www.census.gov/prod/2011pubs/p70-126.pdf.

Kumpfer, K. L. (2014). Family-based interventions for the prevention of substance abuse and other impulse control disorders in girls. Invited Spotlight Article, *ISRN Addiction,* 308789. doi:10.1155/2014/308789.

Kumpfer, K. L., & Alvarado, R. (2003). Family-strengthening approaches for the prevention of youth problem behaviors. *American Psychologist, 58,* 6–7.

Kumpfer, K. L., & Brown, J. (2012, September 22). *New way to reach parents: A SFP DVD. Western States Substance Abuse Annual ATOD conference, Boise, ID.*

Kumpfer, K. L., & DeMarsh, J. P. (1986). Family environmental and genetic influences on children's future chemical dependency. In S. Ezekoye, K. L. Kumpfer, & W. Bukoski (Eds.), *Childhood and chemical abuse: Prevention and intervention.* New York, NY: Haworth.

Kumpfer, K. L., & Hansen, W. (2014). Family-based prevention programs (Ch. 8). In W. Hansen & L. Scheier (Eds.), *Parenting and teen drug use.* Oxford: Oxford University Press.

Kumpfer, K. L., & Johnson, J. L. (2011). Enhancing positive outcomes for children of substance-abusing parents. In A. Johnson (Ed.), *Addiction medicine: Science and practice* (pp. 1307–1329). New York, NY: Springer. ISBN 978-1-4419-0338-9.

Kumpfer, K. L., Alvarado, R., Smith, P., & Bellamy, N. (2002). Cultural sensitivity and adaptation in family-based prevention interventions. *Prevention Science, 3*(3), 241–246. doi:10.1023/A:1019902902119.

Kumpfer, K. L., Alvarado, R., & Whiteside, H. O. (2003). Family-based interventions for substance abuse prevention. *Substance Use and Misuse, 38*(11-13), 1759–1789. PMID: 14582577.

Kumpfer, K. L., Pinyuchon, M., de Melo, A., & Whiteside, H. (2005). Cultural adaptation process for international dissemination of the Strengthening Families Program (SFP). *Evaluation and Health Professions, 33*(2), 226–239.

Kumpfer, K. L., Magalhães, C., & Xie, J. (2012). Cultural adaptations of evidence-based family interventions to strengthen families and improve children's outcomes. *European Journal of Developmental Psychology, 9*(1), 104–116.

Kumpfer, K. L., Smith, P., & Franklin Summerhays, J. (2008). A wake -up call to the prevention field: Are prevention programs for substance use effective for girls? *Substance Use and Misuse., 43*(8), 978–1001.

Lamb, M. E. (1997). Fathers and child development: An introductory overview and guide. In M. E. Lamb (Ed.), *The Role of the father in child development* (3rd ed., pp. 1–18). New York, NY: Wiley.

Lamb, M. E. (Ed.). (2004). *The role of the father in child development* (4th ed.). New York, NY: Wiley.

Lamb, M. E. (2010). *The role of the father in child development* (5th ed.). Hoboken, NJ: Wiley.

Lamb, M. E., & Lewis, C. (2011). The role of parent-child relationships in child development. In M. H. Bornstein & M. E. Lamb (Eds.), *Developmental science: An advanced textbook* (6th ed., pp. 469–517). New York, NY: Taylor & Francis.

Lang, K., & Zagorsky, J. L. (2001). Does growing up with a parent absent really hurt? *Journal of Human Resources, 36*, 253–273.

Lawrence, C. R., Carlson, E. A., & Egeland, B. (2006). The impact of foster care on development. *Development and Psychopathology, 18*(01), 57–76.

Livingston, G., & Parker, K. (2011). *A tale of two fathers: More are active, but more are absent.* Washington, DC: Pew Research Center.

Loveland-Cherry, C. J. (2000). Family interventions to prevent substance abuse: Children and adolescents. *Annu Rev Nurs Res, 18*, 195–218.

Manning, W., & Lamb, K. A. (2003). Adolescent well-being in cohabiting, married, and single-parent families. *Journal of Marriage and the Family, 65*(4), 876–893.

Martin, J. A., Hamilton, B. E., Ventura, S. J., Osterman, M. J. K., & Mathews, T. J. ((2013). *Births: Final data for 2011.* National Vital Statistics Reports; Vol. 62 no 1. Hyattsville, MD: National Center for Health Statistics. 2013. Available from http://www.cdc.gov/nchs/data/nvsr/nvsr62/nvsr62_01.pdf.

Martinez, G. M., Daniels, K., & Chandra, A. (2012). *Fertility of men and women aged 15–44 years in the United States: National survey of family growth, 2006–2010.* Hyattsville, MD: National Center for Health Statistics. National health statistics reports; no 51. Retrieved from http://www.cdc.gov/nchs/data/nhsr/nhsr051.pdf.

Mather, M. (2010). *U.S. children in single-mother families.* Washington, DC: Population Reference Bureau. Retrieved from http://www.prb.org/pdf10/single-motherfamilies.pdf.

McLanahan, S., & Sandefur, D. (1994). *Growing up with a single parent.* Cambridge, MA: Harvard University Press.

McLanahan, S. (2004). Diverging destinies: How children are faring under the second demographic transition. *Demography, 41*(4), 607–627.

McLanahan, S., & Jacobsen, W. (2015). Diverging destinies revisited: Families in an era of increasing inequality. *National Symposium on Family Issues., 5*, 3–23.

McLean, C. A., & Campbell, C. M. (2003). Locating research informants in a multi-ethnic community: Ethnic identities, social networks and recruitment methods. *Ethnicity and health, 8*(1), 41–61.

McLanahan, S., Donahue, E., & Haskins, R. (2005). Introducing Special Issue on Marriage and Child Wellbeing. *The Future of Children, 15*, 3–12.

Miller, T. A., & Hendrie, D. (2008). *Substance abuse prevention: Dollars and cents: A cost-benefit analysis.* Rockville, MD: Center for Substance Abuse Prevention (CSAP), SAMHSA. DHHS Pub. No 07-4298.

Moore, B. A., Fazzino, T., Garnet, B., Cutter, C. J., & Barry, D. T. (2011). Computer-based interventions for drug use disorders: A systematic review. *J Subst Abuse Treat, 40*(3), 215–223. doi:10.1016/j.jsat.2010.11.002.

Morrison, D. R. (2000, March). *The costs of economic uncertainty; Child well-bring in cohabitating and remarried unions following parental divorce.* Paper presented at the Annual Meeting of the Population Association of America, Los Angeles, CA.

Moynihan, D. P. (1965). *The Negro family: The case for national action.* Washington, DC: United States. Dept. of Labor, Office of Policy Planning and Research.

Minuchin, S. (1974). *Families and family therapy.* Cambridge, MA: Harvard University Press.

Parker, K. (2011, Jan 13). *A portrait of stepfamilies.* Pew Research Center report. Retrieved from http://pewsocialtrends.org/2011/01/13/a-portrait-of-stepfamilies/

Petrie, J., Bunn, F., & Byrne, G. (2007). Parenting programmes for preventing tobacco, alcohol or drugs misuse in children under 18: A systematic review. *Health Education Research, 22*(2), 177–191. doi:10.1093/her/cyl061.

Phinney, J. (1996). When we talk about American ethnic groups, what do we mean? *American Psychologist, 51*, 917–918.

Popenoe, D. (2009). *Families without fathers: Fathers, marriage and children in American society.* New Brunswick, NJ: Transaction Books.

Putmam, R. D. (2015). *Our kids: The American dream in crisis.* New York, NY: Simon & Schuster.

Reno, J., & Riley, R. W. (2000). *Working for children and families: Safe and smart after-school programs*. Washington, DC: US Department of Education. Retrieved from http:www. www2. ed.gov/offices/OESE/archives/pubs/parents/SafeSmart/green.

Resnick, M., Bearman, S., Blum, W., Bauman, E., Harris, K., Jones, J … Udry, L. (1997). Protecting adolescents from harm. *Journal of the American Medical Association, 278 (10)*, 823–832.

Rodnium, J. (2007). Causes of delinquency: The Social Ecology Model for Thai youth. Unpublished dissertation, Department of Health Promotion and Education, University of Utah, Salt Lake City, UT.

Rowe, M., Coker, D., & Pan, B. (2004). A comparison of fathers' and mothers' talk to toddlers in low-income families. *Social Development, 13*(2), 278–291.

Rubin, D. M., O'Reilly, A. L., Luan, X., & Localio, A. R. (2007). The impact of placement stability on behavioral well-being for children in foster care. *Pediatrics, 119*(2), 336–344.

Sassler, S., Cunningham, A., & Lichter, D. T. (2009). Intergenerational patterns of union formation and relationship quality. *Journal of Family Issues, 30*(6), 757–786.

Schinke, S. P., Fang, L., & Cole, K. C. (2011). Preventing substance abuse among Black and Hispanic adolescent girls: Results from a computer-delivered, mother-daughter intervention approach. *Subst Use Misuse, 46*(1), 35–45.

Shattuck, R. M., & Kreider, R. M. (2013). *Social and economic characteristics of currently unmarried women with a recent birth, 2011*. Retrieved from http://www.census.gov/prod/2013pubs/acs-21.pdf.

Simms, M. D., Dubowitz, H., & Szilagyi, M. A. (2000). Health care needs of children in the foster care system. *Pediatrics, 106*(Supplement 3), 909–918.

Smokowski, P. R., David-Ferdon, C., & Bacallao, M. (2009). Acculturation and health in minority adolescents. *Special issue of the Journal of Primary Prevention., 30*(3/4), 209–475.

Tobler, N. S., & Kumpfer, K. L. (2000). *Meta-analyses of family approaches to substance abuse prevention*. CSAP, Rockville, MD: Report prepared for SAMHSA.

Tobler, N., & Stratton, H. (1997). Effectiveness of school based drug prevention programs: A meta-analysis of the research. *Journal of Primary Prevention, 18*, 71–128.

Trost, G., Kerr, M., Ward, S., & Pate, R. (2009). *Physical activity and determinants of physical activity in obese and non-obese children*. Brisbane, Queensland, Australia: School of Human Movement Studies, The University of Queensland.

Umana-Taylor, A. J., Diversi, M., & Fine, M. A. (2002). Ethnic identity and self-esteem of Latino adolescents: Distinctions among the Latino populations. *Journal of Adolescent Research, 17*, 303–327. doi:10.1177/0743558402173005.

United States Census Bureau (2011a). *Unmarried and single Americans Week Sept. 18-24, 2011*. Retrieved from http://www.census.gov/newsroom/releases/archives/facts_for_features_special_editions/cb11-ff19.html.

United States Census Bureau (2011b). *Children's living arrangements and characteristics*. Washington, DC: Author. Retrieved from http://www.census.gov/statab/.

United States Census Bureau (2012). *America's families and living arrangements: 2012*. Retrieved from http://www.census.gov/hhes/families/data/cps2012.html.

United Nations Children's Fund. (2007). *Child poverty in perspective: An overview of child well-being in rich countries*. Innocenti Report Card, 7, UNICEF Innocenti Research Centre, Florence.

United Nations Office of Drugs and Crime. Vienna. (UNODC) (2009). *Guide to implementing family skills training programmes for drug abuse prevention*. Electronic Document. https://www.unodc.org/documents/prevention/family-guidelines-E.pdf.

United Nations Office of Drugs and Crime (UNODC. (2010). *Compilation of evidence-based family skills training programmes* (p. 128). Austria: UN Vienna. Retrieved from http://www.coe.int/t/dg3/children/corporalpunishment/positive%20parenting/UNODCFamilySkillsTraining Programmes.pdf.

Ventura, J., Abma, C., Mostter, D., & Henslaw, K. (2008). *Pregnancy rates by outcome for the United States, 1990-2004*. National Vital Statistics Reports, *56* (15). Hyttsville, M.D.: National Center for Health Statistics.

Watson, J. (2005). *Active engagement: Strategies to increase service participation by vulnerable families*. Ashfield, NSW: Centre for Parenting & Research.

Wingood, G. M., Card, J. J., Er, D., Solomon, J., Braxton, N., Lang, D., ... DiClemente, R. J. (2011). Preliminary efficacy of a computer-based HIV intervention for African-American women. *Psychology and Health, 26,* (2), 223–234.

Zhou, M. (2009). How neighbourhoods matter for immigrant children: The formation of educational resources in Chinatown, Koreatown and Pico Union, Los Angeles. *Journal of Ethnic and Migration Studies, 35*(7), 1153–1179.

Part III
Children and Adolescent
Psychological Wellness

Chapter 5
Childhood Stress and Resilience

Andrew J. Barnes

5.1   Introduction

Stress is defined as an event or situation that is unpredictable and/or not controllable and is perceived as having social–emotional significance as a threat to a person's survival. Children differ in their responses to stress, influenced both by constitutional factors (such as threshold to stimuli) and psychosocial context (such as threat appraisal). Stressors such as severe social adversity, abuse, trauma, neglect, or maltreatment directly impact 1 in 7 US children, leading to abnormal brain development, altered physiological regulation, and chronic adult illness (Felitti et al., 1998; Middlebrooks & Audage, 2008). High levels of severe stress during childhood negatively impact the body (Garner et al., 2012; Shonkoff et al., 2012); lead to problems with achievement, behavior, and health (Gunnar, Morison, Chisholm, & Schuder, 2001; Obradovic, Bush, Stamperdahl, Adler, & Boyce, 2010); and are associated with greater risk of suicide (Barnes, Eisenberg, & Resnick, 2010; McGowan et al., 2009) .

Acute stress activates the sympathetic autonomic nervous system (SAM), which responds within seconds, and the hypothalamic–pituitary–adrenal (HPA) system, which responds within 20–30 min, to prepare the body to deal with the perceived threat. This results in signals from the brain's limbic system to prepare target organs for "fight or flight" via norepinephrine and epinephrine (SAM) and cortisol (HPA). Negative hormone feedback loops and the parasympathetic nervous system act as biological "brakes" on these responses, so that they are normally deactivated soon after a threat has passed (Berntson & Cacioppo, 2007). Oxytocin, a hormone

A.J. Barnes, M.D., M.P.H. (✉)
Division of General Pediatrics and Adolescent Health, Department of Pediatrics, University
of Minnesota Medical School, University of Minnesota,
717 Delaware St SE, Suite #370H, Minneapolis, MN 55414, USA
e-mail: DrBarnes@umn.edu

© Springer Science+Business Media New York 2016   85
M.R. Korin (ed.), *Health Promotion for Children and Adolescents*,
DOI 10.1007/978-1-4899-7711-3_5

released from the posterior pituitary, is also increased by acute stress and possibly aids recovery by increasing social bonding and reducing anxiety (Heinrichs, Baumgartner, Kirschbaum, & Ehlert, 2003) .

Children experience a range of stressors throughout their lives, some of which are mild or even positive (e.g., moving to a new home, making new friends, mastering a new skill, solving a problem), and some of which are more intense or negative (e.g., the death of a parent, a natural disaster, medical procedures, major injury or illness). The physiological response to stress is generally proportional to its degree, such that high levels of negative stress can cause physical symptoms such as headaches due to elevated blood pressure, poor concentration due to elevated cortisol, or belly pain due to increased gastric acid production in the stomach. Normally, even when the body responds in these more disruptive ways to negative life events, such stress is thought of as "tolerable" because its effects are buffered by protective factors—such as nurturing adults or self-regulation skills—that bring the body back into balance and mitigate the impact of stress.

However, when negative stress is unrelenting and/or severe, especially in the absence of protective factors, the HPA and SAM systems become overloaded and begin to change to compensate—such stress is termed "toxic." In such cases, these stress response systems can become overactive, underactive, or both; this leads to changes in brain architecture and normal physiology, increasing the risk of long-term problems with learning, behavior, and health. Examples of "toxic stress" include child abuse and maltreatment, untreated parental psychiatric and substance abuse disorders, extreme poverty, and exposure to violence within the family and/or community. These are also referred to as "adverse childhood experiences" (ACEs). Other stressor-related factors that have complex influences on children's' responses to stress include the developmental timing and the specific nature of an ACE (i.e., unfamiliar stressors and/or multiple ACEs lead to poor outcomes). Negative stress of a lesser degree that nevertheless occurs at a chronic, daily level also contributes to stress-related problems (Odgers & Jaffee, 2013).

5.2   The Impact of Stress on Children

Functionally, stress can impinge on children's emotions, behavior, health, and socialization (Forkey, Gillespie, Pettersen, Spector, & Stirling, 2014). These effects are often seen as regression to younger-aged behavior, mood changes, somatic complaints, or activity-level changes and vary according to a child's level of development. Among preschool-aged children, signs of stress include lower than usual self-regulation (e.g., recurrence of thumb-sucking in a child who stopped doing so months ago or bed-wetting in a child who has been continent for a year or more); increased levels of age-typical anxieties and fears (e.g., of separation, the dark, "monsters"); or lower threshold for tantrums. School-aged children can act more verbally and/or physically aggressive at home and/or school, be more irritable or "edgy," be more "clingy" with caregivers, or have lower than usual levels of concentration. Younger adolescents often have somatic complaints (headaches, stomachaches); sleeping difficulties; appetite changes; and decreased performance in academics and/or extracurricular activities. Older adolescents can become less social or have less interest in typical activities, have more risk-taking behavior than usual, or be more irritable than usual.

Toxic stress during childhood negatively impacts the "programming" of interdependent biological systems—including the sympathetic nervous system (Massin, Withofs, Maeyns, & Ravet, 2001), cognitive systems (Stevens, Lauinger, & Neville, 2009), hormonal functioning (Gunnar et al., 2001; Roisman et al., 2009), and immune–inflammatory regulation (Danese et al., 2008; McDade et al., 2005; Miller & Chen, 2007; Miller, Chen, & Cole, 2009; Shirtcliff, Coe, & Pollak, 2009). This occurs because chronic overactivation of the SAM and HPA systems leads to altered physiological "set points" that can predispose to stress-related physical and mental health conditions, which is termed allostasis (McEwen, 1998).

The timing of stress has important implications for its long-term consequences. Many chronic conditions of childhood, such as asthma (Chen et al., 2006) and hypertension (Shankaran et al., 2006), often have their roots in early exposure to toxic stress. Prenatal stress upon a mother increases the risk for her child to have restricted intrauterine growth and thus to be born with a lower than average weight, which is associated with chronic adult conditions predisposing to cardiovascular disease and metabolic problems such as type 2 diabetes (Barker, Osmond, Forsen, Kajantie, & Eriksson, 2005). Childhood health conditions can also be worsened by stress, such as asthma and eczema (Wright, Cohen, & Cohen, 2005), type 1 diabetes (Hanson, Henggeler, & Burghen, 1987), irritable bowel syndrome (Bennett et al., 1998), and juvenile rheumatoid arthritis (Schanberg et al., 2000). Most chronic pain conditions (e.g., migraine headaches or recurrent abdominal pain) are intrinsically linked with children's responses to stress (Compas & Thomsen, 1999; Powers, Gilman, & Hershey, 2006). Children's sleep problems are also strongly linked to family stress (Sadeh, Raviv, & Gruber, 2000).

The mental health consequences of toxic stress include anxiety and mood disorders that can emerge during childhood and persist into adolescence and adulthood (Heim, 1999). Adjustment disorders, post-traumatic stress disorder, and reactive attachment disorder are conditions that can emerge during childhood that are directly attributable to stress. Disorders that emerge during adulthood that have strong links to ACEs include drug use, antisocial behavior and conduct problems, and depressive symptoms (Schilling, 2007).

Stress is also associated with premature degeneration of the body, because it shortens the length of chromosomal telomeres—the DNA on the ends of chromosomes that gets removed as cells age or get damaged. While environmental stressors such as UV radiation have long been implicated in telomere shortening, it is now clear that severe psychosocial stress can do so as well, through uncertain mechanisms. For example, mothers of the most severely chronically ill children who perceived extremely high levels of stress had telomeres that were shortened the equivalent of 10 years of aging, compared to the mothers of healthy children who had low levels of stress (Epel, 2004). For adults who experienced trauma during childhood, telomere length decreases as a function of the number and severity of trauma (Shalev et. al., 2012). Even prenatal stress can significantly shorten children's telomere length (Shalev, 2013), as well as alter HPA function (Tollenar, 2010) and lower immune responsiveness to vaccinations (O'Connor, 2013).

5.3   Protective Factors

Factors both internal and external to the child contribute to the impact of stress. Child-level variables that are constitutional and likely not as amenable to intervention or change include temperamental characteristics such as sensitivity to stimuli, high negativity of mood, and low levels of behavioral inhibition. Other factors within the child that might be more easily altered include cognitive appraisal and locus of control—for example, whether a situation is viewed by the child as controllable or not. Sex may play a role as well, in that girls seem to show more internalizing stress symptoms (such as anxiety and depression) than do boys, who tend to show more externalizing signs (such as aggression).

Family, community, and environmental factors form the context in which the child experiences stress as well. High levels of social support and parenting quality help children build resilience to stress, whereas family disruption and harsh parenting predispose children to stress-related difficulties. Cultural differences and communities also exert powerful effects on children's adjustment, as do peers, immigration, war, natural disaster, and famine. For example, a child with a transgender identity might experience severe stigmatization and social stress in one culture, whereas the same child might be seen as merely different or even as a blessing to the community in another. Similarly, children who suffer from a disaster will have more negative stress-related outcomes if they are also living in a region with high levels of violence.

The interaction of a child's dispositional reactions to stress with his or her external environment is complex and has been termed "biological sensitivity to context" (Boyce and Ellis, 2005) or "differential susceptibility" (Pluess and Belsky, 2012). Research in this area has revealed that children who are highly stress reactive are more vulnerable to negative behavioral and health outcomes than children who are less so, but only when external factors are highly negative (e.g., high ACEs). On the other hand, these same "sensitive" children have a greater likelihood of enjoying positive outcomes under conditions of high support and lower levels of stress.

As children grow, their ways of mitigating stress generally become less externally regulated and more internally regulated. Competence in dealing with stress is ideally modeled, nurtured, and taught by caregivers who encourage their children to deal well with stress in an ongoing, developmentally sensitive way from the time of infancy, contributing to a child's degree of resilience.

5.4 Resilience to Stress

Resilience is operationalized as high developmental competence, good functioning, and positive outcomes in the face of high adversity and negative experiences that usually threaten or derail development (i.e., stress). Studies of individual differences in outcomes in children exposed to toxic stress converge on several characteristics common to those with very positive outcomes (Masten, 2001; Sapienza and Masten, 2011):

- Connections and secure attachment with responsive, caring adults
- Nurturing, authoritative parenting
- Positive connections with school
- Positive peer relationships
- Spiritual faith in a higher power
- Sense of purpose and meaning in life
- Intelligence and problem-solving skills
- Self-regulation and executive function skills
- Positive self-image
- Motivation toward self-efficacy and achievement

Some of these factors, such as intelligence, may be less malleable than others. As such, interventions that aim to promote resilience tend to focus on attachment and caregiving and/or self-regulation, which may be more amenable to change.

5.5 Resilience-Promoting Interventions

Stress-buffering preventive interventions aimed at increasing resilience in children can be universal, selected, or indicated. Universal interventions—those designed to prevent stress-related conditions and promote resilience to stress in the community as a whole, regardless of level of risk—can be delivered in a wide variety of venues, including school health and family education classes. Clinicians engage in this when doing prenatal classes or anticipatory guidance as part of routine well-child visits starting during infancy. Such interventions can include teaching parents to interpret and respond supportively to "baby body language" in the context of learning about their child's temperament, as well as how to handle toddlers' tantrums and use positive parenting strategies. For older children and adolescents, these efforts include educating caregivers and youth about individual differences and bullying, teaching about interpersonal communication and positive peer relationships, fostering connections to school and community organizations, and encouraging involvement in extracurricular activities. These interventions help to build the strong, nurturing relationships and self-regulatory skills that are fundamental to the development of resilience.

Selected (or targeted) interventions aim to prevent the onset of problems in at-risk youth with threats to their development due to high levels of stress and adversity.

Such risks may be identifiable on a demographic basis and/or through screening measures. These include large-scale programs such as home visits to low-SES pregnant mothers, parenting classes for families with children in Head Start, and early intervention for children who are homeless/highly mobile.

Indicated interventions (or treatments) are aimed at children who have developed symptomatic problems or conditions that are due to, or influenced by, toxic stress. These include evidence-based programs such as Parent–Child Interaction Therapy (Funderberk and Eyberg, 2011) as well as highly individualized therapy specific to the child that address his or her unique strengths to aid in overcoming risk.

5.5.1 Attachment and Caregiving

All children will experience stress—be it grief, loss, transition, illness, poverty, or disaster—in the context of important adults in their lives also experiencing stress. Promoting children's adaptive adjustment in the face of any adversity must thus take into account the stress reactions of important adults in their lives. In order to meet children's needs during times of crisis and to teach them how to recover well from future crises, caregivers must cultivate their own competence in meeting stressful life events with equanimity. Caregivers need to learn to "roll" with children's normative emotional–behavioral distress, guiding and reassuring with love—while not encouraging avoidant coping (i.e., overprotection), being dismissive of children's negative feelings and thoughts, or permitting the child to suffer without support. Encouraging awareness, acceptance, and problem-solving engagement using reflective listening and empathetic language is a critical skill for adults to use when helping children under duress thrive by establishing an atmosphere of safety and restoring a sense of equilibrium. A number of interventions have demonstrated efficacy in enhancing these processes to promote resilience.

High-quality adoption and foster care is very well established as an intervention for children who have been maltreated, neglected, and/or have lived within extremely disrupted families with very low-quality or inconsistent caregiving. In studies of Romanian orphans, those placed into a foster home by age 24 months show more secure and organized attachment, and better interpersonal relationships, by preschool age than children who remain institutionalized in a sterile orphanage environment or those are placed into foster care at later ages (Gunnar, 2001).

Similarly targeted interventions, such as Multidimensional Treatment Foster Care for Preschoolers (MTFC-P), Positive Parenting Program (Triple-P), and the Incredible Years (Webster-Stratton et al., 2001), aim to improve parenting quality by training families of very young children to use contingency management and behavioral modification strategies (Fisher and Kim, 2007; Sanders, 1999; Brotman et al., 2007). Such programs prevent or decrease stress among caregivers of these high-risk children, and children whose families participate in these programs show improved social–emotional development and behavior and reduced disruptive behavior. Biologically, these children also normalize their cortisol rhythms and HPA reactivity (Bruce, 2013).

A specific example of one such intervention is Attachment and Biobehavioral Catch-up (ABC). This is a ten-session program for birth, foster, and adoptive parents of toddlers and preschoolers who have experienced neglect, maltreatment, or other early trauma (Dozier, 2008). The intervention aims to address three key issues common to this group of children by teaching their caregivers to provide nurturing care unconditionally, even with children who apparently do not often elicit it or who "push away" the caregiver; respond to children's positive and negative behaviors in a timely and appropriate way to help them "co-regulate" their social–emotional interactions; and behave in a non-threatening, non-frightening, peaceful, and calm manner with their children. In a randomized controlled trial, the ABC program improved high-risk children's secure, organized attachment behavior and normalized their diurnal cortisol secretion greater than a control condition (a family educational program about child development).

Other therapies focus on helping children recover from their reactions to stress by helping them learn self-regulation skills to deal more effectively with the resulting negative thoughts, feelings, and behaviors. One such example, Trauma Focused Cognitive–Behavioral Therapy (TF-CBT), is indicated for children who show signs of PTSD (Cohen et al., 2004). It involves narrative reframing and direct discussion of the trauma and stressful life events experienced by the child, teaching the child to identify negative cognitive distortions and self-correct them with more balanced alternatives, and practicing relaxation and physiological self-regulation to reduce distress. For younger children, TF-CBT includes caregiver training in these techniques, whereas older children and adolescents can benefit from individual or group work.

5.5.2 Self-Regulation

The control of one's own mind and body is central to the process of resilience. Children's natural movement toward greater self-mastery and autonomy in orchestrating the interactions between their cognition, emotion, and physiology begins during infancy and drives the development of self-regulation throughout early childhood, which continues even beyond adolescence (Sussman Gertz & Culbert, 2009). Cognitive aspects of self-regulation include executive function—also referred to as effortful control—encompassing self-monitoring and self-talk, alertness (e.g., starting a complex task), attention (e.g., following directions), and inhibition (e.g., delaying gratification). Emotional self-regulation includes motivation, reward seeking, and avoidance of discomfort. Physiological self-regulation includes interoception (e.g., responsiveness to internal hungry or full signals) and functional control of selected autonomic functions (e.g., sweating). These domains of self-regulation are related and interdependent, and there are individual differences within and between these domains. Some children may be highly regulated with respect to some domains such as switching attention between tasks but poorly regulated in others such as control of breathing; similarly, some children are well regulated in some contexts (e.g., with peers) and less in others (e.g., with teachers). Helping children capitalize on strengths in one area of self-regulation can often help them to strengthen or generalize their skills to other areas for which they may be relatively more limited, in turn helping to drive resilience processes and overall competence.

Executive function is increasingly a target of targeted and selective intervention for youth at risk (Riggs et al., 2006; Diamond 2011). Directly training the brain in these domains, e.g., by playing memory games on a computer, has so far been of minimal impact in studies that have attempted to produce a generalizable improvement in children's self-regulation. A number of educational curricula improve academic readiness and achievement, in part by improving executive function and cognitive and/or emotional self-regulation, such as Tools of the Mind (Vygotsky, 1980), PATHS (Riggs et al., 2006), the Chicago Schools Readiness Project (Raver et al., 2011), and the Incredible Years.

Aerobic exercise and sports training can improve cognitive aspects of self-regulation such as creativity and cognitive flexibility and emotional aspects such as persistence. While physical activity in general can be beneficial for building resilience, certain kinds of physical activity that include focused attention training, such as yoga or martial arts, seem to produce greater benefits on self-regulation in children (Diamond, 2011). Yoga is a physical activity that utilizes postures, breathing techniques, focused attention, and self-control to foster resilience. It is helpful for stress management and cognition (Noggle, 2012; Chaya, 2012) and stress-associated health problems such as asthma (Jain, 1991) and irritable bowel syndrome (Kuttner, 2006).

Other programs that bolster resilience through self-regulation include meditation and/or relaxation training. This is a consciously directed process of quiet, calm, nonjudgmental attentiveness to one's own thoughts and feelings as they ebb and flow. One common and oft-studied type of meditation, mindfulness-based stress reduction has salutary effects on stress-reactive cognition and physiology (Davidson et al., 2003). In children and adolescents, meditation helps with general stress reduction and prosocial behaviors, cognitive and emotional regulation, sleep problems, and pain conditions (Broderick, 2009, 2014; Diamond, 2011).

Similar to (and often part of) meditation or relaxation training as well as yoga, diaphragmatic breathing can work quite well for acute stress reduction and alleviation of children's stress-related problems such as sleep disturbance and anxiety (Olness, 2009). Children can be coached to alter the breathing cycle so that inhalation pushes out the abdominal wall, and slow, rhythmic exhalation allows the abdominal wall to relax. Children younger than school age can be learn this technique as a game of bubble blowing (which requires controlled exhalation) or blowing out imaginary birthday candles, and older children can benefit from paced breathing (e.g., being taught to breathe in for a silent count of three and out for a silent count of five) and/or visually aided pacing (e.g., with an expanding/collapsing Hoberman sphere toy). Related techniques, such as progressive muscle relaxation and autogenic training, can be taught directly to older children and through story to younger children.

Biofeedback is a method of psychophysiological training that uses a computer to provide visual or auditory feedback (positive reinforcement) to a child of their biological signals of stress (such as heart rate variability, muscle tension, peripheral skin temperature, or levels of perspiration), so that as the child downregulates physiologically (e.g., by activating parasympathetic nervous system pathways that serve as "breaks" on the fight-or-flight response), he or she can see or hear the results immediately and thus entrain or condition new "automatic" responses. Commercially available packages that use biofeedback games with high-definition graphics can be quite engaging for children as they learn to "be the boss" of their stress in this way (Culbert and Kajander 2007).

Clinical hypnosis utilizes focused attention (often in combination with mental imagery and/or relaxation) to produce a heightened ability to incorporate therapeutic suggestions. In children and adolescents, it is especially critical to emphasize that all hypnosis is in fact self-hypnosis, because no one in hypnosis can be made to follow suggestions or "be controlled" against their will—quite the contrary, as children most often develop a sense of self-mastery and competence from regular practice of self-hypnosis (Kohen & Olness, 2011). Stages of hypnosis include induction, deepening, therapeutic suggestions, re-alerting, and de-briefing; these stages are highly consistent with children's everyday natural experiences and thus can be easily individualized and tailored to the child's developmental level (Sugarman & Wester, 2013). For example, infants with colic might be engaged in hypnotic experiences aimed at stress reduction, such as swaddling and rocking; preschool-aged children do so via fantasy play; and adolescents often access hypnotic states while daydreaming. Childhood conditions that are stressful, exacerbated, and/or caused by stress are very responsive to hypnosis and similar cognitive–behavioral interventions, including various recurrent pain conditions (Eccleston et al., 2012) including chronic abdominal pain and irritable bowel syndrome (Vlieger et al., 2012) and chronic headache (Olness and Kohen, 1984). Self-regulation training through hypnosis is also effective for alleviating stress and pain due to invasive medical procedures (Uman et al., 2008).

Formal cognitive–behavioral therapy (CBT), usually delivered individually but sometimes in a group format for children under stress (e.g., due to trauma or maltreatment), is also an effective way to enhance self-regulation. This consists of various techniques that teach children to identify feelings and thoughts in stressful situations, changing perception of negative thoughts through cognitive reframing, and to respond with appropriate adaptive behaviors. Programs that are referred to as CBT often incorporate many of the aforementioned interventions. There is little evidence to compare various formats of such interventions or the effective components of them (Forman-Hoffman et al., 2013; Fraser et al., 2013).

5.6 Conclusion

Stress, both acute and chronic, causes changes to the mind and body that can have negative, lasting effects on physical and mental health. Extremely negative or traumatic childhood experiences thus literally get under the skin, directly impacting children's behavior, cognition, and physiology. Some children seem more susceptible to this than others. However, this vulnerability is based on complex interactions between children's individual biological differences and the timing, context, and type of the stress they experience. Fortunately, it is this susceptibility itself that also enables children to respond exquisitely well to positive influences and take advantage of opportunities for recovery, healing, and growth. This capacity, termed resilience, is the tendency of a dynamic system—whether a child, a family, a school, a neighborhood, or a community—to adapt successfully to highly adverse experiences. Resilience processes can be external to the child, such as nurturing adults, and internal to the child, such as self-regulation. These factors buffer or blunt children's biological and psychological stress responses, restoring biological homeostasis and preserving developmental competence, in turn preventing problems and promoting lifelong social–emotional development, mental health, and physical well-being. There is a growing body of programs and interventions—some targeting caregivers, some directly working with children—that can bolster such resilience, restoring typical function in all domains and promising better outcomes for children suffering adversity than would have been predicted.

Web Resources

For Families
American Academy of Child and Adolescent Psychiatry: Facts for Families
http://www.aacap.org/cs/root/facts_for_families/facts_for_families
American Academy of Pediatrics: Healthy Children
http://www.healthychildren.org/English/healthy-living/emotional-wellness/pages/
    Helping-Children-Handle-Stress.aspx
For Practitioners and Professionals
The National Child Traumatic Stress Network
www.nctsn.org
The AMBIT Network for Research and Practice in Child Trauma
http://www.cehd.umn.edu/fsos/projects/ambit/default.asp
The Center for the Developing Child
http://developingchild.harvard.edu

References

Barker, D. J., Osmond, C., Forsen, T. J., Kajantie, E., & Eriksson, J. G. (2005). Trajectories of growth among children who have coronary events as adults. *The New England Journal of Medicine, 353*(17), 1802–1809. doi:10.1056/NEJMoa044160.

Barnes, A. J., Eisenberg, M., & Resnick, M. D. (2010). Suicide and self-injury among children and youth with chronic health conditions. *Pediatrics, 125*(5), 889–895.

Bennett, E. J., Piesse, C., Palmer, K., Badcock, C. A., Tennant, C. C., & Kellow, J. E. (1998). Functional gastrointestinal disorders: Psychological, social, and somatic features. *Gut, 42*(3), 414–420.

Berntson, G. G., & Cacioppo, J. T. (2007). Integrative physiology: homeostasis, allostasis, and the orchestration of systemic physiology (Chapter 19). In J. T. Cacioppo, L. G. Tassinary, & G. G. Berntson (Eds.), *Handbook of psychophysiology* (3rd ed., pp. 433–452). New York, NY: Cambridge University Press.

Boyce, W. T., & Ellis, B. J. (2005). Biological sensitivity to context: I. An evolutionary-developmental theory of the origins and functions of stress reactivity. *Development and Psychopathology, 17*(2), 271–301.

Broderick, P., & Metz, S. (2009). Learning to BREATHE: A pilot trial of a mindfulness curriculum for adolescents. *Advances in School Mental Health Promotion, 2*(1), 35–46. http://doi.org/10.1080.

Broderick, P. C., & Frank, J. L. (2014). Learning to BREATHE: An intervention to foster mindfulness in adolescence. *New Directions for Youth Development, 2014*(142), 31–44. http://doi.org/10.1002/yd.20095.

Brotman, L. M., Gouley, K. K., Huang, K. Y., Kamboukos, D., Fratto, C., & Pine, D. S. (2007). Effects of a psychosocial family-based preventive intervention on cortisol response to a social challenge in preschoolers at high risk for antisocial behavior. *Archives of General Psychiatry, 64*(10), 1172–1179. Retrieved from http://doi.org/64/10/1172.

Bruce, J., Gunnar, M. R., Pears, K. C., & Fisher, P. a. (2013). Early adverse care, stress neurobiology, and prevention science: Lessons learned. *Prevention Science, 14*, 247–256. http://doi.org/10.1007/s11121-012-0354-6.

Chaya, M. S., Nagendra, H., Selvam, S., Kurpad, A., & Srinivasan, K. (2012). Effect of yoga on cognitive abilities in schoolchildren from a socioeconomically disadvantaged background: A randomized controlled study. *Journal of Alternative and Complementary Medicine, 18*(12), 1161–1167. Retrieved from http://doi.org/10.1089/acm.2011.0579.

Chen, E., Hanson, M. D., Paterson, L. Q., Griffin, M. J., Walker, H. A., & Miller, G. E. (2006). Socioeconomic status and inflammatory processes in childhood asthma: The role of psychological stress. *The Journal of Allergy and Clinical Immunology, 117*(5), 1014–1020. doi:S0091-6749(06)00290-9 [pii].

Cohen, S., Doyle, W. J., Turner, R. B., Alper, C. M., & Skoner, D. P. (2004). Childhood socioeconomic status and host resistance to infectious illness in adulthood. *Psychosomatic Medicine, 66*(4), 553–558. http://doi.org/10.1097/01.psy.0000126200.05189.d3.

Compas, B. E., & Thomsen, A. H. (1999). Coping and responses to stress among children with recurrent abdominal pain. *Journal of Developmental and Behavioral Pediatrics: JDBP, 20*(5), 323–324.

Culbert, T., & Kajander, R. (2007). *Be the boss of your stress.* Minneapolis: Free Spirit Publishing.

Danese, A., Moffitt, T. E., Pariante, C. M., Ambler, A., Poulton, R., & Caspi, A. (2008). Elevated inflammation levels in depressed adults with a history of childhood maltreatment. *Archives of General Psychiatry, 65*(4), 409–415. doi:10.1001/archpsyc.65.4.409.

Davidson, R. J., Kabat-Zinn, J., Schumacher, J., Rosenkranz, M., Muller, D., Santorelli, S. F., … Sheridan, J. F. (2003). Alterations in brain and immune function produced by mindfulness meditation. *Psychosomatic Medicine, 65*(4), 564–570.

Diamond, A., & Lee, K. (2011). Interventions shown to aid executive function development in children 4 to 12 years old. *Science, 333*(6045), 959–964. Retrieved from http://doi.org/10.1126/science.1204529.

Dozier, M., Peloso, E., Lewis, E., Laurenceau, J. P., & Levine, S. (2008). Effects of an attachment-based intervention on the cortisol production of infants and toddlers in foster care. *Development and Psychopathology, 20*(3), 845–859. http://doi.org/10.1017/S0954579408000400.

Eccleston, C., Palermo, T. M., de C Williams, A. C., Lewandowski, A., Morley, S., Fisher, E., & Law, E. (2012). Psychological therapies for the management of chronic and recurrent pain in children and adolescents. *Cochrane Database of Systematic Reviews (Online), 12*, CD003968. http://doi.org/10.1002/14651858.CD003968.pub3; 10.1002/14651858.CD003968.pub3

Epel, E. S., Blackburn, E. H., Lin, J., Dhabhar, F. S., Adler, N. E., Morrow, J. D., & Cawthon, R. M. (2004). Accelerated telomere shortening in response to life stress. *Proceedings of the National Academy of Sciences of the United States of America, 101*(49), 17312–17315. http://doi.org/10.1073/pnas.0407162101.

Felitti, V. J., Anda, R. F., Nordenberg, D., Williamson, D. F., Spitz, A. M., Edwards, V., … Marks, J. S. (1998). Relationship of childhood abuse and household dysfunction to many of the leading causes of death in adults. The Adverse Childhood Experiences (ACE) Study. *American Journal of Preventive Medicine, 14*(4), 245–258. doi:10.1016/S0749-3797(98)00017-8.

Fisher, P. A., & Kim, H. K. (2007). Intervention effects on foster preschoolers' attachment-related behaviors from a randomized trial. *Prevention Science, 8*(2), 161–170. doi:10.1007/s11121-007-0066-5.

Forkey, H., Gillespie, R. J., Pettersen, T., Spector, L., & Stirling, J. (2014). In M. D. Dowd (Ed.), *The medical home approach to identifying and responding to exposure to trauma.* Elk Grove Village, IL: American Academy of Pediatrics.

Forman-Hoffman, V. L., Zolotor, A. J., McKeeman, J. L., Blanco, R., Knauer, S. R., Lloyd, S. W., … Viswanathan, M. (2013). Comparative effectiveness of interventions for children exposed to non-relational traumatic events. *Pediatrics, 131*(3), 526–539. 10.1542/peds.2012-3846

Fraser, J. G., Lloyd, S., Murphy, R., Crowson, M., Zolotor, A. J., Coker-Schwimmer, E., & Viswanathan, M. (2013). A comparative effectiveness review of parenting and trauma-focused interventions for children exposed to maltreatment. *Journal of Developmental and Behavioral Pediatrics: JDBP, 34*(0), 353–68. http://doi.org/10.1097/DBP.0b013e31828a7dfc.

Funderburk, B. W., & Eyberg, S. (2011). Chapter 12j. Parent–child interaction therapy. In J. C. Norcross & D. K. Freedheim (Eds.), *History of psychotherapy: Continuity and change* (2nd ed., pp. 415–420). Washington, DC: American Psychological Association.

Garner, A. S., Shonkoff, J. P., Siegel, B. S., Dobbins, M. I., Earls, M. F., Garner, A. S., … AAP Committee on Psychosocial Aspects of Child and Family Health, Committee on Early Childhood, Adoption, and Dependent Care, and Section on Developmental and Behavioral Pediatrics. (2012). Early childhood adversity, toxic stress, and the role of the pediatrician: translating developmental science into lifelong health. *Pediatrics, 129*(1), e224-31. doi:10.1542/peds.2011-2662

Gunnar, M. R. (2001). Effects of early deprivation: Findings from orphanage-reared infants and children. In C. A. Nelson & M. Luciana (Eds.), *Handbook of developmental cognitive neuroscience* (pp. 617–629). Cambridge, MA: MIT Press.

Gunnar, M. R., Morison, S. J., Chisholm, K., & Schuder, M. (2001). Salivary cortisol levels in children adopted from Romanian orphanages. *Development and Psychopathology, 13*(3), 611–628.

Hanson, C. L., Henggeler, S. W., & Burghen, G. A. (1987). Model of associations between psycho-social variables and health-outcome measures of adolescents with IDDM. *Diabetes Care, 10*(6), 752–758.

Heim, C., & Nemeroff, C. B. (1999). The impact of early adverse experiences on brain systems involved in the pathophysiology of anxiety and affective disorders. *Biological Psychiatry, 46*(11), 1509–1522. http://doi.org/S0006-3223(99)00224-3.

Heinrichs, M., Baumgartner, T., Kirschbaum, C., & Ehlert, U. (2003). Social support and oxytocin interact to suppress cortisol and subjective responses to psychosocial stress. *Biological Psychiatry, 54*(12), 1389–1398. doi:S0006322303004657 [pii].

Jain, S. C., Rai, L., Valecha, A., Jha, U. K., Bhatnagar, S. O., & Ram, K. (1991). Effect of yoga training on exercise tolerance in adolescents with childhood asthma. *The Journal of Asthma, 28*(6), 437–442.

Kohen, D. P., & Olness, K. O. (2011). *Hypnosis and hypnotherapy with children* (4th ed.). New York, NY: Routledge, Taylor & Francis Group.

Kohen, D. P., Olness, K. N., Colwell, S. O., & Heimel, A. (1984). The use of relaxation-mental imagery (self-hypnosis) in the management of 505 pediatric behavioral encounters. *Journal of Developmental and Behavioral Pediatrics, 5*(1), 21–25.

Kuttner, L., Chambers, C. T., Hardial, J., Israel, D. M., Jacobson, K., & Evans, K. (2006). A randomized trial of yoga for adolescents with irritable bowel syndrome. *Pain Research & Management. Journal de La Societe Canadienne Pour Le Traitement de La Douleur, 11*(4), 217–223.

Massin, M. M., Withofs, N., Maeyns, K., & Ravet, F. (2001). The influence of fetal and postnatal growth on heart rate variability in young infants. *Cardiology, 95*(2), 80–83. doi:47350 [pii].

Masten, A. S. (2001). Ordinary magic. Resilience processes in development. *The American Psychologist, 56*(3), 227–238.

McDade, T. W., Leonard, W. R., Burhop, J., Reyes-Garcia, V., Vadez, V., Huanca, T., & Godoy, R. A. (2005). Predictors of C-reactive protein in Tsimane' 2 to 15 year-olds in lowland

Bolivia. *American Journal of Physical Anthropology, 128*(4), 906-913. doi:10.1002/ajpa.20222.

McEwen, B. S. (1998). Stress, adaptation, and disease. Allostasis and allostatic load. *Annals of the New York Academy of Sciences, 840*, 33–44.

McGowan, P. O., Sasaki, A., D'Alessio, A. C., Dymov, S., Labonte, B., Szyf, M., … Meaney, M. J. (2009). Epigenetic regulation of the glucocorticoid receptor in human brain associates with childhood abuse. *Nature Neuroscience, 12*(3), 342-348. doi:10.1038/nn.2270

Middlebrooks, J. S., & Audage, N. C. (2008). *The effects of childhood stress on health across the lifespan.* Atlanta, GA: Centers for Disease Control and Prevention, National Center for Injury Prevention and Control.

Miller, G., & Chen, E. (2007). Unfavorable socioeconomic conditions in early life presage expression of proinflammatory phenotype in adolescence. *Psychosomatic Medicine, 69*(5), 402–409. doi:10.1097/PSY.0b013e318068fcf9.

Miller, G., Chen, E., & Cole, S. W. (2009). Health psychology: Developing biologically plausible models linking the social world and physical health. *Annual Review of Psychology, 60*, 501–524. doi:10.1146/annurev.psych.60.110707.163551.

Noggle, J. J., Steiner, N. J., Minami, T., & Khalsa, S. B. (2012). Benefits of yoga for psychosocial well-being in a US high school curriculum: A preliminary randomized controlled trial. *Journal of Developmental and Behavioral Pediatrics, 33*(3), 193–201. doi:10.1097/DBP.0b013e31824afdc4.

Obradovic, J., Bush, N. R., Stamperdahl, J., Adler, N. E., & Boyce, W. T. (2010). Biological sensitivity to context: The interactive effects of stress reactivity and family adversity on socio-emotional behavior and school readiness. *Child Development, 81*(1), 270–289. doi:10.1111/j.1467-8624.2009.01394.x.

O'Connor, T. G., Winter, M. A., Hunn, J., Carnahan, J., Pressman, E. K., Glover, V., … Caserta, M. T. (2013). Prenatal maternal anxiety predicts reduced adaptive immunity in infants. *Brain, Behavior, and Immunity, 32*, 21–28. doi:10.1016/j.bbi.2013.02.002

Odgers, C. L., & Jaffee, S. R. (2013). Routine versus catastrophic influences on the developing child. *Annual Review of Public Health, 34*, 29–48. doi:10.1146/annurev-publhealth-031912-114447.

Olness, K. (2009). Self-control and self-regulation: Normal development to clinical conditions (Chapter 46). In W. B. Carey, A. C. Crocker, W. L. Coleman, E. R. Elias, & H. M. Feldman (Eds.), *Developmental-behavioral pediatrics* (4th ed., pp. 453–459). Philadelphia, PA: Saunders Elsevier.

Pluess, M., & Belsky, J. (2012). Conceptual issues in psychiatric gene-environment interaction research. *The American Journal of Psychiatry, 169*(2), 222–223. doi:10.1176/appi.ajp.2011.11111614. author reply 223.

Powers, S. W., Gilman, D. K., & Hershey, A. D. (2006). Headache and psychological functioning in children and adolescents. *Headache, 46*(9), 1404–1415. doi:HED583 [pii].

Raver, C. C., Jones, S. M., Li-Grining, C., Zhai, F., Bub, K., & Pressler, E. (2011). CSRP's impact on low-income preschoolers' preacademic skills: Self-regulation as a mediating mechanism. *Child Development, 82*(1), 362–378. http://doi.org/ 10.1111/j.1467-8624.2010.01561.x.

Riggs, N. R., Greenberg, M. T., Kusche, C. A., & Pentz, M. A. (2006). The mediational role of neurocognition in the behavioral outcomes of a social-emotional prevention program in elementary school students: Effects of the PATHS curriculum. *Prevention Science, 7*(1), 91–102. http://doi.org/10.1007/s11121-005-0022-1.

Roisman, G. I., Susman, E., Barnett-Walker, K., Booth-LaForce, C., Owen, M. T., Belsky, J., … Network, N. E. C. C. R. (2009). Early family and child-care antecedents of awakening cortisol levels in adolescence. *Child Development, 80*(3), 907–920. doi:10.1111/j.1467-8624.2009.01305.x.

Sadeh, A., Raviv, A., & Gruber, R. (2000). Sleep patterns and sleep disruptions in school-age children. *Developmental Psychology, 36*(3), 291–301.

Sanders, M. R. (1999). Triple P-positive parenting program: Towards an empirically validated multilevel parenting and family support strategy for the prevention of behavior and emotional problems in children. *Clinical Child and Family Psychology Review, 2*(2), 71–90.

Sapienza, J. K., & Masten, A. S. (2011). Understanding and promoting resilience in children and youth. *Current Opinion in Psychiatry, 24*(4), 267–273. http://doi.org/10.1097/YCO.0b013e32834776a8.

Schanberg, L. E., Sandstrom, M. J., Starr, K., Gil, K. M., Lefebvre, J. C., Keefe, F. J., ... Tennen, H. (2000). The relationship of daily mood and stressful events to symptoms in juvenile rheumatic disease. *Arthritis Care and Research: The Official Journal of the Arthritis Health Professions Association, 13*(1), 33-41.

Schilling, E. A., Aseltine Jr, R. H., & Gore, S. (2007). Adverse childhood experiences and mental health in young adults: A longitudinal survey. *BMC Public Health, 7*, 30. 1471-2458-7-30

Shalev, I. (2012). Early life stress and telomere length: Investigating the connection and possible mechanisms: A critical survey of the evidence base, research methodology and basic biology. *BioEssays: News and Reviews in Molecular, Cellular and Developmental Biology, 34*(11), 943–952. doi:10.1002/bies.201200084

Shalev, I., Entringer, S., Wadhwa, P. D., Wolkowitz, O. M., Puterman, E., Lin, J., & Epel, E. S. (2013). Stress and telomere biology: a lifespan perspective. *Psychoneuroendocrinology, 38*(9), 1835–1842. http://doi.org/10.1016/j.psyneuen.2013.03.010.

Shankaran, S., Das, A., Bauer, C. R., Bada, H., Lester, B., Wright, L., ... Poole, K. (2006). Fetal origin of childhood disease: intrauterine growth restriction in term infants and risk for hypertension at 6 years of age. *Archives of Pediatrics & Adolescent Medicine, 160*(9), 977-981. doi:160/9/977 [pii]

Shirtcliff, E. A., Coe, C. L., & Pollak, S. D. (2009). Early childhood stress is associated with elevated antibody levels to herpes simplex virus type 1. *Proceedings of the National Academy of Sciences of the United States of America, 106*(8), 2963–2967. doi:10.1073/pnas.0806660106.

Shonkoff, J. P., Garner, A. S., & Committee on Psychosocial Aspects of Child and Family Health, Committee on Early Childhood, Adoption, and Dependent Care, & Section on Developmental and Behavioral Pediatrics. (2012). The lifelong effects of early childhood adversity and toxic stress. *Pediatrics, 129*(1), e232–46. doi:10.1542/peds.2011-2663.

Stevens, C., Lauinger, B., & Neville, H. (2009). Differences in the neural mechanisms of selective attention in children from different socioeconomic backgrounds: An event-related brain potential study. *Developmental Science, 12*(4), 634–646. doi:10.1111/j.1467-7687.2009.00807.x.

Sugarman, L. I., & Wester, W. C., II (Eds.). (2013). *Therapeutic hypnosis with children and adolescents* (2nd ed.). Carmarthen, Wales: Crowne House.

Sussman Gertz, D., & Culbert, T. (2009). Pediatric self-regulation (Chapter 91). In W. B. Carey, A. C. Crocker, W. L. Coleman, E. R. Elias, & H. M. Feldman (Eds.), *Developmental-behavioral pediatrics* (4th ed., pp. 911–922). Philadelphia, PA: Saunders Elsevier.

Tollenaar, M. S., Jansen, J., Beijers, R., Riksen-Walraven, J. M., & de Weerth, C. (2010). Cortisol in the first year of life: Normative values and intra-individual variability. *Early Human Development, 86*(1), 13–15.

Uman, L. S., Chambers, C. T., McGrath, P. J., & Kisely, S. (2008). A systematic review of randomized controlled trials examining psychological interventions for needle-related procedural pain and distress in children and adolescents: An abbreviated Cochrane review. *Journal of Pediatric Psychology, 33*(8), 842–854. http://doi.org/10.1093/jpepsy/jsn031.

Vlieger, A. M., Rutten, J. M., Govers, A. M., Frankenhuis, C., & Benninga, M. A. (2012). Long-term follow-up of gut-directed hypnotherapy vs. standard care in children with functional abdominal pain or irritable bowel syndrome. *The American Journal of Gastroenterology, 107*(4), 627–631. doi:10.1038/ajg.2011.487

Vygotsky, L. S. (1980). *Mind in society: The development of higher psychological processes.* Cambridge, MA: Harvard University Press.

Webster-Stratton, C., Mihalic, S., Fagan, A., Arnold, D., Taylor, T., & Tingley, C. (2001). *The incredible years: parent, teacher and child training series* (Blueprints for violence prevention series, Vol. 11). Boulder, CO: Center for the Study and Prevention of Violence, Institute of Behavioral Science, University of Colorado.

Wright, R. J., Cohen, R. T., & Cohen, S. (2005). The impact of stress on the development and expression of atopy. *Current Opinion in Allergy and Clinical Immunology, 5*(1), 23–29. doi:10.1097/00130832-200502000-00006.

Chapter 6
Child Mental Health: Recent Developments with Respect to Risk, Resilience, and Interventions

Eliot Goldman, Joan Stamler, Kimberly Kleinman, Sarah Kerner, and Owen Lewis

6.1 Introduction

It is estimated that between 10 and 20 % of children and adolescents in the United States experience significant emotional and behavioral disorders in any given year (Kieling et al., 2011). It is also estimated that 75–80 % of these children do not receive appropriate interventions (Kataoka, Zhang, & Wells, 2002). Common youth disorders such as anxiety, behavioral disorders, severe mood disorders, and substance abuse (Merikangas et al., 2010; Nock et al., 2013) come with an enormous human and economic cost to the health care, education, and justice systems that is estimated at 247 billion dollars annually (Perou et al., 2013). Overall, the prevalence

E. Goldman, Ph.D. (✉)
Department of Psychiatry, Columbia University Medical Center, Columbia University,
14 Rye Ridge Plaza, Suite 244, Rye Brook, NY 10573, USA
e-mail: egoldmanphd@gmail.com

J. Stamler, Ph.D.
Teachers College Columbia University, 90 Hudson Street #3F, New York, NY 10013, USA
e-mail: jstamler@ix.netcom.com

K. Kleinman, Ph.D. • S. Kerner, Psy.D
Department of Pediatric Psychiatry, Columbia University Medical Center, New York-Presbyterian Hospital, 3959 Broadway, 6th Floor North, New York, NY 10032, USA
e-mail: kek9041@nyp.org; sak9099@nyp.org

O. Lewis, M.D.
Department of Psychiatry, Columbia University,
11 East 87th Street, New York, NY 10128, USA
e-mail: Owlewismd@gmail.com

© Springer Science+Business Media New York 2016
M.R. Korin (ed.), *Health Promotion for Children and Adolescents*,
DOI 10.1007/978-1-4899-7711-3_6

of these severe disorders is higher than most common physical conditions such as asthma or diabetes (Merikangas et al., 2010). During the past several years, epidemiologists have emphasized a trend toward increasing rates of youth emotional and behavioral difficulties (Sourander, Niemela, Santalahti, Helenius, & Piha, 2008).

Researchers note a "large generational increase" of rates of psychopathology among American college-age youth during the past several decades (Twenge et al., 2010) that seems to reflect higher rates of psychopathology among youths in general. A number of explanations have been offered for these increased rates, including better systems of identification and reporting (Perou et al., 2013), as well as the ongoing influence of key risk factors on children's mental health. These include the effects of income inequality and poverty (Essex et al., 2006; Yoshikawa, Aber, & Beardslee, 2012), fragmentation of family, and community support systems, as well as parental mental health problems (Barker, Copeland, Maughan, Jaffee, & Uher, 2012; Fatori, Bordin, Curto, & de Paula, 2013; Harper, 2012). In addition, childhood experiences of trauma, deprivation, and chronic stress often lead to increased vulnerability to substance use, depression, and other emotional and behavioral difficulties (Grasso, Greene, & Ford, 2013; Perry, 2008). In this sense children of poverty, living with chronic stress in difficult circumstances, are especially at risk.

Layne and colleagues (Layne et al., 2009; Layne, Briggs, & Courtois, 2014) have developed an intriguing conceptual frame regarding the effect of these variables. They describe a *risk factor caravan* which serves to define how clusters of "various risk factors tend to co-occur, accumulate in number, accrue and cascade forward in their harmful effects, and 'travel' with their host across development." This conceptualization is useful as it encompasses multiple risk factors previously described such as adverse events, chronic stress, cognitive and social challenges, as well as inadequate access to care that accompany the developing child over time (Layne et al., 2009).

This chapter will describe and attempt to unpack elements of this "risk factor caravan" that impinge on children's behavioral and emotional health. There is special emphasis on emerging research in the field of chronic stress, trauma, and poverty as especially powerful factors that influence child development and mental health. In addition, we will describe protective factors such as individual characteristics, family relationships, and community support, with a particular focus on school settings in terms of their potential to foster resilience in dealing with these challenges. Finally we review current promising prevention efforts and possible future directions for program development and interventions.

6.2 Risk Factors in Children's Mental Health

6.2.1 Role of Childhood Adversity

Overall, there is an abundant body of research that suggests that multiple adversities in childhood are associated with increased risk for behavioral and emotional symptoms and impairment in childhood. These adversities include an overlapping set of difficulties that include chronically difficult and stressful life situations related to poverty, community violence, and family dysfunction as well as victimization through abuse. In terms of poverty, recent data indicates that over 20 % of children under the age of 18 are living below the federal poverty line. In addition, another 20 % of children are "'near poor'," living in households with incomes between 100 and 120 % of the federal poverty line (Aber & Chaudry, 2010). Poverty is a critical risk factor for many of the same emotional and behavioral disorders noted in relation to adverse, chronically stressful childhood experiences. For example, children exposed to poverty are at higher risk for poor cognitive outcomes in school performance, antisocial behaviors, and emotional difficulties (Luby et al., 2013). Higher rates of suicide risk and general social adjustment have been noted as well (Yoshikawa et al., 2012). In addition, economic hardship is often associated with depression in parents and marital conflict which may be related to significant child behavioral difficulties (Yoshikawa et al., 2012).

Similar cognitive and affective difficulties have been noted in children who have been victimized. For example, children who have been victimized have been found to have lower levels of executive functioning, attention and concentration in comparison with their same age, non-victimized peers (D'Andrea, Ford, Stolbach, Spinazzola, & van der Kolk, 2012), as well as elevated levels of depression (Weder et al., 2014). Specifically, child sexual abuse has been associated with lower visual and verbal memory scores (Savitz, van der Merwe, Stein, Solms, & Ramesar, 2007).

6.2.2   Effect of Cumulative Risk

During the past decade, researchers have focused on the cumulative effect of these multiple adversities through the study of cumulative and chronic stress, multiple abuse episodes, and a range of adverse childhood experiences (Grasso et al., 2013). A key study in this area has examined the effect of "adverse childhood experiences" (ACEs) on health outcomes. The ACE study involved a large-scale epidemiological examination of the influence of stressful social problems on health-related behaviors and morbidity among a large study group (approximately 17,000 adults) (CDC, 2015; Felitti, 2009; Felitti et al., 1998). For the purposes of the study, ACEs were defined as the child experiencing emotional, physical or sexual abuse, or growing up in a household where someone had been an alcoholic, a drug user, mentally ill, or suicidal, or where the mother was treated violently, or a household member had been imprisoned during the participants' childhood or the child's parents were divorced. Results indicated a widespread presence of these experiences in participants' lives as two-thirds of the participants recorded at least one ACE incident. Overall, researchers found that as the number of reported ACEs increased, the risk for a wide range of chronic, serious health problems increased as well. In addition, as the number of reported ACEs increased, there was a cumulative increase of risk for behavioral and emotional difficulties such as depression, suicide risk, and substance use. For example, in comparison to a person with an ACE score of 0, those with an ACE score of 4 or more were twice as likely to be smokers, 12 times more likely to have attempted suicide, 7 times more likely to be an alcoholic, and 10 times more likely to have injected street drugs (CDC, 2015). The data strongly suggest that adult difficulties that reflect serious emotional problems may often have originated in childhood trauma (Dube et al., 2003).

While the original ACE study involved groundbreaking research definitively connecting childhood stress and trauma with significant risk for poor health and mental health outcomes, the study relied on retrospective reports by adults regarding childhood events. As a result, several limitations of the original ACE project have been highlighted. These include concerns regarding the accuracy and validity of adult retrospective reports, the use of a limited list of adverse events that do not include many significant childhood adversities, and limited information regarding the cumulative effect of multiple adverse events (Layne et al., 2014). A number of recent studies have sought to modify the original study paradigm in an attempt to correct and expand ACE research. For example, a study which focused on the immediate effect of ACEs on youth involving a chart review of approximately 700 children and adolescents at an urban pediatric clinic suggested that, as was true of the original ACE study, two-thirds of the youth had experienced one or more ACEs and 12 % had experienced four or more events. In this study, increased ACE scores correlated with significantly increased risk of learning difficulties, behavioral problems, and obesity (Burke, Hellman, Scott, Weems, & Carrion, 2011). As noted, some have argued that ACE categories are not sufficiently descriptive of the difficulties faced by traumatized youth. Based on youth feedback, it was suggested that single and chronic events such as single-parent homes, exposure to violence, personal victimization, bullying, economic hardship, and discrimination be included in ACE research (Wade, Shea, Rubin, & Wood, 2014). An expanded list of 20 adverse experiences was utilized with an adolescent study population (Layne, Greeson, et al., 2014), and results were consistent with prior ACE-related research. Specifically, a significant relationship existed between adverse childhood events and high-risk behaviors such as delinquency, impaired attachment, substance abuse, and sexual promiscuity. In addition, as noted in earlier studies, there was evidence of the cumulative effect of trauma as each additional type of trauma and loss exposure significantly increased the likelihood of high-risk adolescent behavioral difficulties and/or functional impairment (Layne, Greeson, et al., 2014).

6.2.3   Developmental Role of Stress

Overall, these studies suggest a common pathway from chronic childhood stress to significant health, emotional, and behavioral problems. Chronic stress can be defined as the ongoing pressure of dealing with difficult life circumstances such as poverty, violence, and family dysfunction among others. Stress becomes toxic and severely damaging when there is "extreme, frequent, or extended activation of the stress response, without the buffering presence of a supportive adult" (Johnson, Riley, Granger, & Riis, 2013). Recent studies have suggested possible explanations for these developmental phenomena that are rooted in physiological responses to chronic stress that affect neurological, genetic, and hormonal systems (Grasso et al., 2013). Perry and colleagues (Gaskill & Perry, 2012) have emphasized a sequential model of brain development, wherein disruptions due to trauma, maternal substance abuse while in utero, or other developmental insults can "result in a cascade of dysfunction from lower regions (where these system originate) up to all of the target areas higher in the brain" (Perry, 2009). The timing of these events is particularly crucial as neurodevelopment occurs in different brain areas at different times which renders the child "more sensitive to organizing or disruptive experiences during these ... [developmentally] sensitive periods" (Perry, 2009). Studies of traumatized children suggest that the onset of childhood trauma results in a brain that is "poorly developed and functionally disorganized, rendering the child poorly able to intellectually, verbally, or emotionally respond to normal experiences let alone dramatic ones" (Gaskill & Perry, 2012).

Awareness of the impact of childhood adversity and cumulative stress has also fueled interest in examining the behavioral effects of gene/environment interactions. This relatively new area of research, behavioral epigenetics, has suggested that genetic changes (epigenetic alternations) occur as a result of exposure to environmental adversity, social stress, and traumatic experiences (Lester, Marsit, & Bromer, 2014; Roth, 2013). For example, epigenetic changes were noted following maltreatment leading to increased risk of depression in children (Weder et al., 2014). In addition, there is evidence that exposure to a variety of stressors in infancy and early childhood results in significant changes to a number of hormonal and neurotransmitter systems (Nemeroff & Binder, 2014).

6.3 Protective/Compensatory Factors

6.3.1 Resilience Framework

Paired with the issue of risk is the concept of resilience, defined as "the process of, capacity for, or outcome of successful adaptation despite challenging or threatening circumstances" (Luthar & Zelazo, 2003; Masten, Best, & Garmezy, 1990). A key element in this conceptualization is that resilience "arises from the operation of common human adaptational systems" (Masten & Powell, 2003); in this sense, adverse childhood experience may do its greatest damage by interfering with the natural development of these adaptive systems. Furthermore, since development is an integrative process over time, earlier patterns of positive adaptation or disruption are likely to affect later stages, with competence (successful negotiation of issues through the use of internal and external resources) in one stage of development creating a foundation for future success and lack of competence compromising successful engagement with similar issues as development proceeds (Yates, Egeland, & Sroufe, 2003). Understanding what those natural processes are and how they may be compromised presents an opportunity to redirect the developmental trajectory of children at risk for poor mental or behavioral health and associated outcomes. These efforts at understanding and intervening encompass both preventing psychopathology and promoting the development of competence—the former by identifying and attempting to eliminate or reduce risk and the latter by identifying and attempting to increase relevant assets and adaptational processes.

Within the resilience framework, some have drawn a distinction between "protective processes," in which "protective factors" benefit only, or to a much greater degree, those exposed to the risk factor, and "compensatory factors," which are of equal benefit to all, regardless of exposure to risk or adversity. In research terms, this corresponds to the difference between interactive or moderated effects (protective) and main effects (compensatory) (Fergusson & Horwood, 2003). While interesting in theory, in practical terms, the distinction may be less critical. The majority of studies document factors commonly found to be correlates of more positive development, whether in low- or high-risk contexts (main effects); however, the implications, and therefore the focus, are often most salient for those at higher risk. A resilience framework has helped to promote a greater emphasis on these positive factors and processes and their role in mitigating poor outcomes for this population.

Several studies have demonstrated the positive effect of specific individual, family, and community factors on the development of children exposed to high risk and adversity.

6.3.1.1 Individual Factors

With regard to individual factors, research underscores the important role of personality traits, temperament, and genetics in cultivating resilience in children and adolescents. Studies highlight both superior intellectual functioning and problem-solving skills (Fergusson & Lynskey, 1996; Masten & Coatsworth, 1998) as well as an "easy temperament" (Masten & Coatsworth, 1998) as protective factors throughout the developmental life span. In addition, high self-efficacy and optimism have been associated with fewer mental health problems (Wille, Bettge, Ravens-Sieberer, & BELLA Study Group, 2008). For example, low novelty seeking and high self-esteem were associated with less externalizing problems in children who had experienced adversity (Fergusson & Horwood, 2003). Similarly, low novelty seeking and low neuroticism were associated with less internalizing problems in children exposed to adversity. Moreover, gender was identified as a protective factor, in that females who experience adversity have less risk of developing externalizing problems, while males who face adversity have been shown to have fewer internalizing problems (Fergusson & Horwood, 2003).

6.3.1.2 Parental Attachment and Family Relations

Stable interpersonal relationships foster healthy development and functioning in children and adolescents, beginning with child–parent relationships and family dynamics. There is a considerable research, demonstrating the importance of forming a secure attachment to parents or other primary caregivers from infancy (Bretherton, 1992;

Levy, Meehan, & Temes, 2014; Yates et al., 2003). These first relationships establish a secure base from which infants and toddlers can confidently explore and interact with the world, which is essential for early developmental tasks, promoting self-regulation, problem solving, and autonomy. Secure relationships set up expectations that adults are to be trusted to fulfill one's needs and to provide nurturance, guidance, and support and serve as models for the development of social skills with others. They also foster emerging perceptions of self-efficacy and self-worth. Secure attachment has been associated with early caregiving relationships characterized by responsiveness, positive effect, contingency, and cooperativeness. In contrast, lack of secure attachment or negative relationships can compromise the development of these same foundational skills and attitudes such that early insecure relationships are associated with conduct, attentional, and other behavioral problems in later childhood (Yates et al., 2003). Poverty and life stress can undermine parental sensitivity during infancy and early childhood and, therefore, compromise secure attachment.

An example of the relation between secure family relationships and emotional health is highlighted in a series of studies on adolescent depression. Mazza, Fleming, Abbott, Haggerty, and Catalano (2010) examined the trajectories of adolescent depression by conducting a longitudinal study of depressive symptomology and related factors in children from second through eighth grade. Results indicated that positive family and interpersonal relations are the strongest protective factors against depression. Moreover, adolescents in this study who felt close to their parents and who had positive perceptions of their parents as being caring, understanding, and attentive to their needs endorsed less depressive symptoms (Mazza, Fleming, Abbott, Haggerty, & Catalano, 2010). Likewise, it has been suggested that the presence of nurturing and supportive relationships with at least one parent may mitigate the effects of family adversity (Jenkins & Smith, 1990; Wolfe & Mash, 2006). Familial resources, such as parental support, authoritative parenting, family cohesion, clear rules and expectations, and positive adolescent–parent relationships, have also been associated with more stable functioning and lower rates of depression (Forehand et al., 1991; Lamborn, Mounts, Steinberg, & Dornbusch, 1991).

6.3.1.3 Community Supports

Research has demonstrated that community supports may also buffer against the development of psychopathology in children and adolescents, as a sense of belonging within the community is crucial. Dugas and colleagues (2012) found that eighth graders who participated in sports teams both in and out of school reported less suicidal ideation. Similarly, findings from Mazza et al. (2010) suggest that religion may play a positive role in the lives of adolescents as a significant inverse relationship was found between participation in religious activities and depressive symptoms. Other studies have indicated that children who cultivate interests outside their family or form positive attachments with a non-related adult figure within their community may be more resilient to the effects of family adversity. Having relationships with school staff and participating in sports clubs or church activities have been noted to foster the development of resiliency and competence in children and adolescents in other studies as well (Wille et al., 2008). Finally, researchers have also highlighted the importance of positive peer relationships in the development of resiliency (Fergusson & Lynskey, 1996; Jenkins & Smith, 1990; Wolfe & Mash, 2006).

6.3.1.4   Role of Schools

Schools are a key setting for children's development of behavioral and cognitive competence. As such, it is critical to identify those factors and processes that help to promote resilience in school, as well as those that might undermine it, especially for otherwise vulnerable students. This is particularly critical as adjustment in school can have a multiplier effect, with problems in early grades, including chronic absenteeism and suspension, setting students up for later involvement in the criminal justice system, and increased rates of school dropout. Increased dropout risk is particularly noteworthy, as school dropout is associated with a host of negative economic and social consequences, including poorer physical and mental health as adults. On the other hand, many of those attributes and attitudes that are associated with school success (self-regulation, social skills, cognitive development, and sense of self-efficacy) are also those associated with overall resilience. Overall, school success in and of itself is a protective factor for positive outcomes as children age into adolescence and beyond (Balfanz & Byrnes, 2012; Rumberger & Rotermund, 2012; Yates et al., 2003).

There is considerable evidence for the benefits of a positive relationship with teachers and other adults in the school throughout the course of schooling. Positive relationships are promoted when teachers are sensitive and caring, when they communicate openly, directly, and coherently, and when they promote positive and realistic expectations for their students and support their autonomy in age-appropriate ways. These positive attachments form a secure base for exploration and development and help promote self-reliance and independence. When students bond with significant adults and identify with them, they internalize their attitudes and values and norms for behavior. Positive relationships with teachers also promote social competence that carries over into new interactions, including those with peers. In addition, secure relationships help foster emotional regulation, which, in turn, helps students accept and persist with new challenges, which is foundational to continued learning and academic success (Bergin & Bergin, 2009; Comer & Poussaint, 1992; Masten & Coatsworth, 1998). Positive student–teacher relationships are also associated with less antisocial behavior, including aggression, drug and alcohol use, violence, early sexual activity, and suicide (Bergin & Bergin, 2009).

When discipline is used positively and situated in a trusting relationship with adults, it can present an opportunity to help children solve a problem, develop self-control, and learn better ways of expressing feelings (Comer & Poussaint, 1992; Greene, 2010). Conversely, there is growing evidence that overly controlling, coercive, and inflexible disciplinary approaches by teachers and schools, such as zealously applied "'zero tolerance policies'," result in high rates of suspension and are harmful to students, particularly those who are already at risk. In fact, school suspension and other similar measures are fraught with profoundly dysfunctional processes and outcomes. Research surveys have indicated consistent patterns of disproportionate punishment for African-American students, including suspensions (Raffaele Mendez & Knoff, 2003), expulsions (Kewel Ramani, Gilbertson, Fox, & Provasnik, 2007), and office discipline referrals (Skiba, Michael, Nardo, & Peterson, 2002). Evidence suggests that this trend plays out on district and state levels as well. A recent comprehensive survey of all Texas middle and high schools (Fabelo et al., 2011) indicated that over 30 % of students had an out-of-school suspension with minority students more likely than whites to face harsh punishments. While factors such as poverty, low academic achievement, violent communities, and difficult family circumstances are highlighted in explaining this trend (Gregory, Skiba, & Noguera, 2010), comprehensive solutions to these problems clearly involve finding reasonable, less severe methods for dealing with students who exhibit disruptive behavior. Further, these rigid discipline policies run counter to two developmental needs of students—the capacity to foster strong and trusting relationships with adults in their schools and positive attitudes toward fairness and justice.

Peer relationships are also important. Association with students who are academically motivated has a positive attitude toward school, and a positive academic self-concept promotes academic achievement. Social support from peers, along with that of adults, promotes a sense of belonging. This feeling of being known and liked in school, along with engagement in academics and extracurricular activities, promotes a sense of school bonding, which is associated with lower levels of dropout and higher rates of achievement (Balfanz & Byrnes, 2012; Bergin & Bergin, 2009).

These studies have highlighted specific individual, family, social, and community resources that may serve as protective factors for children and adolescents who experience adversity. In addition, there is growing evidence that just as multiple risk factors increase the likelihood of negative development, multiple protective factors can help to promote competence in multiple domains (Yates et al., 2003).

6.4   Prevention and Intervention

As we continue to learn more about the etiology, characteristics, and trajectory of child and adolescent development, we will be better equipped to determine how these factors should be prioritized to both prevent and alleviate these diverse mental health problems. However, what is already recognized is that efforts should address identified risk factors as well as efforts made to fortify factors that have been shown to protect children and adolescents at risk for emotional and behavioral difficulties. In this sense, there are key roles for families, schools, and other community-based organizations. The sections that follow are not intended to be a comprehensive review of specific programs, but rather are meant to highlight the kinds of approaches that have met with success, as represented by intervention practices and models that have already shown promise.

6.4.1 Early Identification

One key practice involves early identification of at-risk youth. Efforts to establish an early warning system of identification by non-mental health professionals that can be implemented across a wide range of child-serving systems have included a set of "early warning signs" (Jensen et al., 2011) as well as tools to enhance early identification specifically for use by primary care clinicians (Zuckerbrot & Steinbaum, 2012). Further, SAMHSA has been instrumental in highlighting the importance of trauma screening, as well as trauma-informed care (SAMHSA, 2014). Efforts by states and local governments to screen for child mental health issues have generally been effective (Minnesota Department of Human Services, 2014), although some concern remains regarding large-scale child mental health screening (Press, 2014).

Within this context, several authors have emphasized the importance of a more specific assessment regarding childhood trauma and loss as well as chronic individual, family, and community stressors (D'Andrea et al., 2012; Greeson et al., 2014). An excellent example of that type of effort involves a trauma-informed assessment of staff, institutional systems, and clients that is part of a *Trauma-Informed Organizational Toolkit* developed by the National Center on Family Homelessness (Guarino, Soares, Konnath, Clervil, & Bassuk, 2009).

6.4.2 Trauma-Informed Programs

Leveraging insights gained in previously referenced studies of childhood trauma and stress, researchers and practitioners have begun to develop "trauma-informed" programs for schools, foster care, shelters, and other child-serving agencies. While the definition of "trauma informed" is somewhat fluid, programs across systems often share the following elements: providing a safe environment, improving parent and/or staff sensitivity and trauma awareness in interactions with children and families, developing child emotional self-regulation, and offering emotional support to parents and staff (Milot, St-Laurent, & Ethier, 2015). This paradigm has been adapted to trauma-informed school initiatives (Perry, 2009; Walkley & Cox, 2013) placing an emphasis on the development of calm, safe, and predictable environments and promoting teachers' emotional attunement and presence in order to model and foster students' emotional regulation. A successful implementation of a trauma-informed school approach has taken root in Spokane, Washington, where Blodgett and colleagues have augmented positive environmental efforts with practices that recognize and respond when children need more in the form of individualized instruction and more explicit skill building to promote behavioral resilience (Blodgett, 2012).

Other trauma-informed programs have been developed for residential care as well as in work with the homeless. Saxe and colleagues (Brown, McCauley, Navalta, & Saxe, 2013; Saxe & Brown, 2012) have emphasized a "Trauma Systems Therapy" model in residential care that attempts to ameliorate both the traumatized child's difficulties in emotional and behavioral self-regulation and a social environment that is unable to help the child self-regulate. In this model, emphasis is placed on building a relationship of trust, sensitivity to communication between staff and youth, and developing a nonthreatening, stable, and predictable residential environment and family involvement. Hodgdon, Kinniburgh, Gabowitz, Blaustein, and Spinazzola (2013) describe a trauma-informed residential program that emphasizes "Attachment, Regulation, and Competency (ARC)" with a concomitant reduction in residents' PTSD symptoms and episodic need for restraints. Finally, the aforementioned *Trauma-Informed Organizational Toolkit* (Guarino et al., 2009) outlines key elements of a trauma-informed approach that has been specifically developed for work with the homeless. However, the approach can serve as a model for other social service agencies.

6.4.3 Family-Based Programs

A developmental perspective suggests that efforts at prevention and intervention should begin in early childhood since earlier patterns of development will shape later adjustment. Specifically, patterns of maladjustment may be easier to correct if identified closer to onset, and maintaining an adaptive trajectory should be easier than having to reroute a child later in life. Moreover, emerging research in neurodevelopment reinforces the impact of early experience (Yates et al., 2003).

A current program with documented benefits involves a Nurse–Family Partnership program. The program provides nurse home visits during pregnancy to first-time mothers, who are primarily low income, unmarried, and teenaged. Nurses visit monthly during pregnancy until the child is 2 years old to teach positive health-related behaviors and competent child care and foster personal maternal development related to family planning, education, and workforce participation. Three randomized control trials in three locations have demonstrated sizable, sustained effects on important child and maternal outcomes. While effects differed across trials, common effects in two or more include reductions in child abuse/neglect and injuries, reduction in mothers' subsequent births during their late teens and early twenties, and improvement in cognitive/educational outcomes for children of mothers with low mental health/confidence/intelligence as measured by grades 1–6 reading/math achievement ("Nurse-Family Partnership," 2014). Positive results were also obtained via "Child FIRST," a home visitation program (Lowell, Carter, Godoy, Paulicin, & Briggs-Gowan, 2011) that targets low-income families with children aged 6–36 months. Based on child and family screening, the program targets children who are at risk of emotional, behavioral, and/or developmental problems. A clinical team works with the child and parents to provide a psychoeducational context for the child's difficulties and encourages positive child–parent interactions. Outcome measures indicate decreased likelihood of parental emotional difficulties and child behavioral difficulties as well as cognitive gains for children (Lowell et al., 2011).

A third successful family intervention is the Triple P (Positive Parenting Program) system. The program works with families with children aged 0–8 with an extensive set of parenting interventions. The program seeks to strengthen parenting skills and prevent dysfunctional parenting, so as to prevent child maltreatment and emotional, behavioral, and developmental problems ("Small Changes, Big Differences," 2015). The Triple P system emphasizes five core principles of positive parenting: (1) ensuring a safe, engaging environment; (2) promoting a positive learning environment; (3) using assertive discipline; (4) maintaining reasonable expectations; and (5) taking care of oneself as a parent. The intervention involves parenting seminars, parent skills training sessions, and individual consultations, which are delivered in relation to the relative severity of the child's behavioral problems and/or family dysfunction (Prinz, Sanders, Shapiro, Whitaker, & Lutzker, 2009). Program results indicate substantial reductions in the rate of child maltreatment, out-of-home placements and hospitalizations, and/or emergency room visits for at-risk children and families (Foster, Prinz, Sanders, & Shapiro, 2008; Prinz et al., 2009).

6.4.4 School-Based Programs

Second to families, schools are children's natural environment and thus a logical and opportune setting for reaching students with varied degrees of risk, resilience, and protective factors. As such, school systems and school personnel play a critical role in modeling, influencing, and supporting children's development (Cowen et al., 1996; Weist, 1997). This is particularly significant for children with mental health needs as access to available and affordable outpatient mental health clinics is often limited (Greenberg et al., 2003). Schools are therefore crucial in early identification of psychopathology and treatment through the implementation of comprehensive, evidence-based interventions.

Mental health services in school can vary greatly and span a continuum ranging from guidance departments to academic- or hospital-affiliated clinics that employ licensed psychologists and psychiatrists. Just as the offered services can vary, so can the needs of individual students and schools. To better understand the varying levels of need in schools, problematic behavior is often organized into a three-tiered approach (Sugai, Sprague, Horner, & Walker, 2000). The primary tier of prevention offers universal interventions (e.g., classroom- or school-wide) that are designed to target the majority of students without serious problem behavior and aim to have an impact on the overall school climate. The secondary tier targets the 5–15 % of students who are identified as "at risk." Targeted intervention at this level is often offered through specialized group interventions. The remaining students with chronic or intense problem behavior (approximately 1–7 %) are served in the tertiary prevention level through specialized, individualized interventions.

Primary tier interventions offer school- or classroom-wide preventive interventions that target all students, particularly the substantial majority of students who are not receiving secondary or tertiary intervention. These services can enhance a school environment and help to foster resilience and student development within their natural environment. There are some tertiary interventions which can be implemented directly by school personnel without outside consultation, such as Positive Behavioral Interventions and Supports (PBIS). PBIS (also often referred to as SWPBS, "school-wide positive behavior supports") are based on applied behavior analysis and offer a framework for helping school staff integrate evidence-based interventions into the academic and social cultures of their schools (Horner & Sugai, 2015). Schools are supported through resources offered by the US Department of Education's Office of Special Education Programs (OSEP, 2015). Other services require slightly more training and are often introduced through an outside consultant or mental health professional who is working with the school. In this way, many of the tertiary interventions can be taught to, and then implemented by, school personnel with ongoing consultation from trained mental health clinicians. Not only does this further train and empower teachers, it also builds teachers' evidence-based skillsets for use with future cohorts, thus reaching more students. A recent meta-analysis of over 200 tertiary school based interventions, which target social emotional learning processes and are delivered by teachers, reflects their effectiveness and positive impact (Durlak, Weissberg, Dymnicki, Taylor, & Schellinger, 2011). Improvements in social emotional skills, conduct problems, and emotional distress attest to the positive impact of these interventions. There has been a significant increase in universal preventive interventions that nourish school environments. While a comprehensive research review of these programs is beyond the scope of this chapter, we will focus on two promising interventions: the Good Behavior Game (Barrish, Saunders, & Wolf, 1969) and Teacher–Child Interaction Training (Lyon et al., 2009) that represent the kind of approaches that have been successful.

6.4.4.1 The Good Behavior Game

The Good Behavior Game (GBG) (Barrish et al., 1969) is an easily implemented group contingency and behavior management technique that functions both as an intervention and as a preventive measure. The GBG is implemented by dividing the classroom into teams that compete to follow predetermined classroom rules (e.g., stay in your seat; raise your hand). The teacher explains that if one of the students breaks a rule, the rule offender will be verbally recognized, and the team will receive a mark on the board (e.g., "Joey you called out; your team gets a point). Daily and weekly team winners (e.g., those with the fewest points) are rewarded with a prize or privilege. As a group contingency, this method lends itself to classroom settings as students not only monitor their own behavior but also the behavior of peers which has a cumulative impact on overall classroom climate. More recent adaptations maintain the group contingency and competition and yet recognize positive behavior (e.g., "Joey, you raised your hand! Your team gets a point!") (Barrish et al., 1969; Darveaux, 1984)

While the GBG is recognized in numerous studies as an effective intervention for improving behavior (Barrish et al., 1969; Bostow & Geiger, 1976; Darch & Thorpe, 1977; Davies & Witte, 2000; Dolan et al., 1993; Kleinman & Saigh, 2011; Lannie & McCurdy, 2007; McCurdy, Lannie, & Barnabas, 2009; Medland & Stachnik, 1972), evidence also suggests that it has an impact beyond disruptive classroom behavior. In this sense it can be generalized to other group settings with a positive impact on long-term psychosocial factors. The GBG has also been promoted as a universal prevention that is associated with improved academic performance (Saigh, 1987), higher scores on standardized achievement tests, greater odds of high school graduation, greater odds of college attendance, and reduced rates of special education (Bradshaw, Koth, Bevans, Ialongo, & Leaf, 2008). For male students, participation in a GBG classroom for 1 year in the first or second grade was shown to reduce rates of drug and alcohol abuse/dependence disorders, regular cigarette smoking, and antisocial personality disorder by young adulthood (Kellam et al., 2008). While the effects are impressive, the implementation is simple, and the GBG is rated as highly acceptable by teachers and students (Kleinman & Saigh, 2011; McCurdy et al., 2009). Due to the prolific evidence base and ease of implementation, the GBG has been promoted as a "universal behavioral vaccine," (Embry, 2002), the Substance Abuse and Mental Health Services Administration (SAMHSA) called the GBG a "best practice" for the prevention of substance abuse and violent behavior, and Weisz, Sandler, Durlak, and Anton (2005) identified the Good Behavior Game as a "treatment that works."

6.4.4.2 Teacher–Child Interaction Training

Although newer, Teacher–Child Interaction Training (TCIT) (Lyon et al., 2009) is another primary tier intervention with an impressive evidence base. TCIT, a universal prevention program implemented in preschool classrooms, was adapted from Sheila Eyberg's Parent–Child Interaction Therapy (PCIT). PCIT is a manualized evidence-based parent training intervention that has enjoyed considerable support in its ability to decrease externalizing symptoms in children aged two to seven through a combination of parent didactics, live coaching, feedback, and daily practice at home (Eyberg, Nelson, & Boggs, 2008; Thomas & Zimmer-Gembeck, 2007). In order to adapt PCIT into a preventive measure that targets multiple children in their natural setting, TCIT was created and implemented in preschool and kindergarten classrooms. TCIT includes the teaching of the PRIDE skills (i.e., *praise* appropriate behavior, *reflect* appropriate speech, *imitate* appropriate behavior/play, *describe* appropriate behavior, and be *enthusiastic*), avoidance of criticism, the use of effective commands, and methods for increasing compliance with commands and modified time-out. Although a relatively new intervention, TCIT has been well received by users and shown positive effects for increasing student skills and decreasing externalizing behavior (Lyon et al., 2009). It has also been shown to enhance positive teacher–child interactions, which might be expected to lead to additional successes in the future as the evidence base continues to develop (Devers, Stokes, Rainear, & Budd, 2012; Lyon et al., 2009).

As Sugai and colleagues (2000) point out, even after the implementation of universal prevention measures, there are tier two and three students who require additional intervention and support. The Incredible Years program (Webster-Stratton & Reid, 2003) for treating externalizing disorders in children and Interpersonal Psychotherapy–Adolescent Skills Training (Young & Mufson, 2003) for treating adolescents with subsyndromal depression are two examples of well-researched secondary tier interventions that have been used in conjunction with school-based clinics.

6.4.4.3 The Incredible Years

The Incredible Years (IY) (Webster-Stratton & Reid, 2003) is a manualized treatment consisting of three training programs (e.g., child, parent, and teacher) that are designed to be used concurrently. Trained facilitators use didactic presentations, videotaped vignettes, problem solving, discussion, and hands-on activities and/or role-plays to structure the session. The IY child program contains classroom or small group lesson plans that aim to strengthen children's social and emotional competencies through feeling identification, problem solving, anger management, and appropriate classroom behavior and social skills. The IY parent program is available to parents with children ranging in age from toddlers to school aged (6–12 years) and is most commonly delivered in a group format. The IY parent group aims to strengthen the parent–child relationship, implement effective discipline strategies, and help parents promote their child's development. The third program, the IY teacher program, aims to help teachers improve classroom management strategies and foster the student's social and emotional development. Traditionally, the IY programs are implemented most often with students who display disruptive behavior problems and have generally been found to be effective (Eyberg et al., 2008; Lyon et al., 2009). Webster–Stratton and colleagues have demonstrated wide success with Head Start children, parents, and teachers (Webster-Stratton, Reid, & Stoolmiller, 2008). Specifically, teachers in the IY program were shown to use more social and emotional teaching strategies as children in the treatment condition demonstrated significant improvements in emotional self-regulation, social competence, and conduct problems compared to control group students (Webster-Stratton et al., 2008).

6.4.5 Interpersonal Psychotherapy–Adolescent Skills Training

Another secondary tier intervention for youth is Interpersonal Psychotherapy–Adolescent Skills Training (IPT-AST). IPT-AST is a school-based prevention program that targets students who have elevated symptoms of depression, but who do not meet sufficient diagnostic criteria to confirm a diagnosis. The intervention is composed of groups of four to six adolescents, aged 12–16, and involves two individual pre-group sessions and eight group sessions. IPT-AST uses both psychoeducation and training in communication and interpersonal problem-solving skills to achieve four goals: (1) reduce depressive symptoms, (2) prevent the onset of a depressive disorder, (3) improve interpersonal functioning by reducing interpersonal conflict and increasing social support, and (4) reduce the stigma of clinical interventions so that youths are more likely to seek help in the future. The group aspect of IPT-AST is a central component of the model because it provides an opportunity for adolescents experiencing similar difficulties to connect with each other and allows them to practice these interpersonal skills in a comfortable and natural context.

Several randomized control trials (RCTs) have demonstrated that IPT-AST is at least as effective as a cognitive behavior group prevention program and more effective than school counseling in reducing depressive symptoms (Horowitz, Garber, Ciesla, Young, & Mufson, 2007; Young, Mufson, & Davies, 2006; Young, Mufson, & Gallop, 2010) and preventing the onset of depression diagnoses (Young et al., 2006; Young et al., 2010). Corollary analyses have also demonstrated the positive impact of IPT-AST on anxiety symptoms and interpersonal functioning (Young, Kranzler, Gallop, & Mufson, 2012; Young et al., 2012).

Finally, for the approximate 1–7 % of students identified as having chronic or intense concerns, tertiary interventions are required and may be delivered by school-based mental health professionals. For students with this level of need, school-based intervention can provide a tailored combination of individual and/or group psychotherapy, psychopharmacology, parent training, school consultation, and case management. Wilson and colleagues have found school-based prevention programs to be most effective when utilizing behavioral or cognitive–behavioral techniques (Wilson, Gottfredson, & Najaka, 2001). School-based mental health clinics are therefore unique in that students can receive full-service psychiatric treatment in their natural setting, thus reducing some of the burden faced by multi-stressed families. School-based clinics also allow students and therapists to implement interventions in vivo, with increased frequency and increased opportunities for observation and consultation, thus increasing generalizability (Rones & Hoagwood, 2000).

While school-based mental health programs offer a convenient, evidence-based alternative to outpatient mental health clinics, they are not without their limitations. Historically, school mental health staff and programs are marginalized or have been perceived as "add-ons" that are not aligned to the academic mission of schools (Weist & Paternite, 2006). Additionally Wu, Katic, Liu, Fan, and Fuller (2010) found that among students with severe mental health difficulties, only 19 % had accessed school-based services. Students more likely to access school-based mental health services were those who participated in extracurricular activities, implying that it may be those students who are already functioning more successfully who are better able to access school-based mental health services. In addition, Greenberg and colleagues (2003) identify a lack of integration and coordination of school-based mental health services with other components of school operations, as well as implementation and evaluation methods that are lacking in scientific rigor. An alternative is a "pathway to care" model (Atkins, Hoagwood, Kutash, & Seidman, 2010; Kutcher & Wei, 2013), wherein schools are the locus for identification and school personnel (e.g., school counselors, social workers) can support effective linkage to dedicated community-based mental health agencies. In this sense there is an attempt to shift schools' focus back to a key function of learning instead of the siloed provision of mental health services (Cappella, Frazier, Atkins, Schoenwald, & Glisson, 2008). These models may present an alternative to school-based clinics that can be implemented on a broader scale, especially where co-located clinics are not an option.

Overall, there seems to be general agreement that school mental health efforts need to be well integrated with school programs, staff capacity, and school culture. Clinics may underperform when they operate in isolation and are not sufficiently integrated with school staff and ongoing school operations (Hoagwood et al., 2007). While studies have emphasized the need for better coordination between schools and community clinics (Atkins et al., 2010; Cappella et al., 2008), efforts to assess specific program elements that bolster coordination (e.g., enhanced early identification of at-risk students and improved access to community care) have been lacking. A promising recent grant program, developed by SAMHSA, has sought to enhance and integrate these capacities through funding both community agencies (SAMHSA 2015b) and local school districts (SAMHSA, 2015a) across the United States. While student need has been well documented, the considerable challenges inherent in developing a fully integrated school mental health model (Atkins et al., 2010; Stephan, Sugai, Lever, & Connors, 2015).

6.5   Conclusion

It is evident that the rate of child mental health difficulties has been rising. Recent research has highlighted the role of childhood adversity and the way in which it compromises healthy development on neurological, behavioral, and emotional levels. There is also a growing understanding of those positive factors and processes that mitigate risk. While more research is needed, there is an opportunity to shape more effective programs and policies through an emerging understanding and awareness of risk and resilience. Although it is beyond the scope of this chapter to make specific recommendations, we will highlight certain patterns in current research findings and programs that we believe can be used to help guide thinking going forward:

- *Early detection*: As noted, the cumulative effects of multiple risk factors in childhood (stress, poverty, family dysfunction) have the potential to have a profound effect on later development and health. Therefore, early detection, via identification of at-risk youth through effective implementation of a system of early warning signs by informed adults, is essential. Recent efforts showing promise have included training for nonmental health professionals such as pediatricians, nurses, teachers, and other school staff.
- *Trauma awareness*: The confluence of increasingly sophisticated neuroscience, genetic, and epidemiological research has highlighted the effect of toxic stress on child development. Promising trends have included a more refined assessment and understanding of the effects of chronic trauma as well as efforts to design interventions to reverse or at least lessen those effects. This burgeoning awareness has led to the adoption of "trauma-informed" approaches across child-serving systems wherein clients' needs and vulnerabilities are taken into account when designing effective interventions. Federal, state, and municipal programs that support this work in a growing number of clinics, agencies, schools, and other child- and family-serving institutions are an especially encouraging sign.

- *Early family supports*: Research and program development has demonstrated that early intervention with families can reduce the risk of abuse, school failure, and a range of emotional, behavioral, and developmental problems. As the first critical resource for children, it is not surprising that efforts to support potentially vulnerable new mothers during pregnancy and in the first few years of a child's life would yield positive results for themselves and their children.
- *Role of positive relationships for positive development*: Stress becomes toxic and severely damaging when the stress response is repeatedly activated "without the buffering presence of a supportive adult" (Johnson et al., 2013). While this starts with families, as noted above, there is a continuing opportunity for supportive relationships with a host of other adults in a child's life to play a profoundly positive role, ameliorating the effects of stress and promoting self-regulatory and social skills, habits of engagement, and a healthy self-image. Evidence for this can be seen in multiple settings, including the extended family and neighborhood, day care, schools, and community-based institutions.
- *School-based interventions*: Our chapter has highlighted the importance of enhanced student support systems and programs that promote a safe and orderly environment and constructive engagement with supportive adults as a way to foster students' emotional and behavioral competencies and school bonding. For students with the highest level of behavioral and emotional difficulty, a national conversation has clearly begun regarding effective alternatives to excessive school discipline and suspensions (Editorial, 2015; Fabelo et al., 2011) as well as the best methods for improving student support mechanisms ("School Mental Health Project," 2015).
- *Improved access and coordination of care*: Mental health service research has begun to delineate the necessary conditions for effective collaboration between schools, community clinics, and other child-serving agencies. This has been accompanied by improved screening, tracking of patient information through electronic medical records, and recent changes to medical insurance practices in the United States, which together will hopefully improve access and efficiency of care.

The incidence and severity of emotional and mental health issues for children are a serious concern, taking a personal and social toll. However, there is also a growing opportunity to develop evidence-based programs and policies to stem this tide and to continue to support research that will expand our collective knowledge of the problems and our ability to design effective responses.

References

Aber, J. L., & Chaudry, A. (2010). Low-income children, their families and the great recession: What next in policy? The Urban Institute. Retrieved from http://www.urban.org/UploadedPDF/412069_low-income_children.pdf.

Atkins, M. S., Hoagwood, K. E., Kutash, K., & Seidman, E. (2010). Toward the integration of education and mental health in schools. *Administration and Policy in Mental Health, 37*(1-2), 40–47. doi:10.1007/s10488-010-0299-7.

Balfanz, R., & Byrnes, V. (2012). *Chronic absenteeism: Summarizing what we know from nationally available data*. Baltimore, MD: Center for Social Organization of Schools, Johns Hopkins University Center for Social Organization of Schools, Johns Hopkins University.

Barker, E. D., Copeland, W., Maughan, B., Jaffee, S. R., & Uher, R. (2012). Relative impact of maternal depression and associated risk factors on offspring psychopathology. *The British Journal of Psychiatry, 200*(2), 124–129.

Barrish, H. H., Saunders, M., & Wolf, M. M. (1969). Good behavior game: Effects of individual contingencies for group consequences on disruptive behavior in a classroom. *Journal of Applied Behavior Analysis, 2*(2), 119–124.

Bergin, C., & Bergin, D. (2009). Attachment in the classroom. *Educational Psychology Review, 21*(2), 141–170.

Blodgett, C. (2012). A review of community efforts to mitigate and prevent adverse childhood experiences and trauma. Review paper. Retrieved from http://ext100.wsu.edu/cafru/wp-content/uploads/sites/65/2015/03/Complex-Trauma-News-Release1-A-Review-of-Community-Efforts-to-Mitigate-and-Prevent-ACEs-Blodgett-Final.pdf.

Bostow, D., & Geiger, O. (1976). Good behavior game: A replication and systematic analysis with a second grade class. *SALT: School Applications of Learning Theory, 8*(2), 18–27.

Bradshaw, C. P., Koth, C. W., Bevans, K. B., Ialongo, N., & Leaf, P. J. (2008). The impact of school-wide positive behavioral interventions and supports (PBIS) on the organizational health of elementary schools. *School Psychology Quarterly, 23*(4), 462–473.

Bretherton, I. (1992). *Attachment and bonding Handbook of social development: A lifespan perspective* (pp. 133–155). New York, NY: Plenum Press.

Brown, A. D., McCauley, K., Navalta, C. P., & Saxe, G. N. (2013). Trauma systems therapy in residential settings: Improving emotion regulation and the social environment of traumatized children and youth in congregate care. *Journal of Family Violence, 28*, 693–703. doi:10.1007/s10896-013-9542-9.

Burke, N. J., Hellman, J. L., Scott, B. G., Weems, C. F., & Carrion, V. G. (2011). The impact of adverse childhood experiences on an urban pediatric population. *Child Abuse and Neglect, 35*(6), 408–413. doi:10.1016/j.chiabu.2011.02.006.

Cappella, E., Frazier, S. L., Atkins, M. S., Schoenwald, S. K., & Glisson, C. (2008). Enhancing schools' capacity to support children in poverty: An ecological model of school-based mental health services. *Administration and Policy in Mental Health, 35*(5), 395–409. doi:10.1007/s10488-008-0182-y.

CDC. (2015). Injury Prevention & Control: Division of Violence Prevention. Retrieved March 29, 2015, from http://www.cdc.gov/violenceprevention/acestudy/.

Comer, J. P., & Poussaint, A. F. (1992). *Raising Black children: Two leading psychiatrists confront the educational, social, and emotional problems facing Black children*. New York, NY: Plume.

Cowen, E. L., Hightower, A. D., Pedro-Carroll, J. L., Work, W. C., Wyman, P. A., & Haffey, W. G. (1996). *School-based prevention for children at risk: The Primary Mental Health Project*. Washington, DC: American Psychological Association.

D'Andrea, W., Ford, J., Stolbach, B., Spinazzola, J., & van der Kolk, B. A. (2012). Understanding interpersonal trauma in children: Why we need a developmentally appropriate trauma diagnosis. *American Journal of Orthopsychiatry, 82*(2), 187–200.

Darch, C. B., & Thorpe, H. W. (1977). The principal game: A group consequence procedure to increase classroom on-task behavior. *Psychology in the Schools, 14*(3), 341–347.

Darveaux, D. X. (1984). The good behavior game plus merit: Controlling disruptive behavior and improving student motivation. *School Psychology Review, 13*(4), 510–514.

Davies, S., & Witte, R. (2000). Self-management and peer-monitoring within a group contingency to decrease uncontrolled verbalizations of children with Attention-Deficit/Hyperactivity Disorder. *Psychology in the Schools, 37*(2), 135–147.

Devers, K., Stokes, T. F., Rainear, C. A., & Budd, K. S. (2012). *In-classroom coaching using a bug-in-the-ear communication system to improve teacher interactions in managing the behavior challenges of preschoolers*. Paper presented at the Association for Behavior Analysis, Seattle, WA.

Dolan, L. J., Kellam, S. G., Brown, C., Werthamer-Larsson, L., Rebok, G. W., Mayer, L. S., … Wheeler, L. (1993). The short-term impact of two classroom-based preventive interventions on aggressive and shy behaviors and poor achievement. *Journal of Applied Developmental Psychology, 14*(3), 317-345.

Dube, S. R., Felitti, V. J., Dong, M., Chapman, D. P., Giles, W. H., & Anda, R. F. (2003). Childhood abuse, neglect, and household dysfunction and the risk of illicit drug use: The adverse childhood experiences study. *Pediatrics, 111*(3), 564–572.

Dugas, E., Low, N. C., Rodriguez, D., Burrows, S., Contreras, G., Chaiton, M., & O'Loughlin, J. (2012). Early predictors of suicidal ideation in young adults. *The Canadian Journal of Psychiatry / La Revue canadienne de psychiatrie, 57*(7), 429–436.

Durlak, J. A., Weissberg, R. P., Dymnicki, A. B., Taylor, R. D., & Schellinger, K. B. (2011). The impact of enhancing students' social and emotional learning: A meta-analysis of school-based universalinterventions.*ChildDevelopment,82*(1),405–432.doi:10.1111/j.1467-8624.2010.01564.x.

Editorial. (2015). Backing away from zero tolerance *The New York Times*. Retrieved from http://www.nytimes.com/2015/03/26/opinion/backing-away-from-zero-tolerance.html.

Embry, D. D. (2002). The good behavior game: A best practice candidate as a universal behavioral vaccine. *Clinical Child and Family Psychology Review, 5*(4), 273–297.

Essex, M. J., Kraemer, H. C., Armstrong, J. M., Boyce, W., Goldsmith, H., Klein, M. H., … Kupfer, D. J. (2006). Exploring risk factors for the emergence of children's mental health problems. *Archives of General Psychiatry, 63*(11), 1246-1256.

Eyberg, S. M., Nelson, M. M., & Boggs, S. R. (2008). Evidence-based psychosocial treatments for children and adolescents with disruptive behavior. *Journal of Clinical Child and Adolescent Psychology, 37*(1), 215–237.

Fabelo, T., Thompson, M., Plotkin, M., Carmichael, D., Marchbanks, M. & Booth, E. (2011). *Breaking school rules: A statewide study of how school discipline relates to students' success and juvenile justice involvement* (pp. 124): Justice Center: Council of State Governments & Public Policy Research Institute

Fatori, D., Bordin, I. A., Curto, B. M., & de Paula, C. S. (2013). Influence of psychosocial risk factors on the trajectory of mental health problems from childhood to adolescence: A longitudinal study. *BMC Psychiatry, 13*, 31. doi:10.1186/1471-244X-13-31.

Felitti, V. J. (2009). Adverse childhood experiences and adult health. *Academic Pediatrics, 9*(3), 131–132. doi:10.1016/j.acap.2009.03.001.

Felitti, V. J., Anda, R. F., Nordenberg, D., Williamson, D. F., Spitz, A. M., Edwards, V., … Marks, J. S. (1998). Relationship of childhood abuse and household dysfunction to many of the leading causes of death in adults. The Adverse Childhood Experiences (ACE) Study. *American Journal of Preventive Medicine, 14*(4), 245-258.

Fergusson, D. M., & Horwood, L. J. (2003). Resilience to childhood adversity: Results of a 12-year study. In S. S. Luthar (Ed.), *Resilience and vulnerability: Adaptation in the context of childhood adversities* (pp. 130–155). New York, NY: Cambridge University Press.

Fergusson, D. M., & Lynskey, M. T. (1996). Adolescent resiliency to family adversity. *Child Psychology & Psychiatry & Allied Disciplines, 37*(3), 281–292.

Forehand, R., Wierson, M., Thomas, A. M., Armistead, L., Kempton, T., & Neighbors, B. (1991). The role of family stressors and parent relationships on adolescent functioning. *Journal of the American Academy of Child & Adolescent Psychiatry, 30*(2), 316–322.

Foster, E., Prinz, R. J., Sanders, M. R., & Shapiro, C. J. (2008). The costs of a public health infrastructure for delivering parenting and family support. *Children and Youth Services Review, 30*(5), 493–501.

Gaskill, R. L., & Perry, B. D. (2012). *Child sexual abuse, traumatic experiences, and their impact on the developing brain Handbook of child sexual abuse: Identification, assessment, and treatment* (pp. 29–47). Hoboken, NJ: Wiley.

Grasso, D., Greene, C., & Ford, J. D. (2013). Cumulative trauma in childhood. In J. D. Julian & C. A. Christine (Eds.), *Treating complex traumatic stress disorders in children and adolescents: Scientific foundations and therapeutic models* (pp. 79–99). New York, NY: Guilford Press.

Greenberg, M. T., Weissberg, R. P., O'Brien, M. U., Zins, J. E., Fredericks, L., Resnik, H., & Elias, M. J. (2003). Enhancing school-based prevention and youth development through coordinated social, emotional, and academic learning. *American Psychologist, 58*(6–7), 466–474.

Greene, R. W. (2010). Collaborative problem solving. In R. C. Murrihy (Ed.), *Clinical handbook of assessing and treating conduct problems in youth* (pp. 193–220). New York, NY: Springer Science + Business Media.

Greeson, J. K., Briggs, E. C., Layne, C. M., Belcher, H. M., Ostrowski, S. A., Kim, S., … Fairbank, J. A. (2014). Traumatic childhood experiences in the 21st century: Broadening and building on the ACE studies with data from the National Child Traumatic Stress Network. *Journal of Interpersonal Violence, 29*(3), 536-556. doi:10.1177/0886260513505217

Gregory, A., Skiba, R. J., & Noguera, P. A. (2010). The achievement gap and the discipline gap: Two sides of the same coin? *Educational Researcher, 39*(1), 59–68.

Guarino, K., Soares, P., Konnath, K., Clervil, R., & Bassuk, E. (2009). Trauma-Informed Organizational Toolkit (pp. 1-96). Retrieved from www.familyhomelessness.org/media/90.pdf.

Harper, G. (2012). Child and adolescent mental health policy. In J. M. Rey (Ed.), *IACAPAP textbook of child and adolescent mental health*. Geneva, Switzerland: IACAPAP. Retrieved from http://iacapap.org/iacapap-textbook-of-child-and-adolescent-mental-health.

Hoagwood, K. E., Olin, S., Kerker, B. D., Kratochwill, T. R., Crowe, M., & Saka, N. (2007). Empirically based school interventions targeted at academic and mental health functioning. *Journal of Emotional and Behavioral Disorders, 15*(2), 66–92.

Hodgdon, H. B., Kinniburgh, K., Gabowitz, D., Blaustein, M. E., & Spinazzola, J. (2013). Development and implementation of trauma-informed programming in youth residential treatment centers using the ARC framework. *Journal of Family Violence, 28*(7), 679–692.

Horner, R. H., & Sugai, G. (2015). School-wide PBIS: An example of applied behavior analysis implemented at a scale of social importance. *Behavior Analysis in Practice, 8*(1), 80–85.

Horowitz, J. L., Garber, J., Ciesla, J. A., Young, J. F., & Mufson, L. (2007). Prevention of depressive symptoms in adolescents: A randomized trial of cognitive-behavioral and interpersonal prevention programs. *Journal of Consulting and Clinical Psychology, 75*(5), 693–706.

Jenkins, J. M., & Smith, M. A. (1990). Factors protecting children living in disharmonious homes: Maternal reports. *Journal of the American Academy of Child & Adolescent Psychiatry, 29*(1), 60–69.

Jensen, P. S., Goldman, E., Offord, D., Costello, E. J., Friedman, R., Huff, B., … Roberts, R. (2011). Overlooked and underserved: "action signs" for identifying children with unmet mental health needs. *Pediatrics, 128*(5), 970–979. doi:10.1542/peds.2009-0367

Johnson, S. B., Riley, A. W., Granger, D. A., & Riis, J. (2013). The science of early life toxic stress for pediatric practice and advocacy. *Pediatrics, 131*(2), 319–327.

Kataoka, S. H., Zhang, L., & Wells, K. B. (2002). Unmet need for mental health care among U.S. children: variation by ethnicity and insurance status. *Am J Psychiatry, 159*(9), 1548–1555. doi:10.1176/appi.ajp.159.9.1548

Kellam, S. G., Hendricks Brown, C., Poduska, J. M., Ialongo, N. S., Wang, W., Toyinbo, P., … Wilcox, H. C. (2008). Effects of a universal classroom behavior management program in first and second grades on young adult behavioral, psychiatric, and social outcomes. *Drug and Alcohol Dependence, 95*(Suppl 1), S5-S28.

KewelRamani, A., Gilbertson, L., Fox, M., & Provasnik, S. (2007). *Status and trends in the education of racial and ethnic minorities (NCES 2007-039)*. Washington, DC: National Center for Educational Statistics, Institute of Education Sciences, U.S. Department of Education.

Kieling, C., Baker-Henningham, H., Belfer, M., Conti, G., Ertem, I., Omigbodun, O., … Rahman, A. (2011). Child and adolescent mental health worldwide: Evidence for action. *Lancet, 378*(9801), 1515-1525. doi:10.1016/S0140-6736(11)60827-1

Kleinman, K. E., & Saigh, P. A. (2011). The effects of the good behavior game on the conduct of regular education New York City high school students. *Behavior Modification, 35*(1), 95–105.

Kutcher, S., & Wei, Y. (2013). Challenges and solutions in the implementation of the School-Based Pathway to Care Model: The lessons from Nova Scotia and beyond. *Canadian Journal of School Psychology, 28*(1), 90–102.

Lamborn, S. D., Mounts, N. S., Steinberg, L., & Dornbusch, S. M. (1991). Patterns of competence and adjustment among adolescents from authoritative, authoritarian, indulgent, and neglectful families. *Child Development, 62*(5), 1049–1065.

Lannie, A. L., & McCurdy, B. L. (2007). Preventing disruptive behavior in the urban classroom: Effects of the Good Behavior Game on student and teacher behavior. *Education & Treatment of Children, 30*(1), 85–98.

Layne, C. M., Beck, C. J., Rimmasch, H., Southwick, J. S., Moreno, M. A., & Hobfoll, S. E. (2009). Promoting "resilient" posttraumatic adjustment in childhood and beyond: "unpacking" life events, adjustment trajectories, resources, and interventions. In D. Brom, R. Pat-Horenczyk, & D. Julian Ford (Eds.), *Treating traumatized children: Risk, resilience and recovery* (pp. 13–47). New York, NY: Routledge.

Layne, C. M., Briggs, E. C., & Courtois, C. A. (2014). Introduction to the special section: Using the trauma history profile to unpack risk factor caravans and their consequences. *Psychological Trauma: Theory, Research, Practice, and Policy, 6*(Suppl 1), S1–S8.

Layne, C. M., Greeson, J. K., Ostrowski, S. A., Kim, S., Reading, S., Vivrette, R. L., … Pynoos, R. S. (2014). Cumulative trauma exposure and high risk behavior in adolescence: Findings from the National Child Traumatic Stress Network Core Data Set. *Psychological Trauma: Theory, Research, Practice, and Policy, 6*(Suppl 1), S40-S49.

Lester, B. M., Marsit, C. J., & Bromer, C. (2014). *Behavioral epigenetics and the developmental origins of child mental health disorders Infant and early childhood mental health: Core concepts and clinical practice* (pp. 161–173). Arlington, VA: American Psychiatric Publishing.

Levy, K. N., Meehan, K. B., & Temes, C. M. (2014). Attachment theory and personality disorders. In A. N. Danquah & B. Katherine (Eds.), *Attachment theory in adult mental health: A guide to clinical practice* (pp. 95–112). New York, NY: Routledge.

Lowell, D. I., Carter, A. S., Godoy, L., Paulicin, B., & Briggs-Gowan, M. J. (2011). A randomized controlled trial of Child FIRST: A comprehensive home-based intervention translating research into early childhood practice. *Child Development, 82*(1), 193–208.

Luby, J., Belden, A., Botteron, K., Marrus, N., Harms, M. P., Babb, C., … Barch, D. (2013). The effects of poverty on childhood brain development: The mediating effect of caregiving and stressful life events. *JAMA Pediatrics, 167*(12), 1135-1142. doi:10.1001/jamapediatrics.2013.3139

Luthar, S. S., & Zelazo, L. B. (2003). Research on resilience: An integrative review. In S. S. Luthar (Ed.), *Resilience and vulnerability: Adaptation in the context of childhood adversities* (pp. 510–549). New York, NY: Cambridge University Press.

Lyon, A. R., Gershenson, R. A., Farahmand, F. K., Thaxter, P. J., Behling, S., & Budd, K. S. (2009). Effectiveness of Teacher-Child Interaction Training (TCIT) in a preschool setting. *Behavior Modification, 33*(6), 855–884. doi:10.1177/0145445509344215.

Masten, A. S., Best, K. M., & Garmezy, N. (1990). Resilience and development: Contributions from the study of children who overcome adversity. *Development and Psychopathology, 2*(4), 425–444.

Masten, A. S., & Coatsworth, J. (1998). The development of competence in favorable and unfavorable environments: Lessons from research on successful children. *American Psychologist, 53*(2), 205–220.

Masten, A. S., & Powell, J. L. (2003). *A resilience framework for research, policy, and practice Resilience and vulnerability: Adaptation in the context of childhood adversities* (pp. 1–25). New York, NY: Cambridge University Press.

Mazza, J. J., Fleming, C. B., Abbott, R. D., Haggerty, K. P., & Catalano, R. F. (2010). Identifying trajectories of adolescents' depressive phenomena: An examination of early risk factors. *Journal of Youth and Adolescence, 39*(6), 579–593.

McCurdy, B. L., Lannie, A. L., & Barnabas, E. (2009). Reducing disruptive behavior in an urban school cafeteria: An extension of the Good Behavior Game. *Journal of School Psychology, 47*(1), 39–54.

Medland, M. B., & Stachnik, T. J. (1972). Good-behavior game: A replication and systematic analysis. *Journal of Applied Behavior Analysis, 5*(1), 45–51.

Merikangas, K. R., He, J. P., Burstein, M., Swanson, S. A., Avenevoli, S., Cui, L., … Swendsen, J. (2010). Lifetime prevalence of mental disorders in U.S. adolescents: Results from the

National Comorbidity Survey Replication--Adolescent Supplement (NCS-A). *Journal of the American Academy of Child and Adolescent Psychiatry, 49*(10), 980-989. doi:10.1016/j.jaac.2010.05.017

Milot, T., St-Laurent, D., & Ethier, L. S. (2015). Intervening with severely and chronically neglected children and their families: The contribution of trauma-informed approaches. *Child Abuse Review.* doi:10.1002/car.2376.

Nemeroff, C. B., & Binder, E. (2014). The preeminent role of childhood abuse and neglect in vulnerability to major psychiatric disorders: Toward elucidating the underlying neurobiological mechanisms. *Journal of the American Academy of Child and Adolescent Psychiatry, 53*(4), 395–397. doi:10.1016/j.jaac.2014.02.004.

Nock, M. K., Green, J. G., Hwang, I., McLaughlin, K. A., Sampson, N. A., Zaslavsky, A. M., & Kessler, R. C. (2013). Prevalence, correlates, and treatment of lifetime suicidal behavior among adolescents: results from the National Comorbidity Survey Replication Adolescent Supplement. *JAMA Psychiatry, 70*(3), 300–310. doi:10.1001/2013.jamapsychiatry.55.

Nurse-Family Partnership. (2014). *Social programs that work.* Retrieved April 26, 2015, from http://evidencebasedprograms.org/1366-2/nurse-family-partnership.

OSEP. (2015). *Positive behavioral intervention and supports.* Retrieved April 23, 2015, from https://www.pbis.org/.

Perou, R., Bitsko, R.H., Blumberg, S.J., Pastor, P., Ghandour, R. M., Gfroerer, J.C., ... Centers for Disease Control and Prevention (CDC). (2013). Mental Health Surveillance Among Children—United States. *Morbidity and Mortality Weekly Report Supplement,* 17, 62(2):1–35.

Perry, B. D. (2008). Child maltreatment: A neurodevelopmental perspective on the role of trauma and neglect in psychopathology. In T. P. Beauchaine & S. P. Hinshaw (Eds.), *Child and adolescent psychopathology* (pp. 93–128). Hoboken, NJ: Wiley.

Perry, B. D. (2009). Examining child maltreatment through a neurodevelopmental lens: Clinical applications of the neurosequential model of therapeutics. *Journal of Loss and Trauma, 14*(4), 240–255.

Press, A. (2014). *Controversy plagues school mental health screening.* The New York Times, Retrieved from http://www.nytimes.com/aponline/2014/01/13/us/ap-us-school-mental-health--screenings.html.

Prinz, R. J., Sanders, M. R., Shapiro, C. J., Whitaker, D. J., & Lutzker, J. R. (2009). Population-based prevention of child maltreatment: The U.S. triple P system population trial. *Prevention Science, 10*(1), 1–12.

Raffaele Mendez, L. M., & Knoff, H. M. (2003). Who gets suspended from school and why: A demographic analysis of schools and disciplinary infractions in a large school district. *Education & Treatment of Children, 26*(1), 30–51.

Rones, M., & Hoagwood, K. (2000). School-based mental health services: A research review. *Clinical Child and Family Psychology Review, 3*(4), 223–241.

Roth, T. L. (2013). Epigenetic mechanisms in the development of behavior: Advances, challenges, and future promises of a new field. *Development and Psychopathology, 25*(4 Pt 2), 1279–1291.

Rumberger, R. W., & Rotermund, S. (2012). The relationship between engagement and high school dropout. In S. L. Christenson, A. L. Reschly, & C. Wylie (Eds.), *Handbook of research on student engagement* (pp. 491–513). New York, NY: Springer Science + Business Media.

Saigh, P. A. (1987). The effects of an academic good behavior game on the spelling achievement of limited English proficiency students. *British Columbia Journal of Special Education, 11*, 73–80.

SAMHSA. (2014). Trauma-Informed Care in Behavioral Health Services. *Treatment Improvement Protocol (TIP) Series 57.* Retrieved from http://www.integration.samhsa.gov/clinical-practice/SAMSA_TIP_Trauma.pdf.

SAMHSA. (2015a). "Now is the Time" Project AWARE Local Educational Agency Grants. Retrieved June 13, 2015, from http://www.samhsa.gov/grants/grant-announcements/sm-14-019

SAMHSA. (2015b). "Now is the Time" Project AWARE-Community Grants. Retrieved June 13, 2015, from http://www.samhsa.gov/grants/grant-announcements/sm-15-012

Savitz, J., van der Merwe, L., Stein, D. J., Solms, M., & Ramesar, R. (2007). Genotype and child-hood sexual trauma moderate neurocognitive performance: A possible role for brain-derived neurotrophic factor and apolipoprotein E variants. *Biological Psychiatry, 62*(5), 391–399. doi:10.1016/j.biopsych.2006.10.017.

Saxe, G., & Brown, A. (2012). Treating traumatic stress in children and adolescents. *Adolescent Psychiatry, 2*(4), 313–322.

School Mental Health Project. (2015). Retrieved May 4, 2015, from http://smhp.psych.ucla.edu/

Minnesota Department of Human Services. (2014). Great Start Minnesota: Early Childhood Mental Health System. Retrieved May 3, 2015, from http://www.dhs.state.mn.us/main/idcplg?IdcService=GET_DYNAMIC_CONVERSION&RevisionSelectionMethod=LatestReleased&dDocName=dhs16_149100

Skiba, R. J., Michael, R. S., Nardo, A. C., & Peterson, R. L. (2002). The color of discipline: Sources of racial and gender disproportionality in school punishment. *The Urban Review, 34*(4), 317–342.

Small Changes, Big Differences. (2015). Retrieved from http://www.triplep.net/glo-en/home/

Sourander, A., Niemela, S., Santalahti, P., Helenius, H., & Piha, J. (2008). Changes in psychiatric problems and service use among 8-year-old children: A 16-year population-based time-trend study. *Journal of the American Academy of Child and Adolescent Psychiatry, 47*(3), 317–327. doi:10.1097/CHI.0b013e318160b98f.

Stephan, S. H., Sugai, G., Lever, N., & Connors, E. (2015). Strategies for integrating mental health into schools via a multitiered system of support. *Child and Adolescent Psychiatric Clinics of North America, 24*(2), 211–231.

Sugai, G., Sprague, J. R., Horner, R. H., & Walker, H. M. (2000). Preventing school violence: The use of office discipline referrals to assess and monitor school-wide discipline interventions. *Journal of Emotional and Behavioral Disorders, 8*(2), 94–101.

Thomas, R., & Zimmer-Gembeck, M. J. (2007). Behavioral outcomes of parent-child interaction therapy and triple P-positive parenting program: A review and meta-analysis. *Journal of Abnormal Child Psychology, 35*(3), 475–495.

Twenge, J. M., Gentile, B., DeWall, C. N., Ma, D., Lacefield, K., & Schurtz, D. R. (2010). Birth cohort increases in psychopathology among young Americans, 1938-2007: A cross-temporal meta-analysis of the MMPI. *Clinical Psychology Review, 30*(2), 145–154. doi:10.1016/j.cpr.2009.10.005.

Wade, R., Jr., Shea, J. A., Rubin, D., & Wood, J. (2014). Adverse childhood experiences of low-income urban youth. *Pediatrics, 134*(1), e13–e20. doi:10.1542/peds.2013-2475.

Walkley, M., & Cox, T. L. (2013). Building trauma-informed schools and communities. *Children & Schools, 35*(2), 123–126.

Webster-Stratton, C., Reid, M., & Stoolmiller, M. (2008). Preventing conduct problems and improving school readiness: Evaluation of the Incredible Years teacher and child training programs in high-risk schools. *Journal of Child Psychology and Psychiatry, 49*(5), 471–488.

Webster-Stratton, C., & Reid, M. J. (2003). *The incredible years parents, teachers and children training series: A multifaceted treatment approach for young children with conduct problems Evidence-based psychotherapies for children and adolescents* (pp. 224–240). New York, NY: Guilford Press.

Weder, N., Zhang, H., Jensen, K., Yang, B. Z., Simen, A., Jackowski, A., … Kaufman, J. (2014). Child abuse, depression, and methylation in genes involved with stress, neural plasticity, and brain circuitry. *Journal of the American Academy of Child & Adolescent Psychiatry, 53*(4), 417-424.

Weist, M. D. (1997). Expanded school mental health services: A national movement in progress. *Advances in Clinical Child Psychology, 19*, 319–352.

Weist, M. D., & Paternite, C. E. (2006). Building an interconnected policy-training-practice-research agenda to advance school mental health. *Education & Treatment of Children, 29*(2), 173–196.

Weisz, J. R., Sandler, I. N., Durlak, J. A., & Anton, B. S. (2005). Promoting and protecting youth mental health through evidence-based prevention and treatment. *American Psychologist, 60*(6), 628–648.

Wille, N., Bettge, S., Ravens-Sieberer, U., & BELLA Study Group. (2008). Risk and protective factors for children's and adolescents' mental health: Results of the BELLA study. *European Child and Adolescent Psychiatry, 17*(Suppl 1), 133–147. doi:10.1007/s00787-008-1015-y.

Wilson, D. B., Gottfredson, D. C., & Najaka, S. S. (2001). School-based prevention of problem behaviors: A meta-analysis. *Journal of Quantitative Criminology, 17*(3), 247–272.

Wolfe, D. A., & Mash, E. J. (2006). *Behavioral and emotional disorders in adolescents: Nature, assessment, and treatment* (Vol. xvi, p. 719). New York, NY: Guilford Publications.

Wu, P., Katic, B. J., Liu, X., Fan, B., & Fuller, C. J. (2010). Mental health service use among suicidal adolescents: Findings from a U.S. National community survey. *Psychiatric Services, 61*, 17–24.

Yates, T. M., Egeland, B., & Sroufe, L. A. (2003). *Rethinking resilience: A developmental process perspective Resilience and vulnerability: Adaptation in the context of childhood adversities* (pp. 243–266). New York, NY: Cambridge University Press.

Yoshikawa, H., Aber, J. L., & Beardslee, W. R. (2012). The effects of poverty on the mental, emotional, and behavioral health of children and youth: Implications for prevention. *American Psychologist, 67*(4), 272–284. doi:10.1037/a0028015.

Young, J. F., Kranzler, A., Gallop, R., & Mufson, L. (2012). Interpersonal psychotherapy-adolescent skills training: Effects on school and social functioning. *School Mental Health, 4*(4), 254–264.

Young, J. F., Makover, H. B., Cohen, J. R., Mufson, L., Gallop, R. J., & Benas, J. S. (2012). Interpersonal psychotherapy-adolescent skills training: Anxiety outcomes and impact of comorbidity. *Journal of Clinical Child and Adolescent Psychology, 41*(5), 640–653.

Young, J. F., & Mufson, L. (2003). *Manual for Interpersonal Psychotherapy-Adolescent Skills Training (IPT-AST)*. New York, NY: Columbia University.

Young, J. F., Mufson, L., & Davies, M. (2006). Impact of comorbid anxiety in an effectiveness study of interpersonal psychotherapy for depressed adolescents. *Journal of the American Academy of Child & Adolescent Psychiatry, 45*(8), 904–912.

Young, J. F., Mufson, L., & Gallop, R. (2010). Preventing depression: A randomized trial of interpersonal psychotherapy-adolescent skills training. *Depression and Anxiety, 27*(5), 426–433.

Zuckerbrot, R. A., & Steinbaum, D. (2012). *Assessment and diagnosis: Depression instruments and interviews, identifying comorbid conditions managing adolescent depression: The complete guide for primary care clinicians* (pp. 1–20). Kingston, NJ: Civic Research Institute.

Chapter 7
Youth Suicide

**Adam G. Horwitz, Kiel J. Opperman, Amanda Burnside,
Neera Ghaziuddin, and Cheryl A. King**

7.1 Introduction

Adolescent death by suicide is a largely preventable tragedy that affects countless families and communities across the globe. While many causes of death for young people (e.g., influenza, pneumonia) have been reduced with improved medical care over the past generations, suicide is now the second leading cause of death among adolescents aged 12–17 in the United States, accounting for over 10,000 deaths between 2000 and 2010. Additionally, adolescence is characterized by drastic

A.G. Horwitz, M.S.
Department of Psychology, University of Michigan,
530 Church Street, Ann Arbor, MI 48109, USA
e-mail: ahor@umich.edu

K.J. Opperman
Department of Psychology, Wayne State University,
5057 Woodward Avenue, 7th Floor, Detroit, MI 48202, USA
e-mail: kiel.opperman@wayne.edu

A. Burnside
Department of Psychology, Loyola University Chicago,
1000 W Sheridan Road, Chicago, IL 60626, USA
e-mail: aburnside@luc.edu

N. Ghaziuddin, M.D. • C.A. King, Ph.D. (✉)
Department of Psychiatry, University of Michigan,
4250 Plymouth Road, Ann Arbor, MI 48105, USA
e-mail: neeraj@umich.edu; kingca@umich.edu

© Springer Science+Business Media New York 2016   125
M.R. Korin (ed.), *Health Promotion for Children and Adolescents*,
DOI 10.1007/978-1-4899-7711-3_7

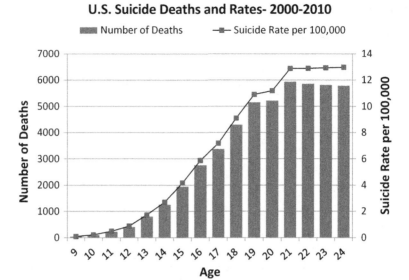

Fig. 7.1 Suicide deaths and rates by age in the United States

increases in the rate of suicide, which eventually level off in early adulthood (see Fig. 7.1; CDC, 2013). In addition to suicide deaths, public health problems are posed by suicidal ideation (i.e., thoughts), suicidal plans, and nonfatal suicide attempts. The rates of suicidal thoughts and behaviors are quite alarming, as according to a nationally representative sample of American high school students, in the past year, 16 % of high school students had serious thoughts of suicide, 13 % made a suicidal plan, 8 % made a suicide attempt, and 2 % made a suicide attempt that necessitated medical attention (CDC, 2012).

Despite these rates of suicidal ideation and suicide attempts, actual death by suicide remains a rare occurrence (3.76 deaths per 100,000 individuals) for this 12–17 age group (CDC, 2013), making death by suicide very difficult to predict. A number of risk and protective factors for suicidal ideation and behavior have been identified across different domains (e.g., demographic, psychological, social/interpersonal) that have allowed researchers and clinicians to identify youth who might be at risk for suicide. This chapter will describe some of these risk and protective factors and provide an overview of the different treatments and interventions that have been developed at global and targeted levels.

7.2   Risk Factors

7.2.1   Demographic

7.2.1.1   Gender

Although death by suicide is hard to predict, a number of risk factors across a variety of domains (e.g., demographic, psychological, social/interpersonal) have emerged as significant predictors of suicidal thoughts and behaviors. With regard to demographic data in the United States, adolescent males (12–17) are nearly three times more likely to die by suicide than females (CDC, 2013). Yet, among high school students, females are more likely to endorse serious thoughts of suicide making a suicidal plan, making a suicide attempt, and making a suicide attempt requiring medical attention (3 % vs. 2 %; CDC, 2012). The disparity between the greater rates of suicidal thoughts and suicide attempts by females and the greater number of suicide deaths by males has been referred to as the "gender paradox" of suicide (Canetto & Sakinofsky, 1998). This paradox can be partially explained by the method used in a suicide attempt. For example, adolescent male suicide deaths are more likely a result of a firearm; female suicides are more often a result of suffocation/hanging. Additionally, females are more likely than males to die by a poisoning/overdose suicide attempt, despite only 2 % of these attempts resulting in death (see Table 7.1). Taken together, females attempt suicide more often than males by less lethal means (e.g., Beautrais, 2003) and thus die by suicide at a lower rate.

7.2.1.2   Race/Ethnicity

Racial and ethnic factors have also been examined with regard to risk for suicide. In the United States, Alaska Natives and American Indians have the highest rates of suicide, followed by Caucasians, Asians/Pacific Islanders, and Blacks/African-Americans. Those identifying as Hispanic have a slightly lower rate of suicide than non-Hispanics (see Table 7.2). The rates of suicide are likely amplified for Alaska Natives and American Indians due to a greater proportion of adolescents living in

Table 7.1 Suicide attempt methods and fatality rates

	Fatal suicide attempts: method used		Fatality rate of method
	Males (%)	Females (%)	(%)
Firearm	47.0	25.0	85.0
Suffocation/hanging	44.5	57.3	69.2
Poisoning/overdose	3.7	11.8	2.4

Data represents fatal suicide attempts of adolescents in the United States from 2000 to 2010 (CDC, 2013); fatality rate data are based on 2001 US data from Vyrostek et al. (2004)

Table 7.2 Suicide rates by race/ethnicity

Race/Ethnicity	Crude rate for suicide (per 100,000)
Alaska Native/American Indian	8.90
White/Caucasian	4.08
Asian/Pacific Islander	2.31
African-American/Black	2.19
Hispanic/Latino	2.69

Data represents completed suicides of youth (12–17) in the United States from 2000 to 2010 (CDC, 2013)

rural or isolated areas, limited employment and educational opportunities, and higher rates of alcohol/substance abuse (Goldston et al., 2008). Despite African-Americans and Blacks having the lowest rate of suicide by race, the rate of suicide attempts among African-American and Black adolescent males doubled between 1991 and 2001 (Joe & Marcus, 2003). Although there are differing rates of suicide across race and ethnicity, there are many variables that correspond to greater suicide risk for individuals across race and ethnicity, in addition to unique factors that warrant special consideration based on cultural, racial, and ethnic differences.

7.2.2 Psychological/Psychiatric

7.2.2.1 Past Suicidal Thoughts, Suicide Attempts, and Non-suicidal Self-Injury

Suicidal ideation is a primary risk factor for adolescent future suicide attempts (e.g., Lewinsohn, Rohde, & Seeley, 1994) and death by suicide (e.g., Brent et al., 1993). Furthermore, there is an incremental association between the severity of suicidal thoughts, characterized by the absence/presence of a method, plan, or intent to act, and risk for future suicide attempts (e.g., Horwitz, Czyz, & King 2015). However, while the vast majority of suicide attempters experience suicidal ideation, there are many adolescents with suicidal ideation that do not go on to make suicide attempts (King et al. 2014; Lewinsohn, Rohde, & Seeley, 1996). In addition to suicidal thoughts, self-injurious behaviors (both suicidal and non-suicidal) are associated with an increased risk for suicide. While those with intent to die during self-injury are more likely to sustain lethal injuries and die by suicide (e.g., Nock & Kessler, 2006), even adolescents with no suicidal intent during self-injury are at an increased risk for making suicide attempts, particularly if the self-injury occurs over a long period of time and is done with a variety of methods (Nock, Joiner, Gordon, Lloyd-Richardson, & Prinstein, 2006). However, the strongest behavioral indicator of a future suicide attempt is a previous suicide attempt (e.g., Brent, Baugher, Bridge, Chen, & Chiappetta, 1999; Lewinsohn et al., 1996). Furthermore, adolescents who have made multiple past attempts are significantly more likely to make a future attempt in comparison to adolescents with one past attempt or only suicidal ideation (e.g., Miranda et al., 2008). Of particular importance, suicide attempts in adolescence carry a long-term risk. In a large longitudinal birth cohort study, those who made a suicide attempt prior to age 18 were 18 times more likely to make a suicide attempt between the ages of 18–25 (Fergusson, Horwood, Ridder, & Beautrais, 2005).

7.2.2.2   Psychiatric Disorders

Carrying a psychiatric diagnosis, while common, is another predictor of suicidal behavior. Psychological autopsy studies have indicated that approximately 80–90 % of adolescents who die by suicide suffer from significant psychopathology (e.g., Brent et al., 1993). Many studies have identified mood disorders (e.g., major depressive disorder, bipolar disorder), disruptive disorders (e.g., attention deficit hyperactivity disorder, conduct disorder), substance use disorders, and anxiety disorders (e.g., generalized anxiety disorder, panic disorder) as psychiatric diagnoses associated with an increased risk of suicide attempts (e.g., Goldston et al., 2009; Lewinsohn et al., 1996; Nock & Kessler, 2006). Shaffer et al. (1996) conducted a case-control psychological autopsy study with the families of 120 adolescents who died by suicide and concluded that mood disorders alone or in combination with conduct disorder or substance abuse characterize the majority of adolescent suicides. Similarly, studies have found that the presence of more than one disorder is associated with an even greater risk for suicide (e.g., Lewinsohn et al., 1996).

7.2.2.3   Alcohol and Other Substance Abuses

Even without a psychiatric diagnosis of a substance use disorder, any use of illegal substances is associated with an increased risk for suicidal behavior. In a longitudinal study, cannabis use in adolescence was associated with later suicidal ideation and suicide attempts, with users being three times more likely to attempt suicide than nonusers (Pedersen, 2008). The use of alcohol in adolescents is also strongly associated with suicidal ideation and attempts. Swahn and Bossarte (2007) found that those reporting preteen alcohol use were at the greatest risk for suicidal ideation and suicide attempts, while those who first drank after the age of 13 were still more likely than nondrinking teens to report suicidal ideation or a suicide attempt. Additionally, in a study by Schilling, Aseltine, Glanovsky, James, and Jacobs (2009), drinking alcohol while feeling down was associated with a significantly greater risk of a future suicide attempt among adolescents not reporting suicidal ideation in the past year. The negative consequences associated with alcohol use are both long term (e.g., depressogenic effects, promotion of adverse life events) and immediate, as active intoxication (e.g., negative effect, impaired thinking, reduced inhibition) can serve as a precipitating influence for a suicide attempt (Brady, 2006).

7.2.3 Social/Interpersonal

7.2.3.1 History of Trauma/Abuse

Physical and sexual abuse in childhood/adolescence is a strong predictor of suicidal behavior. In a longitudinal community study, Silverman, Reinherz, and Giaconia (1996) reported that compared to non-abused children, those who were either physically or sexually abused had significant impairments in functioning at ages 15 and 21 with greater rates of suicidal ideation and suicide attempts. Similarly, adolescents reporting physical abuse were two times more likely to report suicidal ideation, three times more likely to have made a suicidal plan, five times more likely to have made a noninjurious suicide attempt, and 11 times more likely to have made an injurious suicide attempt (Bensley, Van Eeenwyk, Spieker, & Schoder, 1999). Furthermore, those who reported a history of both physical abuse and sexual abuse/molestation were significantly more likely to report suicidal behaviors than those reporting either nonsexual abuse or molestation alone.

7.2.3.2 Bullying/Victimization

Bullying behaviors are prevalent in the United States, as a study examining a representative sample of adolescents in grades 6–10 found that roughly 30 % of adolescents are involved with bullying — 13 % were categorized as a bully, 11 % were categorized as being a victim, and 6 % were categorized as both bullying others and being a victim of bullying (Nansel et al., 2001). Involvement with bullying, whether as a victim or perpetrator, is associated with an increased risk for suicidal thoughts and behavior (e.g., Kaminski & Fang, 2009; Nickerson & Slater, 2009). Klomek, Marrocco, Kleinman, Schonfeld, and Gould (2008) found that high school students who reported experiencing frequent peer victimization were more prone to suicidal thoughts and attempts compared to non-victimized students. While much attention is typically paid to the victims of bullying, the perpetrators also report more suicidal ideation and suicidal behaviors (e.g., Kaltiala-Heino, Rimpelä, Marttunen, Rimpelä, & Rantanen, 1999; Winsper, Lereya, Zanarini, & Wolke, 2012). Moreover, those who report being both a victim and perpetrator of bullying, often referred to as "bully victims," are at the greatest risk. For instance, a recent study of 130,908 adolescent students indicated 22 % of bully perpetrators, 29 % of victims of bullying, and 38 % of those who both bully others and are victims of bullying report suicidal thoughts or a suicide attempt in the past year (Borowsky, Taliaferro, & McMorris, 2013), highlighting the associated risk of involvement with bullying in any form.

7.2.3.3   Exposure to Suicide

Exposure to suicide, whether via peer, family member, acquaintance, or even in the media, is associated with an increased risk for suicide among adolescents. A large Canadian study tracked adolescents and found that having a classmate die by suicide and/or personally knowing someone who died by suicide was associated with increased risks of suicidal thoughts and suicide attempts, particularly for those in early adolescence (Swanson & Colman, 2013). Furthermore, entertainment/political celebrity suicides have a particularly strong influence for a copycat effect, as real-life suicides are four times more likely to produce a copycat effect as compared to fictional stories (Stack, 2000). However, it is important to note that the threat posed by fictional depictions of suicide also carries influence in suicide risk, as was evidenced by a 17% increase in self-poisonings in England emergency departments during the week following a depicted overdose on a popular show (Hawton et al., 1999).

7.3   Protective Factors

7.3.1   Social Connectedness

Durkheim (1897) introduced the study of the relationship between suicide and social connectedness over a century ago with his social integration theory, stating that individuals who are more connected through social groups and structures are less likely to die by suicide. This theory has been substantiated by research on the protective effects of social connectedness against suicidal behavior, yet for adolescents, different types of social connectedness (e.g., family, school, peer) yield distinct protective capacities (King & Merchant, 2008). For instance, a study by Kaminski, Puddy, Hall, Cashman, Crosby, and Ortega (2010) indicated that family and school connectedness reduced the risk of suicidal thoughts and behavior, whereas peer connectedness had no association, despite other studies suggesting peer factors such as low levels of friendship support and peer rejection are associated with an increased risk for suicidal thoughts and behaviors (e.g., Prinstein, Boergers, Spirito, Little, & Grapentine, 2000). It may be that while the lack of peer connectedness is a clear risk factor for suicide, peer connectedness as a protective factor may be dependent upon the type of influence the peers have on the individual. Additionally, gender may have a role in the protective capabilities of peer connectedness, as Bearman and Moody (2004) found that girls, and not boys, were at increased risk for suicidal ideation if they were socially isolated from peers or had intransitive friendships.

7.3.2   Religiosity/Spirituality

Religiosity and spirituality have been identified and promoted as protective factors against suicidal ideation and behavior. However, there are many facets of religion and spirituality that may either explain or confound this protective effect, and research findings have been mixed. For instance, some studies have suggested a protective effect of public, but not private religiosity (e.g., Robins & Fiske, 2009), whereas others have identified private religiosity as a protective factor (e.g., Nonnemaker, McNeely, & Blum, 2003). A lack of consensus in the measurement of private versus public religiosity may be a factor in the discrepant results across studies. While increased social support via involvement in a religious group is a potential confounding variable, religious attendance has been linked with a decreased likelihood of a suicide attempt, even when controlling for levels of social support (Rasic et al., 2009). Religious and spiritual participation may serve a particularly protective function in adolescence, as a study by Nkansah-Amankra, Diedhiou, Agbanu, Agbanu, Opoku-Adomako, and Twumasi-Ankrah (2012) found that religious and spiritual activity participation was associated with reduced suicidal behaviors in adolescence, but less so in adulthood.

7.3.3   Coping Skills

The use of effective coping skills has also been identified as a significant protective factor against suicidal ideation and behavior. For example, Khurana and Romer (2012) found that the use of problem solving, emotional regulation, support seeking, and acceptance each independently predicted a reduction in suicidal ideation over a 1-year period. Furthermore, a study by Gould et al. (2004) indicated that high school students without serious suicidal thoughts or behavior were significantly more likely to endorse help-seeking coping and were less likely to endorse drugs and alcohol as coping strategies, in comparison to students endorsing suicidal thoughts or behavior. A number of studies examining suicidal adolescents have indicated that the development of improved coping and problem-solving skills has resulted in a reduced risk for future suicidal thoughts (e.g., Piquet & Wagner, 2003; Rudd et al., 1996). The modifiability of coping strategies, through appropriate social learning or modeling, and its effectiveness in reducing risk for suicidal ideation and behavior, has made coping/problem-solving skills training a key component to a number of psychological interventions and therapies.

7.4   Prevention/Intervention Strategies

Given the social and economic costs of suicide, a number of prevention and intervention strategies have been developed. The public health approach to suicide prevention often entails a population-based or universal focus, which aims to prevent the initial onset of suicidal behaviors. Such primary prevention strategies may include efforts to promote positive social relationships in the community, as well as reducing access to firearms or illegal substances. Other strategies, commonly referred to as selected prevention strategies (Gordon, 1983), intervene with groups of individuals that are known to be at elevated risk. These might include efforts to reduce risk in family survivors of suicide, adolescents who are victims of sexual trauma or peer bullying, or adolescents who have early signs of depression and alcohol abuse. Finally, indicated strategies or treatments are generally targeted at individuals who are at high risk or already engaging in suicidal behaviors. Taken together, universal, selected, and indicated prevention approaches form a comprehensive strategy for suicide prevention. A number of prevention/intervention strategies, both at the population and individual levels, are discussed.

7.4.1 Universal and Selected Prevention Strategies

7.4.1.1 Gatekeeper Training

Gatekeeper training is a public health approach to suicide prevention designed to educate community members to identify those at risk for suicide, respond appropriately, and refer for clinical services (Gould & Kramer, 2001). Gatekeepers include professionals such as doctors, nurses, social workers, or psychologists, as well as various community members that have interactions with children and adolescents, such as coaches, police, clergy members, counselors, teachers, or student peers (Swanke & Dobie Buila, 2010). As those that are at the highest risk for suicide often do not seek help, gatekeeper training is designed to teach the identification of proven risk factors and appropriate risk management (Gould & Kramer, 2001). In addition, gatekeeper training works to reduce stigmatizing attitudes and encourage linkage to treatment (Mann et al., 2005). Several studies have demonstrated the effectiveness of training programs to improve gatekeeper knowledge of risk factors and efficacy to intervene with at-risk youth (e.g., Wyman et al., 2008). Yet, despite these improvements in attitudes and knowledge, these programs have not yet demonstrated effects on suicidal behaviors (York et al., 2013). Further research is needed to determine the impact of gatekeeper training specifically on reducing youth suicidal behaviors, particularly in community settings (Isaac et al., 2009).

7.4.1.2 Awareness/Psychoeducation

There have been a number of public education campaigns seeking to increase suicide-risk recognition, increase help-seeking behaviors, and reduce stigma and barriers. However, very few have been systematically evaluated. Additionally, public campaigns tend to focus on broader issues, such as depression or mental health stigma, as opposed to suicide specifically (Mann et al., 2005). A review of curriculum-based educational programs indicated that while these programs are able to increase knowledge and improve attitudes regarding mental illness and suicide, there was insufficient evidence to say that these programs had an effect on the rates of suicide (Guo & Harstall, 2002). Similarly, a meta-analysis by Robinson, Cox, Malone, Williamson, Baldwin, Fletcher, and O'Brien (2013) concluded school-based suicide prevention programs show little evidence for reducing suicidal thoughts or behaviors. Continued research is necessary to assess for the feasibility and effectiveness of public education/awareness-based programs, with an emphasis on assessing for changes in suicide-specific outcomes.

7.4.1.3 Media Guidelines

The risks associated with exposure to suicide, particularly through the mass media channels of television and newspapers, have precipitated a number of guidelines for the news media (Gould, Jamieson, & Romer, 2003). In fact, one of the stated goals of the US Surgeon General's 2012 National Strategy for Suicide Prevention was to promote responsible media reporting of suicide and accurate portrayals of suicide and mental illness in the entertainment industry (U.S. Department of Health and Human Services, 2012). These guidelines include avoiding sensationalist headlines that focus on the suicide, avoiding the details or method used in the suicide, and reporting on suicide as a public health issue rather than in a fashion similar to a crime. It is encouraged to use newsworthy suicides as an opportunity to educate the public regarding the complexity of suicide, the role of mental illness and substance abuse, as well as potentially the warning signs and avenues for help seeking (for full guidelines, see reportingonsuicide.org). Only a few studies have evaluated the impact of implementing media guidelines, but have yielded promising results (e.g., Etzersdorfer & Sonneck, 1998). However, difficulties in generating awareness and adherence to these guidelines have made the evaluation process challenging (Pirkis, Blood, Beautrais, Burgess, & Skehan, 2006). Well-controlled additional evaluations of media guidelines in suicide reporting are warranted to definitively determine their effectiveness across large populations.

7.4.1.4 Means Restriction

Means restriction involves reducing accessibility to highly lethal means for suicide through adaptations in the environment (Yip et al., 2012). Since accessibility influences the choice of suicidal method, prevention techniques aimed at restricting access to lethal means have demonstrated reduced rates of suicide (e.g., Hawton, 2007). Firearms are the most lethal method of suicide for all age groups, and guns in the home are associated with a nearly fivefold increased risk for suicide across the life span (Kellermann, Rivara, Somes, & Reay, 1992). Among adolescents, firearms account for nearly 42 % of suicide deaths (CDC, 2013). A pilot study for the National Violent Death Reporting System found that among youth who died by firearm suicide, 82 % used a gun belonging to a family member (Harvard Injury

Control Research Center, 2007). States with the least restrictive gun laws have significantly higher rates of firearm suicide, and restricting access to firearms through the implementation of widespread policy and legislation (such as laws requiring safe in-home storage of firearms) has been associated with an overall decrease in youth firearm-related suicides (e.g., Slater, 2011; Webster, Vernick, Zeoli, & Manganello, 2004). Means restriction efforts are not limited to firearms, as restriction efforts such as placing barriers on jump sites and modifying the type of exhaust emitted from automobiles have also been shown to reduce the rate of suicide deaths (e.g., Perron, Burrows, Fournier, Perron, & Ouellet, 2013; Shelef, 1994).

The success of firearm means restriction in preventing death by suicide is predicated on the assumption that the imminent suicidal crisis will subside or that the youth will choose to substitute with a less lethal method (Hawton, 2007). Some studies have found that while the enactment of harsher gun laws lowers rates of firearm suicide, rates of suicide using alternative methods subsequently increase (e.g., Cheung & Dewa, 2005). It is important to note that means restriction does not necessarily reduce the rate of suicide attempts or lower an individual's intent to die. In fact, some campaigns discourage efforts to restrict means with very low lethality, as it may be substituted with a more lethal alternative (Harvard Injury Control Research Center, 2012). Despite the potential for method substitution, a number of collective reviews in the means restriction literature have encouraged the application of means restriction as a method of suicide prevention (e.g., Daigle, 2005; Mann et al., 2005; Sarchiapone, Mandelli, Iosue, Andrisano, & Roy, 2011).

7.4.2 Screening to Identify High-Risk Groups

7.4.2.1 Pediatric/PCP Screening

The US Surgeon General's 2012 National Strategy for Suicide Prevention (U.S. Department of Health and Human Services, 2012) called for suicide screening across a range of medical settings, particularly by primary care physicians. The goal of suicide screening is to identify individuals at elevated risk for suicide that may have potentially gone unnoticed and refer them to the appropriate care. Primary care physicians are in a unique position to serve as early identifiers and possess the potential to ultimately intervene and prevent suicide (Luoma, Martin, & Pearson, 2002). A strong push has been made to increase education for primary care physicians surrounding the warning signs for adolescent suicide and providing the necessary tools to appropriately intervene (Taliaferro & Borowsky, 2011). Some preliminary studies assessing the implementation of suicide-risk questions in the primary care setting have had positive results. For example, when two questions concerning (1) a wish to be dead and (2) thoughts of suicide (with follow-up questions for affirmative responses) were added to an existing psychosocial screening template in three primary care clinics, there was nearly a fourfold increase in suicide case detections and referral rates for outpatient behavioral health-care centers (Wintersteen, 2010). However, it is important to note that an increase in referral rates does not necessarily correspond to changes in clinical and/or suicide-related outcomes (Asarnow et al., 2011). Further evaluative research is necessary to assess whether these programs effectively reduce the rate of suicide for adolescents.

7.4.2.2 Emergency Department Screening

The emergency department (ED) is an underutilized setting for detecting suicide risk and offers many advantages in conjunction with screening in primary care clinics. An estimated 1.5 million adolescents in the United States rely on the ED as their usual source of health care, and adolescents with greater levels of risk for suicidal behavior (e.g., risky behavior, a history of physical/sexual abuse, higher depression scores) are more likely to use the ED as their usual source of care (Wilson & Klein, 2000). Furthermore, ED settings provide an opportunity to screen male adolescents, who are less likely to regularly seek services from a primary care physician (Marcell, Klein, Fischer, Allan, & Kokotailo, 2002). A study by O'Mara, Hill, Cunningham, and King (2012) surveyed parent and adolescent attitudes in a pediatric emergency department and found support among both parents and adolescents for suicide-risk screening in the ED as part of routine clinical care. Moreover, King, O'Mara, Hayward, and Cunningham (2009) demonstrated the feasibility of such screening to detect suicide-risk factors in youth who present with nonpsychiatric chief complaints. Given the time constraints and triage process of the ED, the development of brief and effective screens for suicide risk is essential to identify and intervene with adolescents who may otherwise go undetected.

7.4.3 Individual Approach

7.4.3.1 Cognitive Behavioral Therapy

Cognitive behavioral therapy (CBT) is a psychotherapeutic approach that addresses dysfunctional processes occurring with an individual's emotions, thoughts, and/or behaviors. CBT is most often utilized in treating depression and anxiety and is occasionally accompanied in treatment by psychotropic medication. Three major studies conducted over the past decade have highlighted important effects of treatment, including the benefit of CBT for adolescents with suicide risk. However, a careful review of these findings is important to understand the strengths and limitations of treatment. The TADS (Treatment for Adolescents with Depression Study; March et al., 2004) is the largest randomized controlled trial study of treatment for adolescent depression. One-third of participants endorsed clinically significant suicidal thoughts at the baseline, though it is important to note that many high-risk adolescents were excluded from this study (e.g., current suicidal plans or intent, serious suicide attempt in the past 6 months). The four treatment arms included CBT alone, fluoxetine alone, CBT + fluoxetine, and placebo pill only. The treatment of depression was associated with a reduction in suicidal thoughts, with the improvement in suicidal ideation most evident for those receiving CBT alone or CBT with fluoxetine (Emslie et al., 2006).

In the TORDIA study (Treatment of Resistant Depression in Adolescents; Brent et al., 2008), a randomized controlled trial that included adolescents who had at least one failed prior trial of a selective serotonin reuptake inhibitor (SSRI), a combined treatment approach of CBT and venlafaxine was associated with the greatest reductions in depression over a 24-week period. However, the protective effect of CBT was not evident on suicide-related adverse events in the study or for those who had a history of non-suicidal self-injury (Asarnow et al., 2009). The TASA study (Treatment of Adolescent Suicide Attempters; Brent et al., 2009) was an open trial (i.e., participants chose treatment not randomly assigned) of adolescents who had attempted suicide in the preceding 90 days. The majority of adolescents chose the CBT + medication group, and scores of depression and suicidal ideation declined over the 6-month study period at rates comparable to non-suicidal depressed adolescents (Vitiello et al., 2009). However, despite this improvement in outcomes with treatment, 12 % of the adolescents in the study made an additional suicide attempt in the 6-month period, one-third of which occurred in the first 4 weeks (Brent et al., 2009). Continued treatment approaches geared toward suicidal adolescents are necessary to further reduce the risk of future suicide attempts and suicide deaths.

7.4.3.2   Multisystemic Therapy

Multisystemic therapy (MST) is an intensive home- and community-based approach designed for children and adolescents with serious emotional disturbance that seeks to address problems across social/ecological systems, such as in the family, school, and community (MST; Henggeler, Schoenwald, Rowland, & Cunningham, 2002). In a study by Huey, Henggeler, Rowland, Halliday-Boykins, Cunningham, Pickrel, and Edwards (2004), adolescents were recruited at a hospital's emergency department and were randomized to either psychiatric hospitalization or MST. The adolescents randomized to the MST condition reported a significant reduction in suicide attempts over a 1-year period in comparison to those who were psychiatrically hospitalized. However, adolescents with a past-year attempt at the baseline were overrepresented in the MST group (allowing for a greater reduction effect), and there were no differences between groups in reported levels of depression, hopelessness, or suicidal ideation at follow-up. Further research is necessary to determine the long-term impacts of MST for adolescents at risk for suicide.

7.4.3.3   Dialectical Behavioral Therapy (DBT; Linehan, 1993)

DBT was originally developed for suicidal adults with borderline personality disorder, but has been adapted for use with adolescents in recent years. DBT focuses on balancing elements such as acceptance and change and flexibility and stability, by critically addressing contrasting viewpoints and looking for truth from multiple perspectives, while also working to improve problem-solving and emotional regulation skills. In a quasi-experimental study of adolescent with borderline-personality features, those receiving an adapted DBT had significantly fewer hospitalizations during a 12-week treatment period than the treatment-as-usual (TAU) group and had significant reductions in suicidal ideation, though no group differences were found with regard to suicide attempts (Rathus & Miller, 2002). However, since this study was not a randomized controlled trial (most severe adolescents were placed in DBT group) and treatment attendance (40 % for TAU, 62 % for DBT) was not particularly strong, the inferences that can be made are limited. A number of other studies (for a review, see MacPherson, Cheavens, & Fristad, 2013) examining DBT in adolescents have indicated improvements from pre- to posttreatment in suicidal ideation and suicidal behavior, as well as other areas of functioning. Nevertheless, the majority of these studies were either open trials or quasi-experimental in design. Randomized controlled trials with adequately sized samples are necessary to fully assess the promising results associated with these preliminary studies of DBT.

7.4.3.4 Suicide-Specific Targeted Interventions

A number of intervention studies have been developed for reducing youth suicidal behavior. For example, the Youth-Nominated Support Team-Version II intervention was developed by King, Klaus, Kramer, Venkataraman, Quinlan, and Gillespie (2009) as a supplement to routine care following psychiatric hospitalization for adolescents. Psychoeducation and consultation were provided for parent-approved adult support persons nominated by the adolescent to provide supportive contact to the adolescent in the 3 months following discharge. Adolescents randomized to this intervention group did not have significantly different one-year outcomes related to suicidal ideation or suicide attempts, though there were modest improvements in functional impairment for non-attempters and a quicker reduction in suicidal ideation for those with multiple past attempts (King, Klaus, et al., 2009). A number of youth suicide interventions were systematically evaluated by Corcoran et al. (2011) for suicidal and self-harm events. While immediate posttest results corresponded with an improvement in suicidal and self-harm events for intervention groups, the follow-up results indicated a reversal, whereby the control group reported fewer suicidal and self-harm events than the intervention group. Additional research, development, and evaluations of suicide-specific interventions are necessary to determine the effectiveness and feasibility of these programs to reduce suicidal behavior in adolescents.

7.5 Future Directions

Suicide is a tragedy that is largely preventable. Many of the prevention and intervention strategies highlighted in this chapter have targeted one or more suicide-risk or protective factors and demonstrated some promising effects, including reductions in suicidal ideation and behavior. Despite the growing body of research across these areas of prevention, only a small number of intensive individually focused strategies have been associated with reductions in actual suicidal behavior. Large-scale and long-term prospective studies are needed to determine how universal and selected strategies might positively alter the developmental trajectories of youth who may be at risk and reduce the onset of suicidal behavior or the likelihood of suicide. Six distinct intervention points that occur along the pathway to suicide have been identified: preventing the initial onset or occurrence of a risk factor, diminishing/removing an emerging risk factor, treating individuals with identifiable mental disorders, halting movement toward co-occurring problems, crisis intervention, and removal of means (King, 1998). The implementation of a full range of evidence-based strategies across multiple intervention points presents the best opportunity to reduce suicide rates. It is encouraged for individuals across disciplines (e.g., psychology, medicine, sociology, public health) and sectors (e.g., health, media, education) to work together and apply current and future research findings to communities at local and national levels in order to reduce the heavy toll that youth suicide currently imposes.

References

Asarnow, J. R., Baraff, L. J., Berk, M., Grob, C. S., Devich-Navarro, M., Suddath, R.,… Tang, L. (2011). An emergency department intervention for linking pediatric suicidal patients to follow-up mental health treatment. *Psychiatric Services, 62*(11), 1303–1309.

Asarnow, J. R., Emslie, G., Clarke, G., Wagner, K. D., Spirito, A., Vitiello, B., …. Brent, D. (2009). Treatment of selective serotonin reuptake inhibitor—Resistant depression in adolescents: Predictors and moderators of treatment response. *Journal of the American Academy of Child and Adolescent Psychiatry, 48*(3), 330-339.

Bearman, P. S., & Moody, J. (2004). Suicide and friendships among American adolescents. *American Journal of Public Health, 94*(1), 89–95.

Beautrais, A. L. (2003). Suicide and serious suicide attempts in youth: A multiple-group comparison study. *American Journal of Psychiatry, 160*(6), 1093–1099.

Bensley, L. S., Van Eeenwyk, J., Spieker, S. J., & Schoder, J. (1999). Self-reported abuse history and adolescent problem behaviors. I. Antisocial and suicidal behaviors. *Journal of Adolescent Health, 24*(3), 163–172.

Borowsky, I. W., Taliaferro, L. A., & McMorris, B. J. (2013). Suicidal thinking and behavior among youth involved in verbal and social bullying: risk and protective factors. *Journal of Adolescent Health, 53*(1 Suppl), S4–S12.

Brady, J. (2006). The association between alcohol misuse and suicidal behaviour. *Alcohol and Alcoholism, 41*(5), 473–478.

Brent, D. A., Baugher, M., Bridge, J., Chen, T., & Chiappetta, L. (1999). Age- and sex-related risk factors for adolescent suicide. *Journal of the American Academy of Child and Adolescent Psychiatry, 38*(12), 1497–1505.

Brent, D. A., Emslie, G. J., Clarke, G., Wagner, K. D., Asarnow, J. R., Keller, M., … Zelazny, J. (2008). Switching to another SSRI or to venlafaxine with or without cognitive behavioral therapy for adolescents with SSRI-resistant depression: The TORDIA randomized controlled trial. *Journal of the American Medical Association, 299*(8), 901–913.

Brent, D. A., Greenhill, L. L., Compton, S., Emslie, G. J., Wells, K., Walkup, J. T., … Turner, B. (2009). The Treatment of Adolescent Suicide Attempters Study (TASA): Predictors of suicidal events in an open treatment trial. *Journal of the American Academy of Child & Adolescent Psychiatry, 48*(10), 987–996.

Brent, D. A., Perper, J. A., Moritz, G., Allman, C., Friend, A., Roth, C., ... Baugher, M. (1993). Psychiatric risk factors for adolescent suicide: A case-control study. *Journal of the American Academy of Child & Adolescent Psychiatry, 32*(3), 521-529.

Canetto, S. S., & Sakinofsky, I. (1998). The gender paradox in suicide. *Suicide & Life-Threatening Behavior, 28*(1), 1–23.

Centers for Disease Control and Prevention. (2012). Youth Risk Behavior Surveillance - United States, 2011. *Morbidity and Mortality Weekly Report, 61*(4).

Centers for Disease Control and Prevention. (2013). Web-based Injury Statistics Query and Reporting System (WISQARS). Retrieved July 8, 2013 from http://www.cdc.gov/injury/wisqars/index.html.

Cheung, A. H., & Dewa, C. S. (2005). Current trends in youth suicide and firearms regulations. *Canadian Journal of Public Health, 96*(2), 131–135.

Corcoran, J., Dattalo, P., Crowley, M., Brown, E., & Grindle, L. (2011). A systematic review of psychosocial interventions for suicidal adolescents. *Children and Youth Services Review, 33*(11), 2112–2118.

Daigle, M. S. (2005). Suicide prevention through means restriction: Assessing the risk of substitution: A critical review and synthesis. *Accident Analysis & Prevention, 37*(4), 625–632.

Emslie, G., Kratochvil, C., Vitiello, B., Silva, S., Mayes, T., McNulty, S., ... March, J. (2006). Treatment for Adolescents With Depression Study (TADS): Safety results. *Journal of the American Academy of Child and Adolescent Psychiatry, 45*(12), 1440–1455.

Etzersdorfer, E., & Sonneck, G. (1998). Preventing suicide by influencing mass-media reporting. The Viennese experience 1980–1996. *Archives of Suicide Research, 4*(1), 67–74.

Fergusson, D. M., Horwood, L. J., Ridder, E. M., & Beautrais, A. L. (2005). Suicidal behaviour in adolescence and subsequent mental health outcomes in young adulthood. *Psychological Medicine, 35*(7), 983–993.

Goldston, D. B., Daniel, S. S., Erkanli, A., Reboussin, B. A., Mayfield, A., Frazier, P. H., & Treadway, S. L. (2009). Psychiatric diagnoses as contemporaneous risk factors for suicide attempts among adolescents and young adults: Developmental changes. *Journal of Consulting and Clinical Psychology, 77*(2), 281–290.

Goldston, D. B., Molock, S. D., Whitbeck, L. B., Murakami, J. L., Zayas, L. H., & Hall, G. C. N. (2008). Cultural considerations in adolescent suicide prevention and psychosocial treatment. *American Psychologist, 63*(1), 14–31.

Gordon, R. S. (1983). An operational classification of disease prevention. *Public Health Reports, 98*(2), 107.

Gould, M. S., Jamieson, P., & Romer, D. (2003). Media contagion and suicide among the young. *American Behavioral Scientist, 46*(9), 1269–1284.

Gould, M. S., & Kramer, R. A. (2001). Youth suicide prevention. *Suicide & Life-Threatening Behavior, 31*(1 Suppl), 6–31.

Gould, M. S., Velting, D., Kleinman, M., Lucas, C., Thomas, J. G., & Chung, M. (2004). Teenagers' attitudes about coping strategies and help-seeking behavior for suicidality. *Journal of the American Academy of Child and Adolescent Psychiatry, 43*(9), 1124–1133.

Guo, B., & Harstall, C. (2002). *Efficacy of suicide prevention programs for children and youth.* Edmonton, AB: Alberta Heritage Foundation for Medical Research.

Harvard Injury Control Research Center. (2007). Youth suicide: Findings from a pilot for the National Violent Death Reporting System. Retrieved June 10, 2013, from http://www.sprc.org/sites/sprc.org/files/library/YouthSuicideFactSheet.pdf.

Harvard Injury Control Research Center. (2012). Means matter: Suicide, guns, and public health Retrieved June 10, 2013, from http://www.hsph.harvard.edu/means-matter/means-matter/saves-lives/

Hawton, K. (2007). Restricting access to methods of suicide. *Crisis: The Journal of Crisis Intervention and Suicide Prevention, 28,* 4–9.

Hawton, K., Simkin, S., Deeks, J. J., O'Connor, S., Keen, A., Altman, D. G., ... Bulstrode, C. (1999). Effects of a drug overdose in a television drama on presentations to hospital for self poisoning: Time series and questionnaire study. *British Medical Journal, 318*(7189), 972–977.

Henggeler, S. W., Schoenwald, S. K., Rowland, M. D., & Cunningham, P. B. (2002). *Mutisystemic treatment of children and adolescents with serious emotional disturbance.* New York, NY: Guilford.

Horwitz, A. G., Czyz, E. K., & King, C. A. (2015). Predicting future suicide attempts among adolescent and emerging adult psychiatric emergency patients. *Journal of Clinical Child and Adolescent Psychology, 44*(5), 751–761.

Huey, S. J., Jr., Henggeler, S. W., Rowland, M. D., Halliday-Boykins, C. A., Cunningham, P. B., Pickrel, S. G., & Edwards, J. (2004). Multisystemic therapy effects on attempted suicide by youths presenting psychiatric emergencies. *Journal of the American Academy of Child & Adolescent Psychiatry, 43*(2), 183–190.

Isaac, M., Elias, B., Katz, L. Y., Belik, S.-L., Deane, F. P., Enns, M. W., & Sareen, J. (2009). Gatekeeper training as a preventative intervention for suicide: A systematic review. *The Canadian Journal of Psychiatry, 54*(4), 260–268.

Joe, S., & Marcus, S. C. (2003). Datapoints: trends by race and gender in suicide attempts among U.S. adolescents, 1991-2001. *Psychiatric Services, 54*(4), 454.

Kaltiala-Heino, R., Rimpelä, M., Marttunen, M. J., Rimpelä, A., & Rantanen, P. (1999). Bullying, depression, and suicidal ideation in Finnish adolescents: School survey. *British Medical Journal, 319*(7206), 348–351.

Kaminski, J. W., & Fang, X. (2009). Victimization by peers and adolescent suicide in three US samples. *The Journal of Pediatrics, 155*(5), 683–688.

Kaminski, J. W., Puddy, R. W., Hall, D. M., Cashman, S. Y., Crosby, A. E., & Ortega, L. A. G. (2010). The relative influence of different domains of social connectedness on self-directed violence in adolescence. *Journal of Youth and Adolescence, 39*(5), 460–473.

Kellermann, A. L., Rivara, F. P., Somes, G., & Reay, D. T. (1992). Suicide in the home in relation to gun ownership. *New England Journal of Medicine, 327*(7), 467–472.

Khurana, A., & Romer, D. (2012). Modeling the distinct pathways of influence of coping strategies on youth suicidal ideation: A national longitudinal study. *Prevention Science, 13*(6), 644–654.

King, C. A. (1998). Suicide across the life span: Pathways to prevention. *Suicide & Life-Threatening Behavior, 28*(4), 328–337.

King, C. A., Jiang, Q., Czyz, E., & Kerr, D. C. R. (2014). Suicidal ideation of psychiatrically hospitalized adolescents has one-year predictive validity for suicide attempts in girls only. *Journal of Abnormal Child Psychology, 42*(3), 467–477.

King, C. A., Klaus, N. M., Kramer, A., Venkataraman, S., Quinlan, P., & Gillespie, B. (2009). The Youth Nominated Support Team for suicidal adolescents -- version II: A randomized control intervention trial. *Journal of Consulting and Clinical Psychology, 77*(5), 880–893.

King, C. A., & Merchant, C. R. (2008). Social and interpersonal factors relating to adolescent suicidality: A review of the literature. *Archives of Suicide Research, 12*(3), 181–196.

King, C. A., O'Mara, R. M., Hayward, C. N., & Cunningham, R. M. (2009). Adolescent suicide risk screening in the emergency department. *Academic Emergency Medicine, 16*(11), 1234–1241.

Klomek, A. B., Marrocco, F., Kleinman, M., Schonfeld, I. S., & Gould, M. S. (2008). Peer victimization, depression, and suicidality in adolescents. *Suicide & Life-Threatening Behavior, 38*(2), 166–180.

Lewinsohn, P. M., Rohde, P., & Seeley, J. R. (1994). Psychosocial risk factors for future adolescent suicide attempts. *Journal of Consulting and Clinical Psychology, 62*(2), 297–305.

Lewinsohn, P. M., Rohde, P., & Seeley, J. R. (1996). Adolescent suicidal ideation and attempts: Prevalence, risk factors, and clinical implications. *Clinical Psychology: Science and Practice, 3*(1), 25–46.

Linehan, M. M. (1993). *Skills training manual for treating borderline personality disorder.* New York, NY: Guilford Press.

Luoma, J. B., Martin, C. E., & Pearson, J. L. (2002). Contact with mental health and primary care providers before suicide: A review of the evidence. *American Journal of Psychiatry, 159*(6), 909–916.

MacPherson, H. A., Cheavens, J. S., & Fristad, M. A. (2013). Dialectical behavior therapy for adolescents: Theory, treatment adaptations, and empirical outcomes. *Clinical Child and Family Psychology Review, 16*(1), 59–80.

Mann, J. J., Apter, A., Bertolote, J., Beautrais, A. L., Currier, D., Haas, A., ... Hendin, H. (2005). Suicide prevention strategies: A systematic review. *Journal of the American Medical Association, 294*(16), 2064–2074.

Marcell, A. V., Klein, J. D., Fischer, I., Allan, M. J., & Kokotailo, P. K. (2002). Male adolescent use of health care services: Where are the boys? *Journal of Adolescent Health, 30*, 35–43.

March, J., Silva, S., Petrycki, S., Curry, J., Wells, K., Fairbank, J.,... Severe, J. (2004). Fluoxetine, cognitive-behavioral therapy, and their combination for adolescents with depression: Treatment for Adolescents with Depression Study (TADS) randomized controlled trial. *Journal of the American Medical Association, 292*(7), 807–820.

Miranda, R., Scott, M., Hicks, R., Wilcox, H. C., Munfakh, J. L. H., & Shaffer, D. (2008). Suicide attempt characteristics, diagnoses, and future attempts: Comparing multiple attempters to single attempters and ideators. *Journal of the American Academy of Child and Adolescent Psychiatry, 47*(1), 32–40.

Nansel, T. R., Overpeck, M., Pilla, R. S., Ruan, W. J., Simons-Morton, B., & Scheidt, P. (2001). Bullying behaviors among US youth: Prevalence and association with psychosocial adjustment. *Journal of the American Medical Association, 285*(16), 2094–2100.

Nickerson, A. B., & Slater, E. D. (2009). School and community violence and victimization as predictors of adolescent suicidal behavior. *School Psychology Review, 38*(2), 218–232.

Nkansah-Amankra, S., Diedhiou, A., Agbanu, S. K., Agbanu, H. L. K., Opoku-Adomako, N. S., & Twumasi-Ankrah, P. (2012). A longitudinal evaluation of religiosity and psychosocial determinants of suicidal behaviors among a population-based sample in the United States. *Journal of Affective Disorders, 139*(1), 40–51.

Nock, M. K., Joiner, T. E., Jr., Gordon, K. H., Lloyd-Richardson, E., & Prinstein, M. J. (2006). Non-suicidal self-injury among adolescents: Diagnostic correlates and relation to suicide attempts. *Psychiatry Research, 144*(1), 65–72.

Nock, M. K., & Kessler, R. C. (2006). Prevalence of and risk factors for suicide attempts versus suicide gestures: Analysis of the National Comorbidity Survey. *Journal of Abnormal Psychology, 115*(3), 616–623.

Nonnemaker, J. M., McNeely, C. A., & Blum, R. W. (2003). Public and private domains of religiosity and adolescent health risk behaviors: Evidence from the National Longitudinal Study of Adolescent Health. *Social Science and Medicine, 57*(11), 2049–2054.

O'Mara, R. M., Hill, R. M., Cunningham, R. M., & King, C. A. (2012). Adolescent and parent attitudes toward screening for suicide risk and mental health problems in the pediatric emergency department. *Pediatric Emergency Care, 28*(7), 626–632.

Pedersen, W. (2008). Does cannabis use lead to depression and suicidal behaviours? A population-based longitudinal study. *Acta Psychiatrica Scandinavica, 118*(5), 395–403.

Perron, S., Burrows, S., Fournier, M., Perron, P.-A., & Ouellet, F. (2013). Installation of a bridge barrier as a suicide prevention strategy in Montréal, Québec, Canada. *American Journal of Public Health, 103*(7), 1235–1239.

Piquet, M. L., & Wagner, B. M. (2003). Coping responses of adolescent suicide attempters and their relation to suicidal ideation across a 2-year follow-up: A preliminary study. *Suicide & Life-Threatening Behavior, 33*(3), 288–301.

Pirkis, J., Blood, R. W., Beautrais, A., Burgess, P., & Skehan, J. (2006). Media guidelines on the reporting of suicide. *Crisis: The Journal of Crisis Intervention and Suicide Prevention, 27*(2), 82–87.

Prinstein, M. J., Boergers, J., Spirito, A., Little, T. D., & Grapentine, W. L. (2000). Peer functioning, family dysfunction, and psychological symptoms in a risk factor model for adolescent inpatients' suicidal ideation severity. *Journal of Clinical Child Psychology, 29*(3), 392–405.

Rasic, D. T., Belik, S.-L., Elias, B., Katz, L. Y., Enns, M., & Sareen, J. (2009). Spirituality, religion and suicidal behavior in a nationally representative sample. *Journal of Affective Disorders, 114*(1-3), 32–40.

Rathus, J. H., & Miller, A. L. (2002). Dialectical Behavior Therapy adapted for suicidal adolescents. *Suicide & Life-Threatening Behavior, 32*(2), 146–157.

Recommendations for reporting on suicide. Retrieved May 28, 2013, from www.reportingonsuicide.org.

Robins, A., & Fiske, A. (2009). Explaining the relation between religiousness and reduced suicidal behavior: Social support rather than specific beliefs. *Suicide & Life-Threatening Behavior, 39*(4), 386–395.

Robinson, J., Cox, G., Malone, A., Williamson, M., Baldwin, G., Fletcher, K., & O'Brien, M. (2013). A systematic review of school-based interventions aimed at preventing, treating, and responding to suicide-related behavior in young people. *Crisis: The Journal of Crisis Intervention and Suicide Prevention, 34*(3), 164–182.

Rudd, M. D., Rajab, M. H., Orman, D. T., Stulman, D. A., Joiner, T. E., Jr., & Dixon, W. (1996). Effectiveness of an outpatient intervention targeting suicidal young adults: Preliminary results. *Journal of Consulting and Clinical Psychology, 64*(1), 179–190.

Sarchiapone, M., Mandelli, L., Iosue, M., Andrisano, C., & Roy, A. (2011). Controlling access to suicide means. *International Journal of Environmental Research and Public Health, 8*(12), 4550–4562.

Schilling, E. A., Aseltine, R. H., Jr., Glanovsky, J. L., James, A., & Jacobs, D. (2009). Adolescent alcohol use, suicidal ideation, and suicide attempts. *Journal of Adolescent Health, 44*(4), 335–341.

Shaffer, D., Gould, M. S., Fisher, P. W., Trautman, P., Moreau, D., Kleinman, M., & Flory, M. (1996). Psychiatric diagnosis in child and adolescent suicide. *Archives of General Psychiatry, 53*(4), 339–348.

Shelef, M. (1994). Unanticipated benefits of automotive emission control: Reduction in fatalities by motor vehicle exhaust gas. *Science of the Total Environment, 146–147*, 93–101.

Silverman, A. B., Reinherz, H. Z., & Giaconia, R. M. (1996). The long-term sequelae of child and adolescent abuse: A longitudinal community study. *Child Abuse & Neglect, 20*(8), 709–723.

Slater, G. Y. (2011). The missing piece: A sociological autopsy of firearm suicide in the United States. *Suicide & Life-Threatening Behavior, 41*(5), 474–490.

Stack, S. (2000). Media impacts on suicide: A quantitative review of 293 findings. *Social Science Quarterly, 81*(4), 957–971.

Swahn, M. H., & Bossarte, R. M. (2007). Gender, early alcohol use, and suicide ideation and attempts: Findings from the 2005 Youth Risk Behavior Survey. *Journal of Adolescent Health, 41*(2), 175–181.

Swanke, J. R., & Dobie Buila, S. M. (2010). Gatekeeper training for caregivers and professionals: A variation on suicide prevention. *Advances in Mental Health, 9*(1), 98–104.

Swanson, S. A., & Colman, I. (2013). Association between exposure to suicide and suicidality outcomes in youth. *Canadian Medical Association Journal, 185*(10), 870–877. doi:10.1503/cmaj.121377.

Taliaferro, L. A., & Borowsky, I. W. (2011). Physician education: A promising strategy to prevent adolescent suicide. *Academic Medicine, 86*(3), 342–347.

U.S. Department of Health and Human Services (HHS), Office of the Surgeon General and National Action Alliance for Suicide Prevention. (2012). *2012 National strategy for suicide prevention: Goals and objectives for action.* Washington D.C: U.S. Department of Health and Human Services.

Vitiello, B., Brent, D. A., Greenhill, L. L., Emslie, G., Wells, K., Walkup, J. T., ... Zelazny, J. (2009). Depressive symptoms and clinical status during the Treatment of Adolescent Suicide Attempters (TASA) study. *Journal of the American Academy of Child and Adolescent Psychiatry, 48*(10), 997–1004.

Vyrostek, S. B., Annest, J. L., & Ryan, G. W. (2004). Surveillance for fatal and nonfatal injuries--United States, 2001. *MMWR Surveillance Summaries, 53*(7), 1–57.

Webster, D. W., Vernick, J. S., Zeoli, A. M., & Manganello, J. A. (2004). Association between youth-focused firearm laws and youth suicides. *JAMA, 292*(5), 594–601.

Wilson, K. M., & Klein, J. D. (2000). Adolescents who use the emergency department as their usual source of care. *Archives of Pediatrics and Adolescent Medicine, 154*(4), 361.

Winsper, C., Lereya, T., Zanarini, M., & Wolke, D. (2012). Involvement in bullying and suicide-related behavior at 11 years: A prospective birth cohort study. *Journal of the American Academy of Child and Adolescent Psychiatry, 51*(3), 271–282.

Wintersteen, M. B. (2010). Standardized screening for suicidal adolescents in primary care. *Pediatrics, 125*(5), 938–944.

Wyman, P. A., Brown, C. H., Inman, J., Cross, W., Schmeelk-Cone, K., Guo, J., & Pena, J. B. (2008). Randomized trial of a gatekeeper program for suicide prevention: 1-year impact on secondary school staff. *Journal of Consulting and Clinical Psychology, 76*(1), 104–115.

Yip, P. S. F., Caine, E., Yousuf, S., Chang, S.-S., Wu, K. C.-C., & Chen, Y.-Y. (2012). Means restriction for suicide prevention. *The Lancet, 379*(9834), 2393–2399.

York, J., Lamis, D. A., Friedman, L., Berman, A. L., Joiner, T. E., McIntosh, J. L., … Pearson, J. (2013). A systematic review process to evaluate suicide prevention programs: A sample case of community-based programs. *Journal of Community Psychology, 41*(1), 35–51.

Chapter 8
Health Concerns Regarding Children and Adolescents with Attention-Deficit/ Hyperactivity Disorder

Alexandria B. Fladhammer, Adrian R. Lyde, Adena B. Meyers, Jeffrey K. Clark, and Steven Landau

8.1 Attention-Deficit/Hyperactivity Disorder

Beginning with the recent publication of the fifth edition of the *Diagnostic and Statistical Manual of Mental Disorders* (American Psychiatric Association, 2013), the psychiatric community discontinued consideration of attention-deficit/hyperactivity disorder (ADHD) as a disruptive behavior disorder (with diagnoses first made in infancy, childhood, or adolescence). Instead, ADHD is now assigned to the neurodevelopmental disorder chapter to reflect presumed brain developmental correlates of ADHD. To create a sense of this new assignment, it is worth knowing the other disorders that are also present in the chapter on neurodevelopmental disorders. These include autism spectrum disorder (ASD), intellectual disability, communication disorders, specific learning disorder, and motor disorders. Even though the formal ADHD diagnostic criteria per se have not changed, ADHD is no longer a constituent in the externalizing group of oppositional-defiant disorder (ODD) and conduct disorder (CD).

From a historical perspective, this neurodevelopmental change is not entirely surprising. It is true that many or most children with ADHD emit disruptive behaviors, and it is true that many or most of these children have symptoms that co-occur (i.e., are comorbid with) ODD and CD. Even so, an examination of medical epidemiological research over the past 100 years suggests that the hallmark characteristics of ADHD (i.e., inattention and impulsivity/hyperactivity) received great attention

A.B. Fladhammer • A.B. Meyers, Ph.D. • S. Landau, Ph.D. (✉)
Department of Psychology, Illinois State University,
Campus Box 4620, Normal, IL 61790, USA
e-mail: fladhammera@gmail.com; abmeyer@ilstu.edu; selandau@ilstu.edu

A.R. Lyde, Ph.D. • J.K. Clark, H.S.D.
Department of Health Sciences, Illinois State University,
Campus Box 5220, Normal, IL 61790, USA
e-mail: arlyde@IllinoisState.edu; jkclark@ilstu.edu

© Springer Science+Business Media New York 2016
M.R. Korin (ed.), *Health Promotion for Children and Adolescents*,
DOI 10.1007/978-1-4899-7711-3_8

immediately following World War I in the midst of a devastating Western European and North American epidemic of *encephalitis lethargica* (Vilensky, Foley, & Gilman, 2007).

At that time, *encephalitis lethargica* was a highly contagious and lethal neurological disease, but there were survivors. Approximately one-third of the children who remitted their early symptoms of this illness developed psychiatric sequelae that included impulsivity and criminal activity. Indeed, delinquency was a common problem that led clinicians of the day to refer to post-illness problems as "moral imbecility" not related to an intellectual deficit. The medical discourse regarding ADHD-related symptoms and *encephalitis lethargica* is interesting, as it may have been the first to draw a causal link between children's behavior and neurological functioning (Rafalovich, 2001) (i.e., the roots of deviance can be explained by organic processes in the brain). This view endures. The first nosological designation of the disorder involved the term "minimal brain damage," and this label persisted until 1980 when attention-deficit disorder (ADD) was added to the psychiatric taxonomy via *DSM-III* (American Psychiatric Association, 1980). The purpose of this chapter is to examine how ADHD is related to health risks and illnesses among children and teens with the disorder. In addition, this chapter will describe the contributions of prevention science to these health-related problems, as well as best practice in school-based prevention and intervention curricula.

As a topic of concern, ADHD children's health has been underrepresented among the foci of research and anecdotal complaints associated with the disorder. To varying degrees, everyone is familiar with ADHD: It is a complex disorder involving age-inappropriate difficulties managing task and setting demands that require attention, motor quiescence, and a reflective cognitive tempo. Because of inattention and hyperactivity/impulsivity, those with ADHD experience problems in the domains of academic functioning, family functioning, and functioning in the peer group. Unfortunately, because the overt behavioral manifestations of the disorder are disruptive, annoying, and stressful to others, risks related to unhealthy behaviors as well as other somatic problems have been routinely ignored. The goal of this chapter is to sensitize school- and clinic-based professionals that the medical health of those with ADHD is an area involving risks as compelling as school failure and antisocial activity.

From an epidemiological perspective, most estimates indicate that between 5 and 8 % of elementary-age children meet formal diagnostic criteria for ADHD, and there is a strong male preponderance among those with the disorder. Neither race nor ethnicity seems to be a correlate of the disorder, and most studies indicate that social class differences are not related to prevalence. Studies that do indicate ADHD may be more common among those in lower social strata tend to be explained by the downward social mobility of parents of children with ADHD. This hypothesis is likely because of the strong intergenerational transmission of ADHD. About one-third of parents of children with ADHD have ADHD themselves, and adults with ADHD are at risk for problems in the workforce.

Those with ADHD are at elevated risk for a host of other problems. Some of these problems may be a direct result of one or more primary symptoms of the disorder (e.g., achievement delays may be attributable to off-task classroom behavior and careless work strategies); some of these problems may be an indirect expression of salient correlates of the disorder (e.g., comorbid conduct disorder may result from stress-provoking child behavior at home leading to coercive family processes during parent-child management confrontations); and some of these problems may result from a failure to develop age-appropriate behaviors (e.g., annoying behavior in the presence of peers may lead to social exclusion that leads to reduced opportunity to develop social skills related to successful peer entry) (Ronk, Hund, & Landau, 2011).

It is beyond the scope of this chapter to describe the range of associated risks conferred to children and teens with ADHD. Suffice it to say that the challenges these individuals experience cross all domains of functioning expected in all settings, including at school, at home, among peers, and in the community.

To better understand the health concerns associated with ADHD, and to intervene effectively, it is necessary to consider a range of risk and protective factors within the individual, family, and broader social environment that may influence health-related behavior and outcomes. The discipline of *developmental psychopathology* may be relevant here, as it focuses on the relation between adaptation and psychopathology and seeks to elucidate how one person can cope and adjust whereas another experiences a maladaptive outcome (see Rutter & Sroufe, 2000). The field of prevention science emphasizes the contribution of multiple risk factors and protective factors in the development of dysfunction and health (Coie et al., 1993). From this perspective, ADHD may be considered one in an array of factors that increases risk for various negative health outcomes. Preventive interventions may improve health outcomes for children with ADHD by increasing protective factors or reducing risk factors at the individual or environmental level.

At the individual level, ADHD is associated with behavioral disinhibition, which can lead to risky behavior and concomitant health problems. Thus, behavioral or pharmacological interventions targeting ADHD core symptoms of hyperactivity/impulsivity and inattention may improve health outcomes for this population. Interventions may also help children and adolescents with ADHD avoid poor health outcomes by promoting protective factors such as responsible decision-making and social skill development. Prevention efforts may also target risk and protective factors within the family (e.g., by increasing parental supervision, reducing the use of physical punishment in order to reduce injuries) or school (e.g., by developing peer group norms that value safe choices and healthy behavior). Prevention programming should also consider macrosystemic factors that contribute to adaptive or maladaptive outcomes. Poverty likely exacerbates health risks among children with ADHD, but policies that provide comprehensive health care, high-quality childcare, and family-friendly employment arrangements may mitigate some of these effects. Similarly, laws and regulations that reduce dangerous distractions (e.g., text messaging) while teens are driving, increase access to contraception, or regulate food and beverage options in and near schools, may help reduce unsafe driving, sexual risk taking, or obesity among all students, including those with ADHD.

8.2   Health Consequences and Correlates of ADHD

The array and severity of health concerns among children and adolescents with ADHD are reflected in the health system expenditures associated with this disorder. Chan, Zhan, and Homer (2002) determined that the health-care cost for a child with ADHD ($1151) is higher than for a child with asthma ($1091) or a typical child in the general population ($712). These costs include outpatient visits, emergency department visits, home health visits, hospital stays, and prescriptions.

Given the dominant theoretical view of ADHD as a disorder involving behavioral disinhibition (e.g., Barkley, 1997), it is not surprising that children and teens with ADHD tend to experience more health problems than typically developing peers. Young people diagnosed with ADHD tend to lack a future orientation, often failing to consider the potential consequences of risky behaviors. Thus, many of their health-related risks are connected to impulsivity and inattention.

The health risks associated with ADHD are exacerbated in the context of psychiatric comorbidity. In their investigation of the health-related quality of life among children and teens with ADHD, Klassen, Miller, and Fine (2004) reported that more than two-thirds had at least one comorbid psychiatric diagnosis (e.g., oppositional-defiant and/or conduct disorder). Comorbid conduct disorder (CD) is especially common among children with ADHD. Waschbusch's (2002) meta-analytic review indicates that children with ADHD and co-occurring CD have symptoms that are not qualitatively different from symptoms found among ADHD-only and CD-only children (i.e., ADHD plus CD is not a distinct disorder); instead, there is a compelling quantitative difference found among those who meet criteria for both ADHD and CD (i.e., their symptoms are much more severe than ADHD- or CD-only cases).

8.2.1   The Preschool and Elementary Years

Impulsivity is associated with health problems among young children with ADHD, with heightened risk in the context of comorbid psychiatric disorders. For instance, children with ADHD are three times more likely than children without ADHD to suffer accidental poisonings (Barkley, 1998). They are also at greater risk for physical injuries (e.g., broken bones and lacerations), particularly if comorbid conduct disorder (CD) is present (Barkley, 2001).

Although stimulant medication often used to treat ADHD has been linked to low appetite and slow weight gain, evidence indicates that a childhood ADHD diagnosis is actually associated with an increased risk of obesity, with covariance estimates within clinical samples ranging from approximately 13 to 58 % (Cortese & Vincenzi, 2012). The etiology for this association remains unknown, but it is possible that ADHD and obesity share genetic and neurobiological functions (e.g., within the dopaminergic system). Further, the impulsivity and inattention associated with ADHD may contribute to weight gain due to abnormal eating patterns. Some studies suggest that individuals with ADHD eat more impulsively, consume foods higher in fat, and exercise less than their peers (see Nigg, 2013, for a review). These unhealthy habits may account for reduced stamina and strength observed among children with ADHD (Harvey & Reid, 1997). The link between ADHD and childhood obesity suggests that children with ADHD may also be at increased risk of developing type II diabetes, although few studies have examined this connection (Nigg, 2013).

In addition to health outcomes associated with poor impulse control and inattention, many children with ADHD also experience health concerns that cannot be directly linked to the primary symptoms of the disorder. For example, impaired sleep is common among children with ADHD, with 50 % of parents reporting that their child has difficulty sleeping (Owens, 2005). These problems include increased restlessness and resistance at bedtime, as well as frequent waking. Quality of sleep is a predictor of any child's attention and memory, and poor sleep increases the risk of school absenteeism. Further, research indicates that individuals who experience sleep problems tend to have poorer quality of life, poorer daily functioning, diminished caregiver mental health, and impaired family functioning (Sung, Hiscock, Sciberras, & Efron, 2008).

Another concern is the risk of sudden death associated with psychostimulant medication use. Gould et al. (2009) reported that, among children with ADHD who experienced unexplained or sudden death, the odds that stimulant medication was used were 6–7 times greater than the odds of dying in a vehicular accident. Excluded from this research study were children who experienced deaths of known causes, such as drug overdoses. Rather, the authors noted concerns associated with stimulant medications, such as increased heart rate and blood pressure (Gould et al., 2009).

In addition to health-related difficulties that children with ADHD personally experience, there are effects on the health of family members. For example, it is well established that the parents of children with ADHD are at risk for their own psychiatric problems, as well as marital discord and higher rates of marital separation and divorce. Further, these parents report they have less time to meet their own needs, fewer family activities, and diminished family cohesion (Klassen et al., 2004). Thus, from a health perspective, ADHD in children can place the entire family at risk.

8.2.2 Middle School and Adolescence

Health risks of ADHD that present in childhood often persist into adolescence. The specific outcomes may change (e.g., impulsivity can lead to accidental poisoning in childhood, but serious auto accidents during the teenage years). Unfortunately, new health problems tend to develop during adolescence. These include eating disorders, other psychiatric illnesses (e.g., depression), alcohol and drug use, unprotected sexual activity, self-injury, early mortality, and suicide (Cortese, Bernardina, & Mouren, 2007; James, Lei, & Dahl, 2004; Nigg, 2013). As with many of the health-related concerns that become problematic in childhood, many of the adolescent-emerging concerns may be a function of the primary symptoms of ADHD (i.e., inattention and hyperactivity/impulsivity).

In their review, Cortese et al. (2007) examined the relationship between ADHD and eating disorders and described a number of studies in which participants with ADHD were significantly more likely than others to binge eat and suffer bulimia. They hypothesized that impulsive and inattentive behavior that is common among those with ADHD may foster disordered eating patterns. Specifically, disinhibited behavior, combined with poor planning and executive functioning deficits, could lead to overconsumption and irregular eating patterns, thus placing youth with ADHD at increased risk for disorders involving binge eating.

As expected, vehicular operation is another risk to health during adolescence. Teens with ADHD are likely to have unsafe driving habits; they are issued more citations than typically developing adolescents and have more accidents (Barkley, Murphy, & Kwasnik, 1996). On average, 40 % of drivers with ADHD have had two serious accidents by the time they reach emerging adulthood, in contrast to 6 % of drivers without ADHD (Barkley, 2002). Again, inattention and impulsivity seem to contribute to unsafe driving habits. Indeed, studies involving computer-based driving simulators have shown that individuals with ADHD evince more scrapes and collisions, erratic steering, and poor steering control, compared to participants without ADHD. These driving errors may also be related to poor motor coordination and slower cognitive processing (Jerome, Segal, & Habinski, 2006).

Substance use is yet another concern that first emerges during adolescence. Lee, Humphreys, Flory, Liu, and Glass (2011) conducted a meta-analysis on the relationship between ADHD and substance use. They determined that adolescents and adults with childhood-onset ADHD were significantly more likely to use nicotine, alcohol, marijuana, cocaine, and other substances compared to those without ADHD. These risky behaviors were not moderated by sex, average age at follow-up, race, community versus clinic sample status, version of *DSM* used for diagnosis, or average length of time between initial contact and follow-up. Lee et al. (2011) asserted that childhood-onset ADHD strongly predicts later substance abuse. Further, August et al. (2006) found that adolescents with ADHD and comorbid ODD/CD reported significantly higher rates of tobacco, alcohol, and substance use than either control or ADHD-only groups. As stated earlier, comorbidity with other disorders (which is seen in approximately 70 % of children with ADHD) significantly increases health risks.

Adolescents with ADHD are also prone to difficulties in their romantic relationships that can lead to negative health outcomes. On average, teens with ADHD have earlier sexual debuts and more sexual partners compared to peers without ADHD (Barkley, 1998). Additionally, adolescents and adults with ADHD are less likely to use contraception. Not surprisingly, this failure to engage in safe sex leads to a higher rate of unplanned pregnancy and sexually transmitted infections (STIs). According to the *Milwaukee Young Adult Outcome Study*, adolescents with ADHD are four times more likely to have an STI and nine times more likely to become parents compared to adolescents without ADHD (Barkley, Fischer, Smallish, &

Fletcher, 2006). Sarver, McCart, Sheidow, and Letourno (2014) examined risky sexual behavior among 115 teens with ADHD, conduct problems, and substance use. Among those with conduct problems, the connection between ADHD and risky sexual behavior was fully mediated by marijuana use. For youth without elevated conduct problems, there was no association between ADHD and risky sexual behavior. It is clear that the numerous and varied health problems associated with ADHD are not independent but interact with and influence one another. Conduct problems in particular, such as ODD and CD, amplify the association between ADHD and risky sexual behavior through an increase in the use of drugs and alcohol. Thus, targeting even one issue (e.g., conduct problems, drug use, and/or alcohol use) could lead to reduction of other health-related risks among those with ADHD.

There are several health risks for adolescents with ADHD that are even more concerning than those previously discussed. Hinshaw et al. (2012) reported that female teens with ADHD are at elevated risk for self-injury and suicide attempts. They found this risk to be significantly higher among those with the ADHD-combined presentation (i.e., those who display both inattentive and hyperactive/impulsive behaviors) as opposed to the predominantly inattentive presentation (i.e., those who only display inattentive behaviors). Hinshaw et al. (2012) hypothesized that impulse-control problems would likely explain the higher rates of self-harm and suicide attempts. Similar studies examining the connection between ADHD and self-injury and suicide attempts found that individuals with ADHD are more likely to commit suicide (Impey & Heun, 2012; James et al., 2004), due in part to an elevated risk of depression (Chronis-Tuscano et al., 2010). Importantly, evidence suggests that severity of inattention rather than depression per se predicts the risk of suicide lethality among clinical samples of participants with depression (Keilp, Gorlyn, Oquendo, Burke, & Mann, 2008).

Finally, several researchers have determined that adolescents and young adults with ADHD are at risk for early mortality. Barkley (2002) hypothesized that impulsivity is the primary culprit. Poor impulse control, which is common among those with ADHD, is associated with cardiovascular disease, cancer, and shorter life expectancy. Similarly, Nigg (2013) suggested that early mortality might be due to elevated smoking, drug use, and accidents. Thus, it is important to note that the impairments commonly associated with ADHD are linked to numerous negative health outcomes, some of which are fatal.

As the primary focus of this chapter is on health-related concerns for children and adolescents with ADHD, little attention is given to the concerns that are most problematic in adulthood. It is important to note that ADHD continues into adulthood for a majority of cases and that adults with ADHD continue to experience negative outcomes including hypertension (Fuemmeler, Ostbye, Yang, McClernon, & Kollins, 2010) and comorbid anxiety and depression (Sobanski, 2006). Further, adults with ADHD experience many difficulties with employment; they are three times more likely to be fired from a job (Barkley, 2002) and change jobs at a rate of 2–3 times within a 10-year period (Barkley, 2002). These problems with employment can lead to lower socioeconomic status and poorer quality of life (de Graaf et al., 2008). Additionally, the health-related concerns that first emerge in childhood and adolescence also persist into adulthood. It is beyond the scope of this chapter to address prevention and intervention related to adults with ADHD, but it is anticipated that addressing negative health outcomes at an early age may help prevent subsequent health difficulties from developing.

8.3   Integrated, School-Based Frameworks to Address the Health Needs of Students with ADHD

As this chapter has described, students with ADHD are at greater risk than peers for co-occurring unhealthy behaviors such as substance abuse and sexual risk taking, plus outcomes such as self-injury and suicide. Treatment approaches to address the core ADHD symptoms of inattention and hyperactivity/impulsivity have been extensively investigated, with psychotropic medication and behavioral intervention strategies emerging as the most commonly used school-based interventions for this population (DuPaul & Stoner, 2014; Barkley et al., 2006). Less attention has been devoted to treating the health consequences of ADHD. Fortunately, a growing body of research demonstrates the effectiveness of a variety of evidence-based interventions (EBIs) that target health concerns relevant to this population. Although most of these interventions were not developed specifically for individuals with ADHD, they may be used as part of a comprehensive service delivery system to address a range of ADHD-related health problems.

Because many of the health risk behaviors associated with ADHD (injury, violence, substance use, unhealthy eating, and inadequate physical activity) begin in childhood and adolescence, schools can play a major role in preventing their initiation and intervening once they occur (CDC, 2014a, 2014b). Although a number of effective school-based programs have been developed to address a range of specific health risk behaviors, many school-based programs and services are uncoordinated and crisis oriented (Domitrovich et al., 2010; EDC, 2001; Fetro in Marx, Wooley, & Northrop, 1998). Furthermore, due to variations in state and local implementation of behavioral, mental, and other health-related EBIs, there is a lack of standardization in what schools provide for students and families. Schools are also challenged to sustain programs and ensure that appropriately trained professionals collaborate when utilizing the most promising EBIs (Becker & Domitrovich, 2011; Vitiello & Sherrill, 2007).

Trends have emerged demonstrating that *integrated* EBI service delivery provides schools a mechanism to blend health and behavioral programs into one service delivery model. "Integration can be both horizontal, occurring within risk levels, and vertical, integrating programs across levels" (Domitrovich et al., 2010, p. 74). Primary benefits of such integration include reduced duplication of services, student progress monitoring, and process evaluation for EBI implementation fidelity (Becker & Domitrovich, 2011). See Domitrovich et al. (2010) for a comprehensive review of the justification and benefits of the EBI integration model.

Addressing the health behavior risks and needs of students with ADHD may best be accomplished via vertical integration of two frameworks for school-based service delivery: coordinated school health (CSH) and multitiered systems of support (MTSS). The first framework, CSH, represents an approach to improving student health and learning by emphasizing the interrelationships among its components: comprehensive health education (e.g., PreK-12 classroom health instruction); health services (e.g., school nurse service provision); healthy school environment (e.g., sanitary physical environment and safe psychosocial environment); physical education; nutrition services; counseling, psychological, and social services; family and community involvement; and health promotion for staff (CDC, 2014c; Marx et al., 1998; Allensworth & Kolbe, 1987). The CSH model aims to improve children's health-related knowledge, attitudes, skills, and behaviors, resulting in better outcomes in the areas of health, education, and social functioning (Kolbe, 2002). Because many risk behaviors such as substance use, violence, and physical inactivity are linked with student disengagement and poor achievement (CDC, 2014d), the benefits of CSH should appeal to all school stakeholders, especially those addressing the needs of students with ADHD.

The second framework to be considered for vertical integration with CSH is called multitiered systems of support (MTSS) (American Institutes for Research, 2013). MTSS is a continuum of tiered support programs and services that are implemented with students at universal (Tier 1), selected (Tier 2), and indicated (Tier 3) levels. Most often implemented as response to intervention (RtI) (Fuchs & Fuchs, 2006) and Positive Behavior Intervention Support (PBIS) (Sugai & Horner, 2002), MTSS programs have demonstrated positive effects on student academic achievement (reading and literacy, specifically) and positive behavior. Due to the organized and data-driven prevention and intervention programs delivered as school-wide, classroom-based, small group, or individual strategies, MTSS provide a population-based structure in which specialized programs may be applied as needed.

Vertical integration of CSH and MTSS is best conceptualized through identifying target student health risk behaviors relevant to its most appropriate CSH component and the appropriate MTSS level. Domitrovich et al. (2010) offer several reasons vertical integration is needed: (1) single interventions may not adequately address multiple factors contributing to health risks among students; (2) integration maximizes student exposure to prevention and intervention programs; (3) fusing strategies may provide synergy among complementary program elements; and (4) integration increases program and professional efficiency and sustainability. Such benefits to all school stakeholders provide incentive to consider vertical integration.

As previously suggested, the ADHD hallmark characteristics of inattention and hyperactivity/impulsivity increase the risk that students with ADHD disproportionately suffer negative health outcomes across the lifespan. However, school and mental health professionals can collaborate to help these compensate by learning health behaviors, plus knowledge, skills, and attitudes that may reduce their health risk.

As an example of how a vertically integrated, school health program might work, consider a second-grade male student with ADHD who is experiencing a high degree of peer rejection due to his aggressive behavior. The student's aggression and disturbed peer relations place him at risk for a variety of negative health outcomes including physical injury, substance use, subsequent depression, and suicide.

Under a vertically integrated school health program, the student would likely experience a universal (MTSS, Tier 1) health education curriculum in his classroom addressing a range of health risk behaviors and social-emotional skills. Such instruction is designed to benefit all students, but may be especially helpful for students with peer difficulties related to ADHD. Through collaboration between family and classroom teacher, the student may also be referred by counseling/psychological and social services (CSH component) to an after-school program where he could receive a selective (MTSS, Tier 2) EBI emphasizing relationship skills and anger/conflict management. If the student's daily social and academic functioning improves with these Tier 1 and Tier 2 supports, no indicated (Tier 3) EBI would be necessary, but if his problems persist, he would be referred for more intensive services.

Many specific EBIs for universal, selected, and indicated levels exist that address the health consequences and correlates that disproportionately affect students with ADHD. Vertical integration is offered as a perspective in which to view the range of distinct universal, selected, and indicated EBIs presented in the next section. However, it is important to note that there are many searchable registries that include a range of health-related, evidence-based programs to address health issues such as substance abuse, violence prevention, and emotional and social competence. Most accommodate delineated searches with a range of participant characteristics or outcome needs. Many registries are supported by federal agencies or other research-based organizations. Programs are often scored with rating levels based on evidence of effectiveness for specific criteria. These registries are useful for professionals or organizations attempting to find appropriate programs for implementation or to support program modification. Although not an exhaustive list, several prominent program registries are described.

The Substance Abuse and Mental Health Services Administration (SAMHSA) operates the National Registry of Evidence-based Programs and Practices (NREPP). It contains more than 300 evidence-based substance abuse and mental health programs and interventions searchable by a wide range of participant or program characteristics (see http://www.nrepp.samhsa.gov/ for more information). Similarly, *Blueprints for Healthy Youth Development* is a searchable database operated by the Center for the Study and Prevention of Violence at the University of Colorado, Boulder. With rigorous scientific standards for establishing program effectiveness (evaluation quality, intervention impact, intervention specificity, and dissemination readiness), programs are categorized as promising or model programs. *Blueprints* has reviewed more than 1200 youth development programs. See http://www.blueprintsprograms.com/ for more information.

8.4   Prevention and Intervention Programs that Address Health Risk Behaviors Among Those with ADHD

Many aspects of effective learning and behavior management strategies that address health risk behaviors manifested by students with ADHD mirror foundational concepts and goals within a CSH approach. The remainder of the chapter highlights examples of EBIs that have successfully addressed the health risk behaviors and health outcomes that were previously attributed to children and teens with ADHD. Even so, there is no known health-related prevention or intervention program designed explicitly for those with ADHD. Table 8.1 denotes each EBI's tier or implementation level as well as the CSH component(s) with which it closely aligns.

Table 8.1 Evidence-based prevention and intervention program aligns with coordinated school health component and tier levels

CSH component	Tier I	Tier II	Tier III
Comprehensive health education	PY/PM	Be Proud Be Responsible	Project Towards No Drug Abuse
	Be Proud Be Responsible		
	Michigan Model for Health		
	Positive Action		
	LifeLines		
	Project Towards No Drug		
	Abuse		
	Fourth R		
	Life Skills		
	LEADS		
Health services			
Healthy school environment	Universal social and emotional learning		
	SANKOFA		
	PY/PM		
	Positive Action		
	Fourth R		
Physical education	Planet Health		Bright Bodies Weight Management
Nutrition services			Bright Bodies Weight Management
Counseling, psychological and social services	Universal social and emotional learning	Incredible Years	Incredible Years
	SANKOFA	Project Towards No Drug Abuse	MST
	Positive Action	CAST	Project Towards No Drug Abuse
	Fourth R		CAST
	Project Towards No Drug Abuse		
	LifeLines		
Family and community involvement		Incredible Years	Incredible Years
			MST
Health promotion for staff			

8.4.1 Social and Emotional Learning and Comprehensive Health Education

It was asserted at the Surgeon General's Conference on Children's Mental Health: "Mental health is a critical component of children's learning and general health. Fostering social and emotional health in children as part of healthy child development must therefore be a national priority" (US Public Health Service, 2000, p. 3). It is unfortunate, however, that as Hoagwood et al. (2007) note, "From a scientific standpoint, the mental health program and educational achievement knowledge bases have arisen in significant isolation from each other" (p. 66).

Recent advances in the field of social and emotional learning (SEL) have begun to bridge gaps between educational programming and mental and physical health. School professionals are increasingly using universal (Tier 1) SEL programs to improve their students' social and emotional skills, academic achievement, and healthy behaviors. SEL integrates "competence promotion and youth development frameworks" (Durlak, Weissberg, Dymnicki, Taylor, & Schellinger, 2011, p. 2) to address risk and protective factors of particular relevance to youth with ADHD, influencing such areas as self-management and self-regulation, responsible decision-making, and social competence. These skills, in turn, have been linked to reductions in aggression, emotional and behavior problems, and—in some cases—lower rates of risky behaviors such as substance use and sexual risk taking. Although these interventions do not target children with ADHD specifically, they facilitate schools' efforts to promote emotional, behavioral, and social skills that are directly related to the key health concerns of this population.

Whereas universal SEL programs are designed to address health-related needs of all students, teachers can also utilize behavioral, self-regulatory, and social relationship intervention strategies with students who exhibit hallmark characteristics of ADHD. For example, to address a student's impaired ability to delay responding to the environmental stimuli, teachers may use appropriate antecedent- consequence-based strategies by posting classroom rules for students to see and review them regularly (antecedent) and overtly praise students when they follow the rules (consequence). Such actions help to create school contexts that support adaptive behavior among children with ADHD (see DuPaul, Weyandt, & Janusis, 2011).

8.4.2 Healthy Eating

Because of the association between ADHD and childhood obesity (see Cortese & Vincenzi, 2012), programs that focus on healthy eating may be indicated. For example, *Planet Health* is a 2-year, school-based, universal (Tier 8.1) EBI for youth ages

12–14 years. The program is designed to increase student caloric expenditure and encourages greater intake of fruits, vegetables, and grains as well as reducing sugar and saturated fat intake. Whereas Gortmaker et al. (1999) found no impact on boys, but it was significant for girls who received this school-based intervention compared to those who did not. This finding is consistent with results from a meta-analysis of school-based interventions targeting obesogenic behaviors and obesity, itself. Girls seem to benefit more than boys from school-based physical activity EBIs (Safron et al., 2011).

Another obesity-related EBI is *Bright Bodies Weight Management*. It is an indicated or Tier 3, 12-month weight management program for obese urban youth ages 5–18. Administered in a clinic or family-based setting, program participants receive nutrition education and engage in behavior modification and exercise to ameliorate obesity and related chronic health problems. Results have revealed that among other positive outcomes, including reduction in total cholesterol (Savoye et al., 2007), participants evinced a 4 % reduction in adiposity and maintained it 12 months after the EBI was over (Savoye et al., 2011).

8.4.3 Injury Prevention, Prosocial Relationships, and Violence

The role of risk factors for child injury has been categorized into three factors, including temperament, estimation of risk in the environment, and parenting (Schwebel & Barton, 2005). Temperament is defined as the child's behavioral style, similar to the concept of personality (Chen & Schmidt, 2015). Studies in this area consistently indicate that aggressive, oppositional, and overactive plus impulsive and under-controlled behavioral styles predict greater risk of unintentional injuries. These characteristics are frequently attributed to those with ADHD. Anecdotally, many parents describe their children with ADHD as "accident prone." Additionally, a child's ability to estimate the level of risk in a given situation (e.g., chasing a ball into the street without looking for traffic) has been shown to impact risk for injury.

It is well established that ADHD and conduct disorder co-occur at a very high rate (Waschbusch, 2002). As such, programs designed to address violence prevention are relevant for many children (especially boys) who present with ADHD. *SANKOFA Youth Violence Prevention Program*—SANKOFA (a word of African origin meaning "to look back in order to move forward")—is a culturally specific, universal (Tier 1) school- or community-based intervention for adolescents aged 13–17 by addressing a range of antisocial behaviors. Quasi-experimental effectiveness studies indicate a reduction in fighting and bullying behaviors, violence-related bystander behavior, and personal victimization at 12-month follow-up after intervention termination (Hines, Vega, & Jemmott, 2004).

Protecting You/Protecting Me (PY/PM) is a 5-year classroom-based, universal (Tier 1) alcohol and vehicle safety program for students in grades 1–5. Although not designed specifically for children and teens with ADHD, many of these students would be needy candidates for such a program. High school students in grades

11–12 may participate in a training program to become mentors to program participants in grades 1–5. *PY/PM* focuses on brain development and how to protect the brain, vehicle safety and emphasizing how to be safe if having to ride with someone who is not alcohol free, and life skills such as decision-making and refusal communication. Among other key findings, results from experimental research demonstrate that *PY/PM* does increase student knowledge and skills related to vehicle safety and the dangers of underage alcohol use (Bell, Padget, Kelley-Baker, & Rider, 2007; Bell, Kelley-Baker, Rider, & Ringwalt, 2005).

Incredible Years® Child Treatment is a well-established selected or indicated (Tier 2 or 3) EBI for children ages 3–11. Administered in small group sessions by therapists or counselors, participants included are those with ADHD, conduct problems, and internalizing issues. *Incredible Years*® has two complementary programs for parents and teachers that address child social skills, conflict resolution, empathy building, problem-solving, and cooperation. These are areas of concern for many children with ADHD. An examination of the school-based *Incredible Years*® treatment program revealed that children whose teachers dispensed the program showed significant improvement in emotional self-regulation and social competence compared to students whose teachers did not participate (Webster-Stratton, Reid, & Stoolmiller, 2009).

Multisystemic Therapy® *(MST*®*)* is an indicated (Tier 3) level EBI for children and youth struggling with serious antisocial behavior contributing to, among other things, criminal activity. Surely, teens with ADHD are viable candidates for such a program because of the high potential presence of comorbid conduct disorder, and it correlates. *MST*® is a community-based, intensive family and adolescent (12–18) treatment that is provided by a master's level therapist. *MST*® uses an ecological perspective to address family, peer, school, and neighborhood structures and factors that contribute to antisocial behavior and other clinical issues (such as substance abuse). *MST*® focuses on improving family relationships (including parenting competency) and developing positive social support networks. *MST*® is designed to be cost effective by reducing the use of hospitalization, residential treatment, and incarceration. Strategic family therapy, structural family therapy, behavioral parent training, and cognitive behavioral therapy treatment approaches are all utilized. *MST*® has been extensively evaluated in efficacy studies that demonstrate a range of positive outcomes. See www.blueprintsprograms.com for a comprehensive reference list.

8.4.4   Substance Use and Sexual Risk Taking

Teens with ADHD are clearly at risk for substance abuse (see Lee et al., 2011) as well as unprotected sex because of co-occurring conduct disorder. Research has identified a number of antecedents to substance use among adolescents. These include aggressiveness, behavioral problems, poor academic performance, and involvement with deviant peers (Poikolainen, 2002). Substance abuse has also been found to co-occur with mood disorders, including major depression (Hovens,

Cantwell, & Kiriakos, 1994; Rohde, Lewinsohn, & Seeley, 1996). Evidence-based prevention and intervention programs have been designed to address these antecedents and support protective factors. As such, a number of school-based EBIs often focus on a variety of behaviors that contribute to student health risks and favorable outcomes. Program designs vary, addressing needs by grade level, geographic setting, or priority at-risk populations.

Positive Action is a well-established universal (Tier 1) EBI. It addresses school climate change and individual student behavior through a classroom curriculum for students aged 5–14. The curriculum teaches students how to engage in positive actions related to physical, intellectual, social, and emotional health, including many aspects of personal behavior (i.e., self-concept, managing self-responsibility, and interpersonal skills). *Positive Action* has scripted lessons organized into six units for each grade level and has substantial evidence of success in violence prevention and illicit drug and alcohol use prevention (Flay, Allred, & Ordway, 2001).

Fourth R: Skills for Youth Relationships is a universal (Tier 1), evidence-based intervention for students between 13 and 17 years old. It promotes healthy and safe behaviors related to dating, bullying, sexuality, and substance use. Experimental research studies have demonstrated reduced physical dating violence and increased condom use 2.5 years after program participation (Crooks, Scott, Ellis, & Wolfe, 2011; Wolfe et al., 2009).

Life Skills Training program is a well-established, universal school-based EBI for middle school students (ages 12–14). Prevention of tobacco, illegal drug and alcohol use, risky driving, HIV/AIDS-related risky behaviors, and violence are all emphasized. This comprehensive program is designed to increase confidence and skills needed to successfully respond to difficult circumstances by focusing one's self-management, social skills, and peer resistance to drug use. Evaluation studies demonstrate both short- and long-term effectiveness up to 10 years (Botvin, Baker, Dusenbury, Botvin, & Diaz, 1995).

Project Towards No Drug Abuse can function as a universal, selected, or indicated substance abuse prevention program for students ages 15–19. Whereas *Project Towards No Drug Abuse* was originally developed for high-risk youth attending alternative high schools, this EBI has been adapted to accommodate the needs of all students. Communication and decision-making skills are emphasized to support resistance to drug use. Multiple program effectiveness studies demonstrate participants' reduced risk of alcohol, tobacco, or illicit drug use, reduced risk of victimization, and reduced weapon carrying (Sun, Skara, Sun, Dent, & Sussman, 2006; Sussman, Sun, McCuller, & Dent, 2003).

Be Proud Be Responsible is a universal or selected EBI primarily addressing the needs of students ages 11–19 living in urban, low socioeconomic environments. *Be Proud Be Responsible* can be implemented as part of a school health curriculum or as small group sessions. Emphasis is placed on skill building to help students develop the self-efficacy necessary to avoid high-risk sexual behavior. Strongest evaluation studies reveal reduced rates of unprotected intercourse, increased rates of condom use, and reduced rates of STIs among participants (Jemmott, Jemmott, Braverman, & Fong, 2005; Jemmott, Jemmott, & Fong, 1998).

8.4.5 Self-Injury and Suicide

Given that adolescents (especially females) with ADHD are at risk for negative affect and depression (Hinshaw et al., 2012), teen suicide is a compelling concern. Suicide is the leading cause of death among youth ages 15–19 years. Ideation and suicide attempts expand the breadth of concern for those at risk. In addition, deliberate self-harm may be an antecedent behavior to suicide and suicide ideation (Chapman & Dixon-Gordon, 2007). Suicidal behaviors are negatively associated with school performance and attendance. Co-occurring risk factors such as depression plus drug use have been found to increase the likelihood of suicide (Thompson, Eggert, Randell, & Pike, 2001).

LifeLines is a universal, school-based suicide-prevention program for students aged 12–18. Quasi-experimental study results show that *LifeLines* participants had an increase in knowledge regarding the facts about suicide and participant beliefs about the inevitability of suicide or the appropriateness of suicide intervention and seeking help. Additionally, friends' thoughts about keeping suicide a secret were changed (Kalafat, Madden, Haley, & O'Halloran, 2007).

LEADS: For Youth (Linking Education and Awareness of Depression and Suicide) is a high school curriculum designed to increase knowledge of depression and suicide, improve knowledge about prevention resources, influence one's perception of depression and suicide, and improve intentions to seek help. A quasi-experimental design was used to evaluate changes in youths' knowledge and perceptions of depression and suicide among students who received the *LEADS* curriculum as opposed to students who did not. Students in the treatment group were more knowledgeable and more likely to agree that depression is a mental illness than students in the comparison group (Leite, Idzelis, Reidenberg, Roggenbaum, & LeBlanc, 2011).

CAST (Coping and Support Training) is a selected and indicated school-based suicide-prevention program for students ages 14–19. *CAST* is a skill-based and social support program delivered in small group sessions. Students who are screened and identified with significant suicide risk may be referred to *CAST* as an indicted level program. Effectiveness study results revealed that CAST participants, compared to *usual care* control group participants at risk for suicide, demonstrated decreased anger, anxiety, hopelessness, and feelings of depression (Eggert, Thompson, Randell, & Pike, 2002). *CAST* has also been shown to enhance and sustain personal control and problem-solving coping in adolescents (Thompson et al., 2001).

8.5 Conclusion

With the latest iteration of the *Diagnostic and Statistical Manual of Mental Disorders,* 5th Edition (APA, 2013), categorizing ADHD among other neurodevelopmental disorders, as opposed to disruptive behavior disorders, those experts who drafted the taxonomy demonstrated their recognition of genetic and biological correlates and sequelae of ADHD. This shift in focus acknowledges that ADHD is a complex disorder; a focus on the behavioral components of ADHD is insufficient in providing the comprehensive help these children need. By focusing on disruptive behaviors only, we neglect the very real and well-documented health problems that are common among children with ADHD. These health concerns vary based on age of the child, but include accidental injuries, obesity, and risky sexual behaviors, plus nicotine, alcohol and illegal drug use, and even early mortality.

Even though health issues among children with ADHD have received limited research attention, they may be more concerning than the behavioral and academic difficulties that are well established in the research literature. Although these health issues have been long neglected, there is substantial research on prevention and intervention programs that can be used to address these concerns. By integrating two school-based service delivery frameworks (coordinated school health and multi-tiered systems of support), we can apply knowledge and resources already amassed to address the health problems experienced by children with ADHD. When schools provide high-quality, evidence-based health and physical education curricula and SEL to all students, they lay the foundation for preventing aggression, risky behavior, and peer relation difficulties and for promoting healthy choices related to diet and physical activity. Vertical integration of these services with selected and indicated EBIs targeting specific areas of health risk, such as substance use, suicide, sexual risk taking, and obesity, will more adequately address the manifold factors that contribute to health problems among those with ADHD and will increase program efficiency and sustainability.

References

Allensworth, D. D., & Kolbe, L. J. (1987). The comprehensive school health program: Exploring an expanded concept. *Journal of School Health, 57*, 409–412. doi:10.1111/j.1746-1561.1987. tb03183.x.

American Institutes for Research. (2013). *What is RTI?* Retrieved from http://www.rti4success. org/whatisrti.

American Psychiatric Association. (1980). *Diagnostic and statistical manual of mental disorders* (3rd ed.). Washington, DC: Author.

American Psychiatric Association. (2013). *Diagnostic and statistical manual of mental disorders* (5th ed.). Arlington, VA: Author.

August, G. J., Winters, K. C., Realmuto, G. M., Fahnhorst, T., Botzet, A., & Lee, S. (2006). Prospective study of adolescent drug use among community samples of ADHD and non-ADHD participants. *Journal of the American Academy of Child and Adolescent Psychiatry, 45*, 824–832. doi:10.1097/01.chi.0000219831.16226.f8.

Barkley, R. A. (1997). Behavioral inhibition, sustained attention, and executive functions: Constructing a unifying theory of ADHD. *Psychological Bulletin, 121*, 65–94. doi:10.1037/0033-2909.121.1.65.

Barkley, R. A. (1998). *Attention-deficit hyperactivity disorder: A handbook for diagnosis and treatment.* New York, NY: Guilford Press.

Barkley, R. A. (2001). Accidents and ADHD. *Economic Neuroscience, 3*, 64–68.

Barkley, R. A. (2002). Major life activity and health outcomes associated with attention-deficit/ hyperactivity disorder. *The Journal of Clinical Psychiatry, 63*, 10–15.

Barkley, R. A., Fischer, M., Smallish, L., & Fletcher, K. (2006). Young adult outcome of hyperactive children: Adaptive functioning in major life activities. *Journal of the American Academy of Child and Adolescent Psychiatry, 49*, 503–513. doi:10.1097/01.chi.0000189134.97436.e2.

Barkley, R. A., Murphy, K. R., & Kwasnik, D. (1996). Motor vehicle driving competencies and risks in teens and young adults with attention deficit hyperactivity disorder. *Pediatrics, 6*, 1089–1095.

Becker, K. D., & Domitrovich, C. E. (2011). The conceptualization, integration, and support of evidence-based interventions in the schools. *School Psychology Review, 40*, 582–589.

Bell, M., Kelley-Baker, T., Rider, R., & Ringwalt, C. (2005). Protecting you/protecting me: Effects of an alcohol prevention and vehicle safety program on elementary students. *Journal of School Health, 75*, 171–177. doi:10.1111/j.1746-1561.2005.tb06667.x.

Bell, M. L., Padget, A., Kelley-Baker, T., & Rider, R. (2007). Can first and second grade students benefit from an alcohol use prevention program? *Journal of Child and Adolescent Substance Use, 16*, 89–107. doi:10.1300/J029v16n03_05.

Botvin, G. J., Baker, E., Dusenbury, L., Botvin, E. M., & Diaz, T. (1995). Long-term follow-up results of a randomized drug abuse prevention trial in a white middle-class population. *Journal of the American Medical Association, 273*, 1106–1112. doi:10.1001/jama.1995.03520380042033.

Centers for Disease Control and Prevention (CDC). (2014a). *Youth risk behavior surveillance system*. Retrieved from http://www.cdc.gov/healthyyouth/yrbs/index.htm.

Centers for Disease Control and Prevention (CDC). (2014b). Youth risk behavior surveillance — United States, 2013. *Morbidity and Mortality Weekly Report, 63*, 1–168.

Centers for Disease Control and Prevention (CDC). (2014c). Components of coordinated school health. Retrieved from http://www.cdc.gov/healthyyouth/cshp/components.htm.

Chan, E., Zhan, C., & Homer, C. J. (2002). Health care use and costs for children with attention-deficit/hyperactivity disorder: National estimates from the medical expenditure survey. *Archives of Pediatrics and Adolescent Medicine, 156*, 504–511. doi:10.1001/archpedi.156.5.504.

Chapman, A. L., & Dixon-Gordon, K. L. (2007). Emotional antecedents and consequences of deliberate self-harm and suicide attempts. *Suicide & Life-Threatening Behavior, 37*, 543–552. doi:10.1521/suli.2007.37.5.543.

Chen, X., & Schmidt, L. A. (2015). Temperament and personality development. In R. Lerner (Ed.), *Handbook of child psychology and developmental science* (Social and emotional development 7th ed., Vol. 3). Hoboken, NJ: Wiley.

Chronis-Tuscano, A., Molina, B. S., Pelham, W. E., Applegate, B., Dahlke, A., Overmyer, M., & Lahey, B. B. (2010). Very early predictors of adolescent depression and suicide attempts in children with attention-deficit/hyperactivity disorder. *Archives of General Psychiatry, 67*, 1044–1051. doi:10.1001/archgenpsychiatry.2010.127.

Coie, J. D., Watt, N. F., West, S. G., Hawkins, J. D., Asarnow, J. R., Markman, H. J. … Long, B. (1993). The science of prevention: A conceptual framework and some directions for a national research program. *American Psychologist, 48*, 1013–1022. doi:10.1037/0003-066X.48.10.1013.

Cortese, S., Bernardina, B. D., & Mouren, M. (2007). Attention-deficit/hyperactivity disorder and binge eating. *Nutrition Reviews, 65*, 404–411. doi:10.1097/YPG.0b013e3283539604.

Cortese, S., & Vincenzi, B. (2012). Obesity and ADHD: Clinical and neurobiological implications. *Current Topics in Behavioral Neurosciences, 9*, 199–218. doi:10.1007/7854_2011_154.

Crooks, C. V., Scott, K., Ellis, W., & Wolfe, D. A. (2011). Impact of a universal school-based violence prevention program on violent delinquency: Distinctive benefits for youth with maltreatment histories. *Child Abuse and Neglect, 35*, 393–400. doi:10.1016/j.chiabu.2011.03.002.

de Graaf, R., Kessler, R.C., Fayyad, J., ten Have, M., Alonso, J., Angermeyer, M., … Posada-Villa, J. (2008). The prevalence and effects of adult attention-deficit/hyperactivity disorder (ADHD) on the performance of workers: Results from the WHO World Mental Health Survey Initiative. *Occupational and Environmental Medicine, 65*, 835–842. doi:10.1097/01.jom.0000166863.33541.39

Domitrovich, C. E., Bradshaw, C. P., Greenberg, M. T., Embry, D., Poduska, J. M., & Ialongo, N. S. (2010). Integrated models of school-based prevention: Logic and theory. *Psychology in the Schools, 47*, 71–88. doi:10.1002/pits.20452.

DuPaul, G. J., & Stoner, G. (2014). *ADHD in the schools: Assessment and intervention strategies* (3rd ed.). New York: The Guilford Press.

DuPaul, G. J., Weyandt, L. L., & Janusis, G. M. (2011). ADHD in the classroom: Effective Intervention strategies. *Theory Into Practice, 50*, 35–42. doi:10.1080/00405841.2011.534935.

Durlak, J. A., Weissberg, R. P., Dymnicki, A. B., Taylor, R. D., & Schellinger, K. B. (2011). The impact of enhancing students' social and emotional learning: A meta-analysis of school-based universal interventions. *Child Development, 82*, 405–432.

EDC (2001). An example of an uncoordinated system. Retrieved from http://www2.edc.org/makinghealthacademic/cshp.asp.

Eggert, L. L., Thompson, E. A., Randell, B. P., & Pike, K. C. (2002). Preliminary effects of brief school-based prevention approaches for reducing youth suicide: Risk behaviors, depression, and drug involvement. *Journal of Child and Adolescent Psychiatric Nursing, 15*, 48–64. doi:10.1111/j.1744-6171.2002.tb00326.x.

Flay, B. R., Allred, C. G., & Ordway, N. (2001). Effects of the Positive Action program on achievement and discipline: Two matched-control comparisons. *Prevention Science, 2*, 71–89.

Fuchs, D., & Fuchs, L. (2006). Introduction to response to intervention: What, why, and how valid is it? *Reading Research Quarterly, 41*, 93–99.

Fuemmeler, B. F., Ostbye, T., Yang, C., McClernon, F. J., & Kollins, S. H. (2010). Association between attention-deficit/hyperactivity disorder symptoms and obesity and hypertension in early adulthood: A population-based study. *International Journal of Obesity, 35*, 852–862. doi:10.1038/ijo.2010.214.

Gortmaker, S., Peterson, K., Wiecha, J., Sobol, A., Dixit, S., Fox, M., & Laird, N. (1999). Reducing obesity via a school-based interdisciplinary intervention among youth. *Archives of Pediatric & Adolescent Medicine, 153*, 409–418. doi:10.1001/archpedi.153.4.409.

Gould, M. S., et al. (2009). Sudden death and use of stimulant medication in youths. *The American Journal of Psychiatry, 166*, 992–1001. doi:10.1176/appi.ajp.2009.09040472.

Harvey, W. J., & Reid, G. (1997). Motor performance of children with attention-deficit hyperactivity disorder: A preliminary investigation. *Adapted Physical Activity Quarterly, 14*, 189–202.

Hines, P. M., Vega, W., & Jemmott, J. (2004). Final report: A culture based model for youth violence risk-reduction. Unpublished manuscript.

Hinshaw, S. P., Owens, E. B., Zalecki, C., Huggins, S. P., Montenegro-Nevado, A. J., Schrodek, E., Swanson, E. N. (2012). Prospective follow-up of girls with attention-deficit/hyperactivity disorder into early adulthood: Continuing impairment include elevated risk for suicide attempts and self-injury. *Journal of Consulting and Clinical Psychology, 80*, 1041–1051. doi:10.1037/a0029451.

Hoagwood, K. E., Olin, S. S., Kerker, B. D., Kratochwill, R. T., Crowe, M., & Sake, N. (2007). Empirically based school interventions targeted at academic and mental health functioning. *Journal of Emotional and Behavioral Disorders, 15*, 66–92. doi:10.1177/10634266070150020301.

Hovens, J. G., Cantwell, D. P., & Kiriakos, R. (1994). Psychiatric comorbidity in hospitalized adolescent substance abusers. *Journal of the American Academy of Child and Adolescent Psychiatry, 33*, 476–483.

Impey, M., & Heun, R. (2012). Completed suicide, ideation, and attempt in attention deficit hyperactivity disorder. *Acta Psychiatrica Scandinavica, 125*, 93–102. doi:10.1111/j.1600-0447.2011.01798.x.

James, A., Lei, F. H., & Dahl, C. (2004). Attention deficit hyperactivity disorder and suicide: A review of possible associations. *Acta Psychiatrica Scandinavica, 110*, 408–415. doi:10.1111/j.1600-0447.2004.00384.x.

Jemmott, J. B., III, Jemmott, L. S., Braverman, P. K., & Fong, G. T. (2005). HIV/STD risk reduction interventions for African American and Latino adolescent girls at an adolescent medicine clinic: A randomized controlled trial. *Archives of Pediatric Adolescent Medicine, 159*, 440–449. doi:10.1001/archpedi.159.5.440.

Jemmott, J. B., Jemmott, L. S., & Fong, G. T. (1998). Abstinence and safer sex HIV risk-reduction interventions for African American adolescents. *Journal of the American Medical Association, 279*, 1529–1536. doi:10.1001/jama.279.19.1529.

Jerome, L., Segal, A., & Habinski, L. (2006). What we know about ADHD and driving risk: A literature review, meta-analysis, and critique. *Journal of the Canadian Academy of Child and Adolescent Psychiatry, 15*, 105–125.

Kalafat, J., Madden, M., Haley, D., & O'Halloran, S. (2007). Evaluation of Lifelines classes: A component of the school-community based Maine Youth Suicide Prevention Project. Report for NREPP. Unpublished manuscript.

Keilp, J. G., Gorlyn, M., Oquendo, M. A., Burke, A. K., & Mann, J. J. (2008). Attention deficit in depressed suicide attempters. *Psychiatry Research, 159*, 7–17. doi:10.1016/j.psychres.2007.08.020.

Klassen, A. F., Miller, A., & Fine, S. (2004). Health-related quality of life in children and adolescents who have a diagnosis of Attention-Deficit/Hyperactivity Disorder. *Pediatrics, 114*, 541–548. doi:10.1542/peds.2004-0844.

Kolbe, L. (2002). Education reform and the goals of modern school health programs. *The State Education Standard, 3*, 4–11.

Lee, S. S., Humphreys, K. L., Flory, K., Liu, R., & Glass, K. (2011). Prospective association of childhood attention-deficit/hyperactivity disorder (ADHD) and substance use and abuse/dependence: A meta-analytic review. *Clinical Psychology Review, 31*, 328–341. doi:10.1016/j.cpr.2011.01.006.

Leite, A., Idzelis, M., Reidenberg, D., Roggenbaum, S., & LeBlanc, A. (2011). *Linking Education and Awareness of Depression and Suicide (LEADS): An evaluation of a school-based suicide prevention curriculum for high school youth*. St. Paul, MN: Wilder Research.

Marx, E., Wooley, S. F., & Northrop, D. (Eds.). (1998). *Health is academic: A guide to coordinated school health programs*. New York: Teacher's College Press.

Nigg, J. T. (2013). Attention-deficit/hyperactivity disorder and adverse health outcomes. *Clinical Psychology Review, 33*, 215–228. doi:10.1016/j.cpr.2012.11.005.

Owens, J. A. (2005). The ADHD and sleep conundrum: A review. *Journal of Developmental Behavioral Pediatrics, 26*, 312–322. doi:10.1097/00004703-200508000-00011.

Poikolainen, K. (2002). Antecedents of substance use in adolescence. *Current Opinion in Psychiatry, 15*, 241–245. doi:10.1097/00001504-200205000-00003.

Rafalovich, A. (2001). The conceptual history of attention deficit hyperactivity disorder: Idiocy, imbecility, encephalitis and the child deviant, 1877–1929. *Deviant Behavior: An Interdisciplinary Journal, 22*, 93–115. doi:10.1080/016396201750065009.

Rohde, P., Lewinsohn, P. M., & Seeley, J. R. (1996). Psychiatric comorbidity with problematic alcohol use in high school students. *Journal of the American Academy of Child & Adolescent Psychiatry, 35*, 101–110.

Ronk, M. J., Hund, A. M., & Landau, S. (2011). Assessment of social competence of boys with attention-deficit/hyperactivity disorder: Problematic peer entry, host responses, and evaluations. *Journal of Abnormal Child Psychology, 39*, 829–840. doi:10.1007/s10802-011-9497-3.

Rutter, M., & Sroufe, L. A. (2000). Developmental psychopathology: Concepts and challenges. *Development and Psychopathology, 12*, 265–295. doi:10.1017/S0954579400003023.

Safron, M. Cislak, A. Gaspar, T. & Luszczynska, A. (2011). Effects of school-based interventions targeting obesity-related behaviors and body weight change: A Systematic umbrella review. *Behavioral Medicine, 37*, 15–25. doi:10.1080/08964289.2010.543194.

Sarver, D. E., McCart, M. R., Sheidow, A. J., & Letourno, E. J. (2014). ADHD and risky sexual behavior in adolescents: Conduct problems and substance use as mediators of risk. *Journal of Child Psychology and Psychiatry, 55*(12), 1345–1353. doi:10.1111/jcpp.12249.

Savoye, M., Nowicka, P., Shaw, M., Yu, S., Dziura, J., Chavent, G. … Caprio, S. (2011). Long-term results of an obesity program in an ethnically diverse pediatric population. *Pediatrics, 127*, 1-9. doi: 10.1542/peds.2010-0697.

Savoye, M., Shaw, M., Dziura, J., Tamborlane, W., Rose, P., Guandalini, C. … Caprio, S. (2007). Effects of a weight management program on body composition and metabolic parameters in overweight children: a randomized control trial. *Journal of the American Medical Association, 297*, 2697-2704. doi:10.1001/jama.297.24.2697.

Schwebel, D. C., & Barton, B. K. (2005). Contributions of multiple risk factors to child injury. *Journal of Pediatric Psychology, 30*, 553–561. doi:10.1093/jpepsy/jsi042.

Sobanski, E. (2006). Psychiatric comorbidity in adults with attention-deficit/hyperactivity disorder (ADHD). *European Archives of Psychiatry and Clinical Neuroscience, 256*, 26–31. doi:10.1007/s00406-006-1004-4.

Sugai, G., & Horner, R. H. (2002). Introduction to the special series on positive behavior support in schools. *Journal of Emotional and Behavioral Disorders, 10*, 130–135.

Sun, W., Skara, S., Sun, P., Dent, C. W., & Sussman, S. (2006). Project Towards No Drug Abuse: Long-term substance use outcomes evaluation. *Preventive Medicine, 42*, 188–192. doi:10.1016/j.ypmed.2005.11.011.

Sung, V., Hiscock, H., Sciberras, E., & Efron, D. (2008). Sleep problems in children with attention-deficit/hyperactivity disorder: Prevalence and the effect on the child and family. *Archives of Pediatrics & Adolescent Medicine, 162*, 336–342. doi:10.1001/archpedi.162.4.336.

Sussman, S., Sun, P., McCuller, W. J., & Dent, C. W. (2003). Project Towards No Drug Abuse: Two-year outcomes of a trial that compares health educator delivery to self-instruction. *Preventive Medicine, 37*, 155–162. doi:10.1016/S0091-7435(03)00108-7.

Thompson, E. A., Eggert, L. L., Randell, B. P., & Pike, K. C. (2001). Evaluation of indicated suicide risk prevention approaches for potential high school dropouts. *American Journal of Public Health, 91*, 742–752. doi:10.2105/AJPH.91.5.742.

United States Department of Health and Human Services (USDHHS), United States Department of Education (USDOE), & United States Department of Justice (USDOJ). (2000). *Report of the Surgeon General's Conference on Children's Mental Health: A National Action Agenda*. Washington, DC: Author.

Vilensky, J. A., Foley, P., & Gilman, S. (2007). Children and encephalitis lethargica: A historical review. *Pediatric Neurology, 37*, 79–84. doi:10.1016/j.pediatrneurol.2007.04.012.

Vitiello, B., & Sherrill, J. (2007). School-based interventions for students with attention deficit hyperactivity disorder: Research implications and prospects. *School Psychology Review, 36*, 287–290.

Waschbusch, D. A. (2002). A meta-analytic examination of comorbid hyperactive-impulsive-attention problems and conduct problems. *Psychological Bulletin, 128*, 118–150. doi:10.1037/0033-2909.128.1.118.

Webster-Stratton, C., Reid, M. J., & Stoolmiller, M. (2009). Preventing conduct problems and improving school readiness: Evaluation of the Incredible Years teacher and child training programs in high-risk schools. *Journal of Child Psychology and Psychiatry, 49*, 471–488. doi:10.1111/j.1469-7610.2007.01861.x.

Wolfe, D. A., Crooks, C., Jaffe, P., Chiodo, D., Hughes, R., Ellis, R., ...& Donner, A. (2009). A school-based program to prevent adolescent dating violence: A cluster randomized trial. *Archives of Pediatrics and Adolescent Medicine, 163*, 692-699. doi:10.1001/archpediatrics.2009.69.

Part IV
Social and Behavioral Wellness in Children and Adolecents

Chapter 9
Preventing Risky Sexual Behavior in Adolescents

Eric R. Walsh-Buhi, Sarah B. Maness, and Helen Mahony

9.1 Introduction

Risky sexual behavior, including having first sexual intercourse at an early age, having a greater number of sexual partners, nonuse of condoms and other pregnancy prevention methods, and use of alcohol or other drugs before sex, contributes to unintended pregnancy and STIs, including HIV/AIDS. According to the Centers for Disease Control and Prevention (CDC) Youth Risk Behavior Surveillance System (YRBSS), nationwide, almost half of high school students have ever had sexual intercourse (CDC, 2012). Although the prevalence of ever having had sexual intercourse decreased between 1991 and 2001 (from 54 to 46 %), it did not change statistically significantly from 2001 (46 %) to 2011 (47 %). Certain subgroups of adolescents remain at high risk. For instance, the prevalence of ever having had sexual intercourse is statistically higher among male (49 %) than female (46 %) adolescents and among black (60 %) and Hispanic (49 %) adolescents than white (44 %) adolescents (CDC, 2012).

Having first sexual intercourse at an early age (i.e., before the age of 13 years) is an indicator of risky sexual behavior. Nationwide, 6 % of adolescents in grades

E.R. Walsh-Buhi, Ph.D. (✉)
Division of Health Promotion and Behavioral Science, Graduate School of Public Health,
San Diego State University, 5500 Campanile Drive, San Diego, CA 92182-4162, USA
e-mail: ebuhi@sdsu.edu

S.B. Maness, Ph.D.
Health and Exercise Science, University of Oklahoma,
1401 Asp Avenue, Norman, OK 73019, USA
e-mail: smaness@ou.edu

H. Mahony, M.P.H.
Department of Community and Family Health, University of South Florida,
13201 Bruce B. Downs Blvd., MDC0056, Tampa, FL 33612, USA
e-mail: hgeorgie@health.usf.edu

© Springer Science+Business Media New York 2016
M.R. Korin (ed.), *Health Promotion for Children and Adolescents*,
DOI 10.1007/978-1-4899-7711-3_9

9–12 have had sexual intercourse for the first time before age 13 years (early sex; CDC, 2012). Similar to the prevalence of ever having had sexual intercourse, the prevalence of having early sex is statistically higher among certain subgroups of adolescents. Overall, the prevalence of having early sex is higher among male (9 %) than female (3 %) adolescents. The prevalence of having early sex is also higher among black (14 %) and Hispanic (7 %) adolescents than white (4 %) adolescents (CDC, 2012).

Having a greater number of sexual partners is also an indicator of risky sexual behavior. Nationwide, 15 % of high school students have had sexual intercourse with four or more persons during their life (CDC, 2012). Overall, the prevalence of having had sexual intercourse with four or more persons was statistically higher among male (18 %) than female (13 %) adolescents. The prevalence of having had sexual intercourse with four or more persons was also higher among black (25 %) and Hispanic (15 %) adolescents than white (13 %) adolescents (CDC, 2012).

Condom use or, more importantly, nonuse of condoms or other effective methods of pregnancy prevention (e.g., birth control pills, the shot [Depo-Provera], NuvaRing, the contraceptive implant [Implanon or Nexplanon], or intrauterine devices [IUDs]) are critical indicators of risky sexual behavior. Among currently sexually active adolescents in the USA, more than half reported that either they or their partner had used a condom during last sexual intercourse; 13 % had not used any method to prevent pregnancy during last sexual intercourse (CDC, 2012). Overall, the prevalence of having used a condom during last sexual intercourse was statistically higher among male (67 %) than female (54 %) adolescents. Female adolescents were also worse off (compared with males) in terms of not having used any method to prevent pregnancy; the prevalence of using no method was higher among female (15 %) than male (11 %) adolescents. While black and Hispanic adolescents have a higher prevalence of early sex and sexual intercourse with four or more persons, compared to their white counterparts, black adolescents appear to use condoms and other methods to prevent pregnancy at greater rates. The prevalence of having used a condom during last sexual intercourse was higher among black (65 %) than Hispanic (58 %) adolescents. The prevalence of using no method to prevent pregnancy was higher among Hispanic (19 %) and black (13 %) adolescents than white (10 %) adolescents and higher among Hispanic (19 %) than black (13 %) adolescents (CDC, 2012).

Lastly, combining alcohol and drug use with sexual intercourse is also risky behavior. Among currently sexually active adolescents, nearly one quarter had drunk alcohol or used drugs before last sexual intercourse (CDC, 2012). Overall, the prevalence of having drunk alcohol or used drugs before last sexual intercourse was statistically higher among male (26 %) than female (18 %) adolescents and among white (23 %) than black (18 %) adolescents.

What do these epidemiologic data mean for adolescent health and well-being? First and foremost, risky sexual behavior can result in unintended pregnancy, which can have negative physical and emotional health, as well as academic and economic consequences on adolescents and their children. Women who become pregnant during adolescence are at higher risk for adverse health outcomes, such as hypertension and anemia, preterm delivery, cesarean section, low birth weight, and infant death (Martin et al., 2010; Matthews & Macdorman, 2010; Youngkin & Davis, 2006). Women who become teen mothers are also at a disadvantage for achievement in school and are less likely to receive a high school diploma; only half of teen mothers earn a high school diploma by the age of 22 years, compared to 90 % of teenagers who do not give birth (Perper, Peterson, & Manlove, 2010). Offspring of teen parents are more likely to experience abuse, to be placed in foster care, and to become pregnant during adolescence themselves (Manlove et al. 2008; Perper et al., 2010). These children are also at greater risk for difficulty with academic achievement, school dropout, and unemployment than those not born to a teenage mother (Hoffman, 2008; Perper et al. 2010). Male children of teenage parents are more than two times more likely to be incarcerated during their lifetimes than male children born to non-teenage mothers (Hoffman, 2008). These consequences also affect society at large. In 2008, teen pregnancy and childbirth cost US taxpayers nearly $11 billion, resulting from healthcare utilization, foster care, and lost tax revenue due to lower economic potential and increased incarceration rates of children born to teen parents (National Campaign, 2011). Second, STIs can lead to both physical and social consequences for adolescents. Each year, untreated STIs cause infertility in at least 24,000 women in the USA, and untreated syphilis in pregnant women results in infant death in up to nearly half of cases (CDC, 2011).

9.2 Sexual Behavior and Behavioral Theory

To decrease risky sexual behavior among adolescents (and, accordingly, to combat the consequences of such behavior), public health professionals, educators, and policy makers in the USA have developed, implemented, and evaluated prevention programs in multiple settings. In fact, over the last 25 years, an entire literature of evidence-based programming to prevent risky sexual behavior has emerged. Such programming is reaching adolescents in a variety of settings, including schools, community settings, and clinical settings. However, before we provide examples of evidence-based programs implemented in each of these settings, we will first provide a critical understanding of the relationship between sexual behavior and behavioral theory. That is, we must first ask the question why do adolescents engage in risky sexual behavior? Having an answer to this question will aid in preventing risky sexual behaviors or, at a minimum, will help readers to understand how certain programs function to prevent risky sexual behavior.

Behavioral theory provides a framework to understand and contextualize social, health, and sexual behavior. In brief, theory attempts to explain why people do or behave the way they do in a variety of situations. Knowing why people behave a certain way sets the stage to inform research and prevention program development and implementation. Elements of prevention programs often sound positive, but a theoretical basis can provide evidence-informed support and structure (Glanz,

Table 9.1 Commonly used theories in sexual behavior-related interventions

Individual level:
Health belief model
Theory of reasoned action
Theory of planned behavior
Transtheoretical model
Information-motivation-behavioral skill model
Protection motivation theory
Interpersonal level:
Social cognitive theory
Community level:
Diffusion of innovations
Ecological:
Social ecological model
Theory of gender and power

Rimer, & Viswanath, 2008). Prevention programs that are most likely to succeed are those that are based on a clear understanding of the health behavior selected for change and the context surrounding this behavior, which theory provides (Glanz et al., 2008). Programs have been found to be more effective if they are based on theory, including programs related to preventing risky sexual behavior (Grol, Bosch, Hulscher, Eccles, & Wensing, 2007).

Health behavior theories, in particular, attempt to explain why individuals engage or fail to engage in particular health-related behaviors (Noar, 2005). Health behavioral theories help us to understand why people believe, think, or do the things they do. Although many theories exist, each theory has unique components that can make one theory more appropriate over another for application in a particular program or study (DiClemente, Salazar, & Crosby, 2011). It is important to critically think about which theory would be most valuable to the particular work in question prior to implementation.

Among programmatic efforts to prevent risky sexual behavior, many evidence-based programs are guided by behavioral theory. Multiple theories have been applied to predict sexual behavior and inform program planning to change risky sexual behavior (Table 9.1). The most commonly used theories overall in health education, health behavior, and preventive medicine include the transtheoretical model, social cognitive theory, and health belief model (Glanz et al., 2008).

Many programs to decrease risky sexual behavior are based on a combination of several behavioral theories. For example, *SiHLE* (*Sisters, Informing, Healing, Living, and Empowering*) utilizes both the social cognitive theory and the theory of gender and power to understand healthy relationships and negotiate safer sex while encouraging cultural and gender pride (DiClemente et al., 2004). Another example is *¡Cuidate!*, which uses social cognitive theory and the theories of reasoned action and planned behavior to support its aims of increasing self-efficacy and behavior change in relation to HIV risk behaviors (OAH, 2012). A full description of these programs and others found to reduce sexual risk behavior are included in the next section.

Although evidence-based, theory-driven programs exist, when studying sexual behavior, many studies have failed to use behavioral theory. One systematic review of self-esteem and sexual behavior indicated that fewer than half of the 38 included studies did not report any theoretical framework (Goodson, Buhi, & Dunsomore, 2006). It is important to focus on the use to theory due to ties to increase evidence-based and contextually supported research. The use of theory also leads to improved intervention outcomes in program planning in sexual health.

Table 9.1 provides a list of commonly used theories in sexual behavior-related interventions. These theories have had previous use in programs focusing on reducing risk sexual behavior, including those focusing on lowering HIV risk (Bandura, 1994; Bertrand, 2004; Fisher, Fisher, Bryan, & Misovic, 2002; Latkin & Knowlton, 2005; Prochaska, Redding, Harlow, Rossi, & Velicer, 1994; Rosenstock, Strecher, & Becker, 1994; Van der Velde & Van der Pligt, 1991; Wingood & DiClemente, 2000), improving condom use (Albarracín, Johnson, Fishbein, & Muellerleile, 2001), reducing sexual assault (Campbell, Dworkin, & Cabral, 2009), and preventing adolescent pregnancy (Raneri & Wiemann, 2007). Reviewing theories and selecting the most appropriate framework prior to program development set the stage for effective intervention related to preventing risky sexual behaviors.

9.3 Settings for and Evidence Supporting Interventions Designed to Prevent Risky Sexual Behavior

The evidence of effectiveness of programs developed to prevent teen pregnancy, births, STIs, or sexual risk behaviors (such as nonuse of condoms or other effective methods of birth control) has been included in reviews conducted by both Kirby (2007) and the Office of Adolescent Health (OAH) (2012). An overview of these programs is displayed in Table 9.2. Eleven of these programs were included for review by both Kirby and OAH and are highlighted in this section. While many of these programs can be implemented in more than one setting, for the purposes here they were categorized as school, community, or clinic setting depending on where they were evaluated. The following programs were evaluated in a school setting: *Aban Aya Youth Project*; *Draw the Line/Respect the Line*; *Reducing the Risk: Building Skills to Prevent Pregnancy, STD, and HIV*; *Safer Choices*; and *Teen Outreach Program (TOP)*. Four programs reviewed by both Kirby (2007) and OAH (2012) were evaluated in community settings: *Making Proud Choices, ¡Cuídate! (Take Care of Yourself), Children's Aid Society-Carrera Program*, and *Teen Health Project: Community-Level HIV Prevention for Adolescents in Low-Income Housing Development. Becoming a Responsible Teen (BART)* and *Sisters, Informing, Healing, Living, and Empowering (SiHLE)* were two programs evaluated in a clinic setting.

There are pros and cons to delivering these programs in the settings presented here: school, community, and clinic. The benefits of a school setting include a broad reach of students as well as consistent delivery of the program if it is taught during

Table 9.2 Evidence-based adolescent pregnancy and/or sexually transmitted infection prevention programs

Program name	Type	Evaluation Setting	Citation (curriculum materials)
Heritage Keepers Abstinence Education	Abstinence	Middle schools and high schools	http://www.heritageservices.org/curriculum/
Making a Difference!	Abstinence	Community based	Select Media http://www.selectmedia.org/programs/difference.html
Promoting Health Among Teens! Abstinence Only	Abstinence	Community based	Select Media http://www.selectmedia.org/programs/phatab.html
Advance provision of emergency contraception	Clinic based	Health clinics	Not curriculum based
Reproductive Health Counseling for Young Men	Counseling	Health clinics	Sociometric Corporation PASHA http://www.socio.com/paspp08.php
Safer Sex	Program for special populations: Sexually active young women who have been diagnosed with an STI	Health clinics	Sociometric Corporation Program Archive on Sexuality, Health, and Adolescent (PASHA) http://www.socio.com/passt27.php
Keepin' it REAL	Mother-adolescent program	Community based	Dr. Colleen Dilorio Department of Behavioral Sciences and Health Education Rollins School of Public Health, Emory University cdilori@sph.emory.edu
All4You!	Program for special populations: alternative schools	High Schools	ETR Associates www.pub.etr.org
Assisting in Rehabilitating Kids (ARK)	Program for special populations: substance-dependent youth	Specialized Settings: residential drug treatment facilities	Dr. Janet S. St. Lawrence, Mississippi State University, Meridian jlawrence@meridian.msstate.edu
Be Proud, Be Responsible, Be Protective!	Program for special populations: pregnant and parenting females	High schools	Select Media http://www.selectmedia.org/programs/protective.html

(continued)

Table 9.2 (continued)

Program name	Type	Evaluation Setting	Citation (curriculum materials)
Project TALC	Programs for special populations: parents living with HIV and their adolescent children	Community based	UCLA Center for HIV Identification, Prevention, and Treatment Services http://chipts.ucla.edu/projects/talc-la/
Respeto/Proteger	Program for special populations: young Latino parents	Community based	Deborah Koniak-Griffin, Ed.D., R.N.C., F.A.A.N.; Janna Lesser, R.N., Ph.D.; Barbara Kappos, M.S.W.; Jerry Tello dkoniak@sonnet.ucla.edu
Riker's Health Advocacy Program	Program for special populations: drug users and youth in correctional facilities	Specialized settings	Sociometric Corporation PASHA http://www.socio.com/passt10.php
SHARP	Program for special populations: high-risk youth in juvenile detention facilities	Specialized setting: juvenile detention facilities	Angela Bryan, Ph.D., University of New Mexico abryan@unm.edu.
Be Proud, Be Responsible!	Sexuality education	After-school program	Select Media http://www.selectmedia.org/programs/items/be-proud.html
What Could You Do?	Sexuality education	Health clinics	Sociometric Corporation Program Archive on Sexuality, Health, and Adolescent (PASHA) http://www.socio.com/passt19.php
Becoming a Responsible Teen	Sexuality education	Health clinics	ETR Associates www.pub.etr.org
Draw the Line, Respect the Line	Sexuality education	Middle schools	ETR Associates www.pub.etr.org
FOCUS	Sexuality education	Specialized setting: marine recruit training	Sociometric Corporation Program Archive on Sexuality, Health, and Adolescent (PASHA) http://www.socio.com/passt22.php
HORIZONS	Sexuality education	Health clinics	Sociometric Corporation PASHA http://www.socio.com/passt29.php
It's Your Game: Keep it Real	Sexuality education	Middle schools	www.itsyourgame.org

(continued)

Table 9.2 (continued)

Program name	Type	Evaluation Setting	Citation (curriculum materials)
Making Proud Choices	Sexuality education	Community based	Select Media http://www.selectmedia.org/programs/choices.html
Promoting Health Among Teens! Comprehensive	Sexuality education	Middle schools	Select Media http://www.selectmedia.org/programs/phatcompr.html
Reducing the Risk	Sexuality education	High schools	ETR Associates www.pub.etr.org
Safer Choices	Sexuality education	High schools	ETR Associates www.pub.etr.org
SiHLE	Sexuality education	Health clinics	Sociometric Corporation PASHA http://www.socio.com/passt23.php
Sisters Saving Sisters	Sexuality education	Health clinics	Select Media http://www.selectmedia.org/
Teen Health Project: HIV Prevention for Adolescents in Low-Income Housing Developments	Sexuality education	Community based	Sociometric Corporation Program Archive on Sexuality, Health, and Adolescent (PASHA) http://www.socio.com/passt25.php
Reach for Health Community Youth Service Learning	Service learning	Middle schools	Sociometric Corporation PASHA http://www.socio.com/paspp10.php
Teen Outreach Program	Youth development/ service learning	High schools and after school	Wyman Center http://wymancenter.org/wyman_top.php.
Aban Aya	Youth development	Middle schools	Sociometric Corporation PASHA http://www.socio.com/passt24.php
Children's Aid Society-Carrera Program	Youth development	Community-based after-school program	Children's Aid Society http://stopteenpregnancy.childrensaidsociety.org/
Project AIM	Youth development	Middle schools	Children's Hospital of LA; Dr. Leslie Clark lclark@chla.usc.edu
Raising Healthy Children	Youth development	Elementary schools	University of Washington, Social Development Research Group http://www.sdrg.org/rhcsummary.asp#3

regular class hours. A community setting has similar pros if the program is taught within a group that meets regularly. However, implementing programs in community settings that youth do not attend regularly could present issues in delivery of the full program (that is, maintaining fidelity to the program model). This same issue presents itself in clinic settings. Programs implemented in clinics often involve fewer sessions than school-based programs because attendance can be more difficult to sustain when providing a program in a location that youth do not visit regularly.

While each program is different, aside from the goal of preventing teen pregnancy, they share many similarities. The majority of the programs are theory based and utilize group sessions to deliver material to youth. Due to similar prevention methods, many of these types of programs are designed to prevent not only teen pregnancy but also HIV/AIDs. Several of the programs described here, including *BART* and *¡Cuídate!*, were specifically designed as HIV prevention programs, but were evaluated and found to be effective in reducing teen pregnancy (OAH, 2012). These programs meet over a predetermined number of sessions in which activities, lectures, and class participations are utilized. Where the programs differ is in the specific methods used to teach pregnancy prevention, the theory and background used to develop the curriculum, and overall goals, such as the encouragement of sexual abstinence, sexual refusal skill training, and/or promotion of condom use. Programs also differ in their target audience. Programs such as the *Aban Aya Youth Project*, *BART*, *¡Cuídate!*, and *SiHLE* were developed specifically for use in minority youth populations. In addition, programs like the *TOP* and *Safer Choices* include community elements, such as the TOP's community service learning component in which youth participate in projects benefiting the communities where they live. Further descriptions of programs are described below.

9.3.1 School Settings

9.3.1.1 Aban Aya Youth Project

Developed based on the theory of triadic influence, the *Aban Aya Youth Project* is an Afrocentric, social development, and classroom-based curriculum focused on reducing high-risk behaviors like violence, antagonism, and substance use and promoting abstinence from sexual activity (Flay, Graumlich, Segawa, Burns, & Holliday, 2004). Aban Aya is a term used in the Ghanaian language to mean social protection and self-determination (Flay et al., 2004). The program also includes the option of adding a school and community-wide component. The social development curriculum (SDC) consists of an intensive four-year program (for youth in grades 5–8) with 16–21 lessons administered per year (OAH, 2012). The lessons in the SDC teach cognitive behavioral skills that can increase self-esteem, help with stress and anxiety, encourage interpersonal relationships, and establish proficiency in decision-making, problem solving, conflict resolution, and goal setting (Flay et al.,

2004). The curriculum strives to change unsafe norms of carrying a weapon, selling drugs, and engaging in high-risk sexual behavior (OAH, 2012). *Aban Aya* contains the following six core components: abstinence; developing behavioral skills; information on contraception; self-efficacy; HIV/AIDS, STI, and sexuality education; and African-American culture, values, and history (OAH, 2012). Teaching methods utilized by the program include small and large-group discussions, lectures, role-plays, videos and games, and quizzes and homework (OAH, 2012).

The evidence for program effectiveness comes from an evaluation conducted by Flay et al. (2004). A randomized controlled trial was carried out in 12 low-income metropolitan schools in Chicago. Study participants were predominately African-American, and all were in fifth grade at the beginning of the evaluation. When the program ended, results showed statistically significant program effects for male participants, but there were no effects for females. Males participating in the program were statistically less likely to report recent sexual intercourse and more likely to report using condoms. While the program was evaluated within schools, the developers note that there is potential for the program to be implemented in community-based settings and with middle school youth of other racial and/or ethnic groups (OAH, 2012).

9.3.1.2 Draw the Line/Respect the Line

Draw the Line/Respect the Line was developed based on social cognitive theory and social inoculation theory, with the goal of reducing the number of youth who initiate sexual intercourse and increasing condom use among those engaging in sex (Coyle, Kirby, Marin, Gómez, & Gregorich, 2004). This program promotes sexual abstinence and provides students in grades six through eight with tools necessary to prevent HIV, STIs, and pregnancy (OAH, 2012). The curriculum consists of 20 lessons that instruct participants on how to create their own sexual limits and how to hold those limits, even when challenged (Coyle et al., 2004).

The first five lessons are for youth in sixth grade and focus on teaching skills for refusal in nonsexual settings (OAH, 2012). Examples of the core content components contained within these five lessons are the concept of limits, drawing and respecting limits, and refusal skills (OAH, 2012). Participants in seventh grade are taught eight lessons that include skills for refusing sexual intercourse and information on the consequences of sex (OAH, 2012). Some core components of the seventh grade curriculum are emotional and social ramifications of having sex, facts about STIs, and facilitating positive attitudes toward abstaining from sex (OAH, 2012). The eighth-grade curriculum consists of seven lessons with a spotlight on practicing the refusal skills learned in earlier lessons and a condom use demonstration (OAH, 2012). Core components include step-by-step instructions on using a condom, overcoming barriers to sticking with limits, and homework activities that encourage parent-to-child discussion of HIV. Lessons use a variety of teaching methods, including small and large-group discussions, paired and small-group practice, stories, and individual activities for youth.

A randomized controlled trial conducted by Coyle et al. (2004) enrolled sixth graders attending public schools in northern California. Participants in the evaluation were predominately Hispanic. Surveys were administered at the start of the program, annually for seventh and eighth grades, and one year after the program ended. Results from the survey administered in the seventh grade showed that, compared to nonprogram participants, male participants were statistically less likely to report ever having had sex and less likely to report having had sex in the previous 12 months. Additionally, males in the program engaged in sexual intercourse less frequently and had fewer partners in the previous 12 months. These findings persisted when the program ended in eighth grade. One year after the program ended, there was still a statistically significant program impact for the outcomes of ever had sex and sexual intercourse in the previous 12 months, but the program effect on the outcomes of frequency of sexual intercourse and number of partners was no longer statistically significant. No program effects were found for females at any time point. *Draw the Line/Respect the Line* can be adapted to be implemented in older youth (grades 7–9) and in nonschool settings (OAH, 2012).

9.3.1.3   Reducing the Risk: Building Skills to Prevent Pregnancy, STD, and HIV

Reducing the Risk promotes attitudes and skills that assist youth in preventing pregnancy, STIs, and HIV (OAH, 2012). The 16-lesson program was designed using social learning theory, social inoculation theory, and cognitive behavioral theory (Kirby, Barth, Leland, & Fetro, 1991). The program emphasizes such skills as communication, decision-making, planning, delay tactics, and refusal strategies (Kirby et al., 1991). Class activities are designed to encourage youth to plan ahead in order to avoid high-risk behaviors (OAH, 2012). The program is designed for youth 13–18 years old, and each of the 16 lessons is 45 min in duration. Lessons are taught sequentially with classes held 2–3 times per week. Important content components include knowledge of pregnancy risk, self-efficacy and refusal skills in high-pressure situations, and teaching proficiency in obtaining information on contraceptive methods through clinic services.

Reducing the Risk has been evaluated three times. The first evaluation, conducted by Kirby et al. (1991), was carried out in 46 high school classrooms in rural and urban communities in northern California. Study participants were a racially and ethnically diverse mix of ninth, tenth, eleventh, and twelfth graders. Eighteen months after completing the program, female participants who were sexually inexperienced at the start of the program were statistically less likely to report having had unprotected sex. There was no difference in this outcome for males. Additionally, there was no statistically significant difference in the outcomes of sexual initiation, recent intercourse, or pregnancy for males or females. Two replication evaluations of this program have also been conducted. The first, by Hubbard, Giese, and Rainey (1998), found that participants in the program were statistically less likely to initiate sex. Participants who were sexually active were found to be more likely to use methods to prevent pregnancy, HIV, and STIs. The most recent replication evaluation, by Zimmerman et al. (2008), also determined that youth in the program were less likely to initiate sex. This study did not find any difference in condom use between program participants and nonparticipants.

9.3.1.4 Safer Choices

The purpose of *Safer Choices* is to reduce pregnancy, STIs, and HIV among high school students through various components such as school organization, curriculum, peer resources and school environment, parent education, and school-community linkages (OAH, 2012). The program was developed based on social cognitive theory, social influence model, and models of school change (Basen-Engquist et al., 2001) and is implemented over a 2-year period. The specific goals of *Safer Choices* are to reduce the number of adolescents engaging in sex and increase condom use among sexually active adolescents (OAH, 2012). The program attempts to accomplish these goals by increasing knowledge about HIV and STIs and promoting positive attitudes toward sexual abstinence and condom use at the multiple levels of individual, school, and community. The curriculum consists of 21 lessons, 11 of which are taught during ninth grade and 10 lessons in the tenth grade. The lessons are interactive and focus on HIV, STIs, condom use, refusal skills, and decision-making skills. Many activities are facilitated by participants nominated by their peers.

The evidence for program effectiveness comes from a randomized controlled trial conducted by Basen-Engquist et al. (2001) that included 20 urban high schools from northern California and southeastern Texas. Results from surveys administered at program completion determined that there were no statistical differences among the outcomes of sex in the previous 3 months or in the number of unprotected sex occasions in the 3 months prior to the survey. One year after program completion, there was still no statistically significant difference in whether participants had engaged in sexual intercourse in the previous 3 months. Program participants were, however, more likely to report having used a condom in the previous 3 months, compared to youth not participating in the program (OAH, 2012).

9.3.1.5 Teen Outreach Program

The *Teen Outreach Program* (*TOP*) is a positive youth development program that emphasizes youth as valuable resources to prevent teen pregnancy, school dropouts, and course failures (OAH, 2012). An important aspect of the *TOP* model is developing positive relationships with adult program facilitators and with other youth participating in the program. The program is implemented through two avenues: Changing Scenes Curriculum and Community Service Learning. There are four levels of Changing Scenes Curriculum, depending on the age group. Level 1 is designed for 12- to 13-year-old youth, while level 2 is for 14-year-olds. Level 3 is for youth 15–16 years old and, level 4 is designed for those who are 17 years of age.

The program consists of three interrelated elements of supervised community service, class discussions about experiences during community service, and class discussions and activities on adolescent social and developmental topics. The *TOP* has goals of increasing healthy behaviors, developing life skills, and establishing a sense of purpose, and it accomplishes these goals through lessons including content on relationships, values, communication and assertiveness, goal setting, and adolescent development and sexual health. Participants in the program must receive a minimum of 25 lessons over 9 months and complete at least 20 h of community service.

The first evaluation of the *TOP*, by Allen, Philliber, and Hoggson (1990), was conducted in 35 different sites in 30 schools across the country among a racially and ethnically diverse group of students in grades 7–12. This evaluation found that females participating in the program were statistically significantly less likely to become pregnant while in the program, compared to females who were not in the program. A replication evaluation conducted by Allen, Philliber, Herrling, and Kuperminc (1997) was carried out in high schools in 25 different sites nationwide. This evaluation also found a statistically significant effect for females in the program. Females were less likely to become pregnant while participating in the program compared to those who did not participate.

9.3.2 Community Settings

9.3.2.1 Making Proud Choices

Making Proud Choices is a program delivered over a 2-week period to reduce the risk of HIV, STIs, and pregnancy (OAH, 2012). The program, which is based on the social cognitive theory, the theory of reasoned action, and the theory of planned behavior (Jemmott, Jemmott, & Fong, 1998), consists of the following eight 1-h modules:

1. Getting to Know You and Steps to Making Your Dreams and Goals Come True
2. The Consequences of Sex: HIV Infection
3. Attitudes and Beliefs about HIV and Condom Use
4. Strategies for Preventing HIV Infection: Stop, Think, and Act
5. The Consequences of Sex: STDs and Correct Condom Use
6. The Consequences of Sex: Pregnancy
7. Developing Condom Use Skills and Negotiation Skills
8. Enhancing Condom Use Skills and Negotiation Skills

Making Proud Choices uses a variety of teaching methods, such as role-plays, small-group activities, and videos.

The evidence of effectiveness for *Making Proud Choices* comes from a randomized controlled trial of African-American youth in sixth and seventh grades (Jemmott et al., 1998). Surveys were administered when the program concluded and 3, 6, and 12 months after the program ended. Three months after the program ended, the youth who participated in the program and who were sexually experienced at the beginning of the program were statistically significantly less likely to have had sex in the previous 3 months. This effect remained at 6 and 12-month post-program completion. This effect was not observed for sexually inexperienced youth at any of the follow-up time points. There was no difference for the outcomes of rate or frequency of sexual intercourse, and this finding persisted 6 and 12 months after the program ended. *Making Proud Choices* can also be implemented with older youth, with non-African-American youth, and in clinic or school settings (OAH, 2012).

9.3.2.2   ¡Cuídate! (Take Care of Yourself)

¡Cuídate! is a culturally specific program designed for Latino youth that highlights aspects of Latino culture, so sexual abstinence and condom use are viewed as culturally appropriate (OAH, 2012). Using social cognitive theory and the theories of reasoned action and planned behavior, the program aims to increase each youth's self-efficacy in communicating and negotiating abstinence and condom use with their partner. By doing this, the program attempts to change attitudes, beliefs, and behaviors and increase self-efficacy of behaviors that reduce the risk of HIV. The program consists of six 1-h modules that are implemented over 2 or more days.

The program is intended for youth aged 13–18 years, and groups can be mixed gender of between 6 and 10 youth (OAH, 2012). The name of the program, *¡Cuídate!* (Take Care of Yourself), highlights a core content component of taking care of oneself, one's partner, family, and community. Another core component is to emphasize Latino cultural values such as familialism and gender norms and show how these values are in agreement with safer sex practices. The program uses a variety of teaching methods, such as small-group discussion, videos, activities, and skill-building tasks.

¡Cuídate! was evaluated in a randomized controlled trial where 684 Latino youth enrolled in the program provided by neighborhood organizations (Villarruel, Jemmott, & Jemmott, 2006). Surveys were administered at 3, 6, and 12 months after program completion. Effectiveness was averaged across the three different time points. Youth participating in the program were statistically less likely to have had sexual intercourse in the previous 3 months and also less likely to have had multiple partners in the previous 3 months. These youth also engaged in fewer days of unprotected sex and were more likely to report consistent condom use compared to youth who were not in the program. However, there was no program effect on condom use at most recent sex or on the proportion of days of sex that were condom protected. The developer notes that *¡Cuídate!* can also be implemented in school and after-school settings.

9.3.2.3   Children's Aid Society-Carrera Program

The *Carrera Program* is a long-term program that holds a holistic view of a youth's development with the goal of avoiding pregnancy (OAH, 2012). It is focused on empowering youth so that they can develop their own personal goals and a desire to have a successful future. Additionally, the program provides sexuality education. While the program is not theory based, youth are viewed as "at promise" instead of "at risk" (Philliber, Kaye, Herrling, & West, 2002). The program consists of the following seven core components: education, job club, family life and sexuality education, self-expression, lifetime individual sports; full medical and dental care, and mental health services (OAH, 2012). The *Carrera Program* also includes a parent family life and sexuality education component in order to increase the parent's ability to discuss important family and sexuality topics with their child.

The program intends to promote the youth's desire to avoid pregnancy and provide opportunities for youth to discover their interests and talents while emphasizing education, employment, and youth development (OAH, 2012). Youth are invited to participate in the program when they are 11–12 years of age and continue in the program until they graduate high school. During the school year, participants attend program sessions Monday through Friday, and each lesson lasts 3 h (Philliber et al., 2002). During the summer, youth attend maintenance meetings.

The *Carrera Program* was evaluated in a randomized controlled trial conducted in New York City (Philliber et al., 2002). Youth were predominately African-American and Hispanic and were between the ages of 13–15 years at the start of the study. Three years after the program began, females were statistically significantly less likely to have become pregnant or sexually active. Sexually experienced females were statistically more likely to report using a condom and a highly effective method of birth control at last sex, compared to nonprogram participants. No program effects were found for boys. The program is intended to be implemented in a community setting with disadvantaged youth ages 11–12 years.

9.3.2.4 Teen Health Project: Community-Level HIV Prevention for Adolescents in Low-Income Housing Development

Teen Health Project promotes the skills necessary for adolescents to enact social change and uses modeling, peer norms, and social reinforcement to continue HIV prevention behavior (OAH, 2012). Guided by diffusion of innovations and social cognitive theory, the core components of the program are adolescent workshops; behavioral skill development; education on contraception, sexuality, HIV/AIDS, and STIs; and community outreach (Sikkema et al., 2005). The adolescent workshops consist of two 3-h workshops that are offered once per week for 2 weeks (OAH, 2012). There are two follow-up sessions offered 4–5 months after the initial workshop that last approximately 2 h each. Another important component of the program is the *Teen Health Project* Leadership Council whereby youth nominate each other to serve as leaders on the council. The council meets once per week in between the first and second follow-up sessions for 90 min, and it continues to meet for 6 months thereafter. HIV prevention messages are presented throughout program activities, project newsletters, community-wide social events, talent shows, concerts, and festivals. By promoting sexual abstinence and condom use among those who are sexually active, the program hopes to maintain HIV prevention behaviors among the youth, their peers, and the entire community (OAH, 2012). The *Teen Health Project* offers parents an opportunity to attend a workshop that provides information about HIV/AIDS and approaches to discussing abstinence and condom use with their children.

The program was evaluated in a randomized controlled trial of ethnically and racially diverse housing developments in Wisconsin, Virginia, and Washington (Sikkema et al., 2005). Three months after completion of the workshops, there was no statistically significant difference among adolescents for the outcome of abstinence (among those who were sexually inexperienced at the beginning of the program). One year after completion of the program, however, youth who participated in the program and were sexually inexperienced at the onset of the program were more likely to have remained abstinent compared to youth who did not participate in the program. These youth were also more likely to report using condoms. The program is intended to be implemented in a community setting with ethnically and racially diverse youth aged 12–17 years.

9.3.3   Clinic Settings

9.3.3.1   Becoming a Responsible Teen

Becoming a Responsible Teen (or *BART*) is designed for use among African-American youth to prevent HIV and pregnancy. Participants are between the ages of 14–18 and engage in interactive group discussions and role-plays that were developed by the youth in the program (OAH, 2012). Created using the information motivation behavior model and social learning theory as a foundation, program participants are taught to educate their peers about the risks of HIV and to practice these skills outside the program meetings. In addition to HIV education, other lessons include information on pregnancy prevention, correct condom use, assertive communication, refusal techniques, self-management, problem solving skills, and abstinence. There are eight 2-hour-long lessons, which are intended to be delivered once per week for 8 weeks. Core content components are comprised of knowledge, attitudes, skills and self-efficacy, perception of risk, social and peer norms, behavioral beliefs, values, intentions, and communication in relation to HIV risk and sexual behavior.

The program was evaluated in randomized controlled trial conducted in a health center in a midsized city in the southern part of the USA (St. Lawrence et al., 1995). Surveys were administered immediately after the program ended and again after 6 and 12 months. Outcomes were averaged across time points. Youth in the program reported fewer occasions of unprotected oral and anal intercourse and used condoms more frequently during vaginal intercourse. No program impacts were observed on the number of sexual partners or the number of unprotected occasions of vaginal intercourse, and there was no change in condom-protected anal intercourse. The 12-month survey point showed that participants were less likely to have had sex in the previous 2 months. While the program was evaluated in a clinic setting, it can also be implemented in nonschool or after-school settings.

9.3.3.2 SiHLE: Sisters, Informing, Healing, Living, and Empowering

SiHLE is a peer-led, social-skill teaching program with the intent of reducing sexual risk behaviors among heterosexual African-American girls who are sexually experienced and who are at high risk of HIV infection (OAH, 2012). Using social cognitive theory and theory of gender and power (DiClemente et al., 2004), the program also addresses relationships, dating, and sexual health by promoting cultural and gender pride in order to provide adolescents with the skills to avoid HIV and other STIs (OAH, 2012). Core content includes increasing knowledge about HIV transmission, teaching how to negotiate abstinence or safer sex behavior, practicing correct condom use, advancing an understanding of the differences between healthy and unhealthy relationships, and increasing self-efficacy by promoting pride in one's culture and gender. The program consists of six lessons that are administered to small groups of 10–12 youth. One 4-hour lesson is taught once per week for 4 weeks, and then one lesson is taught at 6 and 12 months afterward (DiClemente et al., 2004).

DiClemente et al. (2004) conducted a randomized controlled trial, in which youth participated in the program in a health center in the southern US Surveys were administered at 6- and 12-month post-program. At the 6-month follow-up, participants were less likely to have become pregnant and more likely to have used condoms consistently during those previous 6 months. Participants were also more likely to use a condom at most recent sex, and a higher percentage engaged in condom-protected intercourse during both the previous 1 month and 6 months. These findings persisted at the 12-month follow-up. The participants also reported fewer episodes of unprotected intercourse during both the previous 1 month and 6 months and were less likely to become infected with chlamydia. These findings were still statistically significant 12-month post-program. No program effect was found for the outcome of consistent condom use in the month prior to the survey. There was no difference in terms of infection with gonorrhea or trichomoniasis at any follow-up time point. Twelve months after the program ended, participants were more likely to report consistent condom use during the previous 1 month and 6 months. Lastly, no program effect on incidence of pregnancy in the previous 6 months was observed at the 12-month follow-up (Table 9.2).

9.4   Recommendations for Future Prevention Programming, Guidance on Developing Effective Programs, and Helpful Resources for Planning Prevention Programs

Evidence-based programs are imperative to ensure that time and resources are efficiently and effectively used in efforts to reduce risky sexual behavior among adolescents. If a program is not evidence based, then there is the potential that the program may not actually be effective in decreasing risky sexual behavior. Evidence-based programs provide the support necessary to invest limited resources toward the prevention of risky sexual behavior among adolescents.

If an existing evidence-based program is not selected for use, there are helpful guidelines to take in to consideration when developing a program with the goal of reducing risky sexual behavior. In order to develop an effective program, it is important to clearly identify the health issues to address within the given community and to select objectives to measure in the implementation of the program. For example, who is affected by the problem, what resources do we currently have, and what resources do we need to address the problem (US DHHS, 2015)?

Resources previously described in this book, including intervention mapping, RE-AIM, and PRECEDE-PROCEED, can also be helpful in the development of sexual health programs. An example of intervention mapping as applied to increasing condom use will be described in detail.

Intervention mapping is a planning framework that was designed to build on PRECEDE-PROCEED but also emphasize the use of theory and empirical data (Bartholomew, Parcel, & Kok, 1998). Intervention mapping contains six steps. Members of the priority population should be involved in planning, especially in steps 3 and 4.

Step 1: Plan and conduct community needs assessment.
Step 2: Create a matrix of proximal program objectives. This matrix will include what participants will learn as part of the program and what changes can be expected as a result.
Step 3: Select theory-based intervention methods and strategies that are based on behavioral theory and existing empirical research.
Step 4: Design and organize the program components and pretest included materials.
Step 5: Specify implementation plans for the program.
Step 6: Evaluate the program.

In terms of risky sexual behavior, Step 1 could involve a community need assessment to discover what sexual risk behaviors are a problem in the given community. As an example, the community need assessment could include identifying a lack of condom use among high school-aged youth in the community.

In Step 2, program planners will need to decide what objectives the program will include. The need to set clear objectives before developing the program is necessary to assess whether the program has reached its goals. In relation to risky sexual behavior, an example of an objective could include "increasing the percentage of youth reporting consistent condom use within the past three months, from 50 to 75 %."

As previously discussed in this chapter, theory is an important component of programs to reduce adolescent sexual risk behavior. Step 3 of intervention mapping involves selecting and applying theory to the program. Steps 4 and 5 involve the development of a curriculum related to sexual behavior and health among youth as well as how this program will be implemented. For instance, will the program be offered as part of a school curriculum? Will the program be offered to a group after-school or in an alternate setting (such as in a community setting or correctional facility)? These steps require buy-in from the community in order to successfully implement a plan for how and where a program will occur.

Lastly, in Step 6, the program should be evaluated to see if objectives were met. Students could be surveyed at time points before and after completing the program to assess the selected objective of consistent condom use within the past three months.

This hypothetical example gives information on how intervention mapping can be applied to a specific issue related to risky sexual behavior. Similarly, the steps RE-AIM and the PRECEDE-PROCEED model can be followed with topic areas specifically related to risky sexual behavior among adolescents. These tools provide guidance within the development of programs to support success.

9.5 Conclusion

Preventing risky sexual behavior among adolescents is a vital public health issue. This chapter has described why this issue is so important, due to high rates of adolescent pregnancy, STIs, and HIV in the USA, as well as the economic costs to society that these issues present. Using behavioral theory to develop programs that prevent risky sexual behavior is critical in creating effective programs that contribute to the reduction of risk behaviors. Examples of these types of programs and their venues were presented and described in detail. Lastly, additional resources were provided to aid in planning and developing programs to reduce risky sexual health behavior among adolescents.

References

Albarracín, D., Johnson, B. T., Fishbein, M., & Muellerleile, P. A. (2001). Theories of reasoned action and planned behavior as models of condom use: A meta-analysis. *Psychological Bulletin, 127*(1), 142–161. doi:10.1037/0033-2909.127.1.142.

Allen, J. P., Philliber, S., Herrling, S., & Kuperminc, G. P. (1997). Preventing teen pregnancy and academic failure: Experimental evaluation of a developmentally based approach. *Child Development, 68*(4), 729–742. doi:10.1111/j.1467-8624.1997.tb04233.x.

Allen, J. P., Philliber, S., & Hoggson, N. (1990). School-based prevention of teen-age pregnancy and school dropout: Process evaluation of the national replication of the Teen Outreach Program. *American Journal of Community Psychology, 18*(4), 505–524.

Bandura, A. (1994). Social cognitive theory and exercise of control over HIV infection. In R. J. DiClemente & J. L. Peterson (Eds.), *Preventing AIDS: Theories and methods of behavioral interventions* (pp. 25–29). New York, NY: Plenum Press.

Bartholomew, L. K., Parcel, G. S., & Kok, G. (1998). Intervention mapping: A process for developing theory- and evidence-based health education programs. *Health Education & Behavior, 25*(5), 545–563.

Basen-Engquist, K., Coyle, K. K., Parcel, G. S., Kirby, D., Banspach, S. W., Carvajal, S. C., & Baumler, E. (2001). Schoolwide effects of a multicomponent HIV, STD, and pregnancy prevention program for high school students. *Health Education and Behavior, 28*(2): 166-185. doi:10.1177/109019810102800204.

Bertrand, J. T. (2004). Diffusion of innovations and HIV/AIDS. *Journal of Health Communication, 9*(Suppl1), 113–121. doi:10.1080/10810730490271575.

Campbell, R., Dworkin, E., & Cabral, G. (2009). An ecological model of the impact of sexual assault on women's mental health. *Trauma, Violence & Abuse, 10*(3), 225–246. doi:10.1177/1524838009334456.

Centers for Disease Control and Prevention. (2011). *10 ways STDs impact women differently from men.* Retrieved from http://www.cdc.gov/nchhstp/newsroom/docs/STDs-Women-042011.pdf.

Centers for Disease Control and Prevention. (2012). Youth risk behavior surveillance—United States, 2011. *Morbidity and Mortality Weekly Report, 61*(4), 1–162.

Coyle, K. K., Kirby, D. B., Marin, B. V., Gómez, C. A., & Gregorich, S. E. (2004). Draw the Line/Respect the Line: A randomized trial of a middle school intervention to reduce sexual risk behaviors. *American Journal of Public Health, 94*(5), 843–851.

DiClemente, R. J., Salazar, L. F., & Crosby, R. A. (2011). *Health behavior theory for public health: Principles, foundations and applications.* Burlington, MA: Jones & Bartlett Learning.

DiClemente, R. J., Wingood, G. M., Harrington, K. F., Lang, D. L., Davies, S. L., Hook, E. W., III., … .Robillard, A. (2004). Efficacy of an HIV prevention intervention for African American adolescent girls: A randomized controlled trial. *Journal of the American Medical Association, 292*(2), 171-179. doi:10.1001/jama.292.2.171.

Fisher, C. M., Fisher, W. A., Bryan, A. D., & Misovic, S. J. (2002). Information-motivation-behavioral skills model-based HIV risk behavior change intervention for inner-city high school youth. *Health Psychology, 21*(2), 177–186.

Flay, B. R., Graumlich, S., Segawa, E., Burns, J. L., & Holliday, M. Y. (2004). Effects of two prevention programs on high-risk behaviors among African American youth: A randomized trial. *Archives of Pediatrics & Adolescent Medicine, 158*(4), 377–384. doi:10.1001/archpedi.158.4.377.

Glanz, K., Rimer, B. K., & Viswanath, K. (2008). *Health behavior and health education: Theory, research and practice.* San Francisco, CA: Jossey-Bass.

Goodson, P., Buhi, E. R., & Dunsomore, S. C. (2006). Self-esteem and adolescent sexual behaviors, attitudes, and intentions: A systematic review. *Journal of Adolescent Health, 38*(3), 310–319. doi:10.1016/j.jadohealth.2005.05.026.

Grol, R. P., Bosch, M. C., Hulscher, M. E., Eccles, M. P., & Wensing, M. (2007). Planning and studying improvement in patient care: The use of theoretical perspectives. *The Milbank Quarterly, 85*(1), 93–138.

Hoffman, S. D. (2008). *Kids having kids: Economic costs and social consequences of teen pregnancy.* Washington, DC: Urban Institute Press.

Hubbard, B. M., Giese, M. L., & Rainey, J. (1998). A replication of Reducing the Risk, a theory-based sexuality curriculum for adolescents. *Journal of School Health, 68*(6), 243–247.

Jemmott, J. B., III, Jemmott, L. S., & Fong, L. S. (1998). Abstinence and safer sex HIV risk-reduction interventions for African American adolescents: A randomized controlled trial. *Journal of the American Medical Association, 279*(19), 1529–1536. doi:10.1001/jama.279.19.1529.

Kirby, D. (2007). *Emerging Answers.* The National Campaign, Retrieved from http://thenational-campaign.org/resource/emerging-answers-2007%E2%80%94full-report.

Kirby, D., Barth, R. P., Leland, N., & Fetro, J. V. (1991). Reducing the risk: Impact of a new curriculum on sexual risk-taking. *Family Planning Perspectives, 23*(6), 253–263.

Latkin, C. A., & Knowlton, A. R. (2005). Micro-social structural approaches to HIV prevention: A socialecologicalperspective.*AIDSCare,17*(Suppl11),S102–S113.doi:10.1080/09540120500121185.

Manlove, J. S., Terry-Humen, E., Minceli, L. A., & Moore, K. A. (2008). Outcome for children of teen mothers from kindergarten through adolescence. In S. Hoffman & R. Maynard (Eds.), *Kids having kids: Economic costs and social consequences of teenage pregnancy*. Washington, DC: Urban Institute Press.

Martin, J. A., Hamilton, B. E., Sutton, P. D., Ventura, S. J., Matthews, T. J., & Osterman, M. J. K. (2010). Births: Final data for 2008. *National Vital Statistics Reports, 59*(1), 1–72. Retrieved from http://www.cdc.gov/nchs/data/nvsr/nvsr59/nvsr59_01.pdf.

Matthews, T., & Macdorman, M. (2010). Infant mortality statistics from the 2006 period linked birth/infant death data set. *National Vital Statistics Reports, 58*(17), 1–32. Retrieved from http://www.cdc.gov/nchs/data/nvsr/nvsr58/nvsr58_17.pdf.

National Campaign to Prevent Teen and Unplanned Pregnancy. (2011). *Counting it up: The public costs of teen childbearing*. Washington, DC. Retrieved from http://www.thenationalcampaign.org/costs/default.aspx.

Noar, S. M. (2005). A health educator's guide to theories of health behavior. *International Quarterly of Community Health Education, 24*(1), 75–92.

Office of Adolescent Health. (2012). *Evidence-based programs (31 programs)*. Retrieved from http://www.hhs.gov/ash/oah/oah-initiatives/teen_pregnancy/resources/db/programs.html.

Perper, K., Peterson, K., & Manlove, J. (2010). *Child trends fact sheet: Diploma attainment among teen mothers*. Washington, DC: Child Trends. Retrieved from http://www.childtrends.org/wp-content/uploads/2010/01/child_trends-2010_01_22_FS_diplomaattainment.pdf.

Philliber, S., Kaye, J. W., Herrling, S., & West, E. (2002). Preventing pregnancy and improving healthcare access among teenagers: An evaluation of the Children's AID Society-Carrera Program. *Perspectives on Sexual and Reproductive Health, 34*(5), 244–251.

Prochaska, J. O., Redding, C. A., Harlow, L. L., Rossi, J. S., & Velicer, W. F. (1994). The transtheoretical model of change and HIV prevention: A review. *Health Education & Behavior, 21*(4), 471–486. doi:10.1177/109019819402100410.

Raneri, L. G., & Wiemann, C. M. (2007). *Social ecological predictors of repeat adolescent pregnancy*. Perspectives on Sexual and Reproductive Health, 39(1), 39-47. doi:10.1363/3903907.

Rosenstock, I. M., Strecher, V. J., & Becker, M. H. (1994). The health belief model and HIV risk behavior change. In R. J. DiClemente & J. L. Peterson (Eds.), *Preventing AIDS: Theories and methods of behavioral interventions* (pp. 5–24). New York, NY: Plenum Press.

Sikkema, K. J., Anderson, E. S., Kelly, J. A., Winett, R. A., Gore-Felton, C., Roffman, R. A., … Brondino, M. J. (2005). Outcomes of a randomized controlled community-level HIV prevention intervention for adolescents in low-income housing developments. *AIDS, 19*(14), 1509–1516.

St. Lawrence, J. S., Brasfield, T. L., Jefferson, K. W., Alleyne, E., O'Bannon, R. E., III, & Shirley, A. (1995). Cognitive-behavioral intervention to reduce African American adolescent's risk for HIV infection. *Journal of Consulting and Clinical Psychology, 63*(2), 221–237.

U.S. Department of Health and Human Services. (2015). Program planning. Retrieved from http://www.healthypeople.gov/2020/tools-and-resources/program-planning.

Van der Velde, F. W., & Van der Pligt, J. (1991). AIDS-related health behavior: Coping, protection motivation, and previous behavior. *Journal of Behavioral Medicine, 14*(5), 429–451. doi:10.1007/BF00845103.

Villarruel, A. M., Jemmott, J. B., III, & Jemmott, L. S. (2006). A randomized controlled trial testing and HIV prevention intervention for Latino youth. *Archives of Pediatrics & Adolescent Medicine, 160*(11), 1187. doi:10.1001/archpedi.160.8.772.

Wingood, G. M., & DiClemente, R. J. (2000). Application of the theory of gender and power to examine HIV-related exposures, risk factors, and effective interventions for women. *Health Education & Behavior, 27*(5), 539–565. doi:10.1177/109019810002700502.

Youngkin, E., & Davis, M. (2006). *Women's health: A primary care clinical guide* (3rd ed.). Upper Saddle River, NJ: Prentice Hall.

Zimmerman, R., Donohew, L., Sionéan, C., Cupp, P., Feist-Price, S., & Helme, D. (2008). Effects of a school-based, theory driven HIV and pregnancy prevention curriculum. *Perspectives on Sexual and Reproductive Health, 40*(1), 42–51. doi:10.1363/4004208.

Chapter 10
Early Gender Development in Children and Links with Mental and Physical Health

May Ling D. Halim, Danielle Bryant, and Kenneth J. Zucker

10.1 Introduction

In early childhood, gender is often center-stage in children's worlds. It is usually the first social category of which children become aware. Children learn that society generally divides the world into male and female, and they learn that society places them into one of these categories. Cognitive theories of gender development posit that this awareness of gender identity spurs children on to pay attention to what gender means and to form gender schemas (Martin, Ruble, & Szkrybalo, 2002). For instance, children quickly learn that "pink is for girls" and "blue is for boys." Further, once children gather and learn well-established gender stereotypes, and form their own gender stereotypes, cognitive theories of gender development posit that they are highly motivated to be "good" members of their gender group. For example, whereas a young girl might have liked all kinds of colors at age 2, by age 4, her whole wardrobe, right down to her socks, might now be pink (Halim et al., 2014).

It is important to note that not all girls eventually wear pink from head-to-toe. Indeed, there is much variability in the gender identification and gender-typing of children. Here, we define *gender identification* as a child's sense of self as a female or male (Zucker & Bradley, 1995). *Gender-typing* is a broader construct that includes gender identification, but also extends to children's concepts or beliefs, preferences, and behaviors that align with expectations of what is appropriate for each gender (Ruble, Martin, & Berenbaum, 2006). There is variability in the levels

M.L.D. Halim, Ph.D. (✉) • D. Bryant, M.A.
Department of Psychology, California State University,
1250 Bellflower Blvd, Long Beach, CA 90840-0901, USA
e-mail: mayling.halim@csulb.edu

K.J. Zucker, Ph.D.
Centre for Addiction and Mental Health, 250 College Street, Toronto, ON, Canada, M5T 1R8
e-mail: ken.zucker@utoronto.ca

© Springer Science+Business Media New York 2016
M.R. Korin (ed.), *Health Promotion for Children and Adolescents*,
DOI 10.1007/978-1-4899-7711-3_10

of gender-typing among children—some are very gender-traditional and some are non-gender-traditional. The aim of this chapter is to examine this variability in gender identification and gender-typing from early to middle childhood and to investigate whether this variability has implications for the mental and physical health of children. We will first discuss developmental trends in gender identification and gender-typing from early to middle childhood. Next, we will discuss psychological theories pertaining to how gender identity and gender-typing might relate to health outcomes. We will then summarize what empirical evidence exists that examines this link between gender and health. Finally, we will discuss future directions and practical implications. Throughout, we will focus on both normative and gender-variant child populations, with the caveat that there is much less known about gender-variant children.

10.2 Developmental Trends in Gender Identification and Gender-Typing

Gender identity, as with other social categories, has multiple dimensions (Ashmore, Deaux, & McLaughlin-Volpe, 2004; Halim & Ruble, 2010). From a developmental perspective, gender identity includes basic gender category knowledge and a sense that one belongs to a gender category (*I'm a girl/boy*) (Kohlberg, 1966). This understanding likely starts as early as 18 months of age and is usually achieved by 30 months of age (Campbell, Shirley, & Caygill, 2002; Zosuls et al., 2009). Gender identity also includes the understanding of *gender constancy,* the understanding that one's gender typically remains relatively permanent across time (a boy will become a man, a woman was a girl) and superficial transformations (boys can play with dolls and remain a boy, girls can wear pants and remain a girl) (Kohlberg, 1966; Slaby & Frey, 1975). In addition to these milestones, gender identity includes the dimensions of *centrality* or *importance* (how important and salient gender is to one's overall self-concept), *evaluation* or private *regard* for one's gender along a positive–negative valence (I am happy to be a girl/boy) (also related to the concept of *felt contentedness* with one's gender), and one's evaluations of how others regard one's gender (I think others regard girls/boys positively) (*public regard*) (Halim, Ruble, & Tamis-Lemonda, 2013). Egan and Perry's (2001) model of gender identity in children also includes the dimensions of *intergroup bias* (attitudes towards the other gender), *felt pressure* for gender conformity from others and from one's self, and *felt typicality* (self-perceptions of how similar one is to same-gender children across activities, personality, and in general). New work also suggests that it is important to examine not only children's perceived similarity to same-gender children, but also to examine children's perceived similarity to *other*-gender children (Martin, Andrews, England, Ruble, & Zosuls, 2016).

Gender-typing is a superordinate category to gender identity and also multidimensional in nature (Huston, 1983). It includes the ways in which children enact and think about gender, in line with social stereotypes. Psychologists have, in fact, outlined a matrix of gender-typing with four constructs (concepts/beliefs, identity/ self-perceptions, preferences, behavioral enactment) crossed by six content areas (biological/categorical sex, activities/interests, personal–social attributes, social relationships, styles/symbols, values regarding gender) (see Ruble et al., 2006). For example, if we only looked at concepts/beliefs crossed with the six content areas, a girl could exhibit gender-typing by showing awareness of gender categories and gender stereotypes, such as that people expect girls to play with dolls, be nice, and wear pink, while learning that society often values males more than females. If we look at other areas of the matrix, children can show gender-typing by not only knowing and exhibiting stereotypes, but also through play behavior, mannerisms, and attitudes towards girls and boys. Overall, gender-typing is a broad construct that includes multiple ways that gender can be thought about and enacted in the every-day life of a child.

10.2.1 Normative Population

10.2.1.1 Gender Identity

In early childhood, during the preschool and kindergarten years, children generally feel very positive about their gender (Halim & Lindner, 2013). Most young children report that being a girl or boy is "very important" to them and also tend to report that they are "very happy" with being a girl or a boy (Ruble, Lurye, & Zosuls, 2007). Further, recent research suggests that this general love of their gender group and gender identity generalizes across multiple ethnic groups. In our study of 246 African American, Chinese-, Mexican-, and Dominican-immigrant 5-year-old children, about a third of the children chose the extreme end of the scale to express their utmost positivity about their gender (Halim, Ruble, Tamis-LeMonda, Shrout, & Amodio, 2012). Overall, 89 % of the children felt positively about their gender and considered gender to be an important aspect of the self, and 11 % evaluated their gender negatively and did not feel it was important. Our work also suggests that there is change in gender identity during this early childhood period. In a longitudinal study of the same children, boys increased in their private regard from age 4–5. Girls already had high levels throughout ages 4 and 5 (Halim et al., 2016). A cross-sectional study on White children from middle-class backgrounds found a trajectory of gender identification that was consistent with our findings, with the most positive regard and centrality at ages 4 and 5 compared to ages 3, 6, and 7 (Ruble, Taylor, et al., 2007).

The trajectory of gender identification in middle childhood is not as clear, as most research on this age group has focused more on connections between gender identity and adjustment, and not on mean levels of gender identification in and of itself (e.g., Egan & Perry, 2001). In addition, different measures and samples have been used in studies examining children in early versus middle childhood, so it is not possible to make strong conclusions about changes in gender identification across these developmental periods. Acknowledging these limitations, however, we can observe some interesting trends. First, overall means of gender contentedness appear to be somewhat more tempered in their positivity among grade-school samples than in preschool/kindergarten samples (Carver, Yunger, & Perry, 2003; Corby, Hodges, & Perry, 2007). The subsequent trajectory of gender identification from Grades 3 or 4 through Grade 8 is murkier. One study showed higher levels of gender contentedness with age (Carver et al., 2003), but another study showed lower levels of gender contentedness with age (Egan & Perry, 2001). Future studies are needed to understand these different results. Both studies included similar children in terms of age groups, ethnic composition, geographic location, and household socioeconomic status. However, at least from early childhood to middle childhood, children appear to be more "rigid" in their gender identification earlier in development.

In middle childhood, there has also been evidence for gender differences in gender identification. Across three samples of White, Black, and Hispanic children, boys showed higher mean levels of gender contentedness in elementary school compared to girls (Carver et al., 2003; Corby et al., 2007; Egan & Perry, 2001). Mean levels indicated that boys were "sort of" to "very" content with being a boy. In contrast, depending on the age group and sample, girls were either between discontent and content with being a girl (Egan & Perry, 2001) or just "sort of" content with being a girl (Corby et al., 2007). Interestingly, this gender difference found in elementary school with boys being more content with their gender compared to girls has not been seen in preschool/kindergarten samples. We speculate, then, that, as a group, girls show more change in their gender identification compared with boys from early to middle childhood, decreasing more in how happy they are with being a girl. Girls' more lukewarm gender identification in middle childhood is an interesting contrast to their strong bias in intergroup attitudes (very positive attitudes towards girls as a group) over boys as a group (Leroux, 2008; Susskind & Hodges, 2007).

This proposed asymmetry in girls' and boys' trajectories of gender identification from early to middle childhood is reflected in the tomboy phenomenon. As many as one-third to two-thirds of girls self-identify as "sort of" or unequivocal tomboys in middle childhood, peaking between ages 7 and 9 (Ahlqvist, Halim, Greulich, Lurye, & Ruble, 2013; Martin & Dinella, 2012). Who are these tomboys? Tomboys tend to show higher levels of male-typed play and activity preferences, have more favorable attitudes towards boys, and play with more boys than do traditional girls (Ahlqvist et al., 2013; Bailey, Bechtold, & Berenbaum, 2002; Martin & Dinella, 2012). In contrast to the prevalence of tomboyhood for girls in elementary school, no equivalent label to "tomboy" is even available for boys. Any close approximation to tomboy (e.g., "sissy") usually has a derogatory connotation (Martin, 1990). Thus, generally, girls and boys do shift from gender rigidity to flexibility in gender identification (positively evaluating being a boy/girl and considering being a boy/girl to be important) as they approach middle childhood. However, girls' gender identification may approach flexibility even more compared to boys, as they have the option to self-identify as tomboys.

10.2.1.2 Gender-Typing

Children's gender-typing also shows a similar shift from gender "rigidity" to more flexibility from early to middle childhood. In early childhood, children show rigid beliefs about gender (e.g., believing that only girls should play with dolls; Signorella, Bigler, & Liben, 1993). At this time, they are also more censorious of gender norm violations (e.g., not wanting to be friends with a boy who wears nail polish; Ruble, Taylor, et al. 2007). Some scholars have even identified certain children as "gender police" (Martin & Ruble, 2010), individuals who track others' conformity to gender norms and remark when conformity is lacking. In addition to rigid beliefs, children also exhibit rigid gender-typed behavior and preferences at this time. It is common to see children engaging in high levels of gender-typed play (Halim et al., 2013). Longitudinal work has also shown that engagement in cross-gender-typed play (e.g., boys playing with kitchen sets) *decreases* across ages 3–5 (Halim et al., 2013). Children increasingly play with same-gender peers as well across this period (Maccoby & Jacklin, 1987; Martin, Fabes, Evans, & Wyman, 1999). Many also tend to increasingly wear gender-stereotypical dress, tending to increase in stereotypicality from ages 3–4, in particular (Halim et al., 2014). Our previous work has shown that about two-thirds of girls at age four tend to exhibit "appearance rigidity," which is when girls demand to wear highly gender-stereotypical clothing with as much frequency as parents will allow (Halim et al., 2014). For example, girls may want to wear pink from head-to-toe and insist on wearing a skirt or a dress every single day, even for physically active occasions or when the weather is cold. These girls also refuse to wear pants, sometimes coming to tears when parents insist on putting on some pants. Young girls from diverse ethnic backgrounds within the USA and from East Asian countries have exhibited this behavior, suggesting that the "pink frilly dress a phenomenon" is robust (Arredondo et al., 2014; Halim et al., 2014). We have discovered that boys, too, show their own kind of appearance rigidity, which was more prevalent than we had expected. Depending on ethnic background, anywhere from 27 to 56% of boys showed appearance rigidity during early childhood, often refusing to wear anything remotely hinting of femininity and preferring superhero decals and sports-themed clothing. Hence, overall, in both beliefs and behaviors, children tend to exhibit gender rigidity during early childhood.

In middle childhood, we start to see a shift towards more gender flexibility as compared to early childhood, especially among girls. In terms of gender beliefs, endorsement and belief in gender stereotypes tends to decrease from age 5 or 6 through age 12 (Blakemore, 2003; Trautner et al., 2005). In elementary school, children are more likely to believe that some girls and some boys do and should be allowed to play with both trucks and dolls. Friendliness towards children who violate gender norms also tends to be higher than in early childhood, at least according to children's self-report (Ahlqvist et al., 2013; Ruble, Taylor, et al., 2007). As children, and particularly girls, get older, their behaviors also tend to adhere less to strict gender norms (Ruble et al., 2006). Overall, research suggests that children, and especially girls, tend to show more gender flexibility in their beliefs and behaviors during middle childhood compared to early childhood.

Hence, across both gender identification and gender-typing more broadly, normative trajectories of gender development chart a course of rigidity during early childhood and more flexibility during middle childhood. There are likely several reasons for this shift from rigidity to flexibility. Cognitive theories of gender development posit that these changes occur in alignment with changes in children's awareness of and understanding about gender and changes in children's general social cognition (Halim, Ruble, & Amodio, 2011). For example, in early childhood, children may strongly identify with their gender as this identification is new and exciting (Tajfel & Turner, 2004). They may be rigid in their behaviors and their beliefs because they do not yet understand that, even if they violate gender norms, their gender remains the same (Kohlberg, 1966). They may keep others in line in following gender norms as well as they lack a sophisticated understanding of individual differences, or within-category variability, and subgrouping (e.g., some girls can be nice and sweet, other girls are not). In middle childhood, their understanding of gender has advanced and their social cognitive skills have grown, possibly contributing to more flexibility. There is some empirical support for these theories (see Martin et al., 2002), but researchers are still gathering more direct evidence for these claims.

10.2.2   Gender-Variant Population

Just as the normative population shows variance in gender identification and gender-typing, gender variation exists within the non-normative population (Martin & Dinella, 2012). Some children might show discontent with their gender; others might question their sexual orientation at some point. In more extreme cases, some children identify outside of the pervasive and persistent historical binary gender categories of "male" and "female," which allow little room for fluctuation. These children are often referred to clinicians and are seen as experiencing *gender dysphoria*. For the purposes of this chapter, we thus define "non-normative" to include those children who may be referred to a clinician based on gender issues, children who may question their heterosexuality, and the small minority of children who express gender attitudes, beliefs, and behaviors that are counter to what the majority of children tend to express. Because this population covers many different types of individuals, it is important to note that discussing the diverse experiences of gender-variant children is challenging.

Before we discuss the developmental trajectories of gender identification and gender-typing of gender-variant children, it is also important to understand how many children might feel atypical about their gender. In one study, when asked if their child "behaves like the opposite sex," about 0–6 % of mothers of boys and 0–12 % of mothers of girls agreed that this was sometimes to very true (Zucker, Bradley, & Sanikhani, 1997). However, in the same sample, when asked whether their child "wishes to be of opposite sex," percentages were lower with 0–2 % of mothers of boys and 0–6 % of mothers of girls agreeing with this statement (Zucker et al., 1997). More recently, one study developed a measure based on Aron, Aron, and Smollan's (1992) Inclusion of Other in the Self Scale. Experimenters showed kindergarten to fourth-grade children from diverse ethnic backgrounds two sets of items, one measuring self-perceived similarity to girls and the other measuring self-perceived similarity to boys across actions, appearance, activities, and general similarity (e.g., "How much are you like girls/boys?") (Martin et al., 2016). Each set depicted different versions of a drawing with a group of girls or boys at one end of a line and a figure representing the child at the other end of the line. The different versions varied in how close (overlapping) or distant the group of girls/boys and the child were from each other, and children pointed to which version best represented the self in relation to the other girls and boys. Using cluster analysis, the following distribution was found: (1) about half of children perceived themselves to be more similar to same-gender compared to other-gender children, (2) 6% perceived themselves to be more similar to the other-gender compared to same-gender children, (3) 30% perceived themselves to be about equally and highly similar to both same- and other-gender children (androgynous), and (4) 17% perceived themselves to be dissimilar to both same- or other-gender children. This study suggests that anywhere from 6 to 23% of children may feel dissimilar to same-gender peers.

In studies examining gender private regard and centrality, 92 3- to 7-year-olds from mostly White, middle-class backgrounds were shown two groups of paper dolls. These children were asked questions like, "Some girls/boys feel proud to be a girl/boy, but other girls/boys do not feel proud to be a girl/boy. Which girls/boys are more like you?" (see Ruble, Taylor, et al., 2007). After selecting a group, children were asked, "Is that really true for you, or just sort of true for you?" in a Harter-type format. About 34% of the sample felt negatively about being a girl or boy (equal percentages of girls and boys). However, only 3% felt *very* negatively about being a girl or boy. In a separate sample, 246 ethnic minority 5-year-olds (Mexican-, Chinese-, Dominican-, and African-American) from low-income households were shown a scale of faces (very sad face to very happy face) and asked, "How do you feel about being a girl/boy?" (Halim, 2012). About 14% felt negatively about being a girl or boy. However, only 7% felt *very* negatively about being a girl or boy. Those who felt very negatively were more likely to be boys and less likely to be Dominican-American. Together, these data suggest that, in early childhood at least, anywhere from 14 to 34% of children feel negatively about being a girl or boy, and anywhere from 3 to 7% feel *especially* negatively about being a girl or boy. Much more research needs to be conducted to understand the prevalence of gender discontent. However, these studies do highlight that the issues we discuss may affect a substantial number of children.

10.2.2.1 Gender Identity

Because of the challenges involved with studying gender-variant populations (e.g., lower prevalence, willingness of communities and families to participate), few research studies have been able to examine the developmental trajectories of gender identification in gender-variant populations with the same fine-grained approach of tracking children from year to year from early to middle childhood. Instead, researchers have generally been interested in the stability of gender identification from childhood to adulthood. That is, do gender-variant adults show different gender identification during childhood compared to gender-normative adults, and, if so, at what age do they diverge?

According to both prospective and retrospective studies, the answer is mixed. In terms of gender dysphoria, children as young as age two may feel incompatible with their assigned gender; however, this does not guarantee a lifetime of gender dysphoria (Steensma, Biemond, de Boer, & Cohen-Kettenis, 2011; Steensma, McGuire, Kreukels, Beekman, & Cohen-Kettenis, 2013). Recent studies following up gender dysphoric children in adulthood found that natal boys showed persistence rates of 12.2 % (Singh, 2012) and 20.3 % (Wallien & Cohen-Kettenis, 2008) and follow-up studies of natal girls showed persistence rates of 12.0 % (Drummond, Bradley, Badali-Peterson, & Zucker, 2008) and 50 % (Wallien & Cohen-Kettenis, 2008). All of these studies showed higher persistence rates than an earlier study of natal boys, where the persistence rate was only 2.2 % Green (1987). Overall, these data suggest that the majority of gender dysphoric children later identify with their assigned biological sex.

If individuals do remain gender dysphoric and wish to pursue life as the other gender, they are referred to as transgender or, in the clinical literature, as transsexual. A large-scale retrospective study conducted on gender-nonconforming transgender students found that the average age of perceiving oneself as "different" in terms of gender was at about age 5 (Rankin & Beemyn, 2012). About a fifth of the individuals surveyed "always" felt different in terms of gender, and 97 % indicated feeling a lack of fit with their gender-normative peers. Similarly, in a sample of 31 male-to-female (MTF) and 24 female-to-male (FTM) transgender youth, 26 (84 %) of the MTF and 16 (67 %) of the FTM youth always wished to be born the other sex (Grossman, D'Augelli, Howell, & Hubbard, 2005). These studies suggest that for gender dysphoric children who later become transgender, the majority identifies with the other sex relatively early in childhood, and identification with the other sex is stable.

Limited research has examined the gender identification of children who question their heterosexuality, and this research is also mixed. Similar to gender dysphoria, some children who question their heterosexuality later identify as homosexual in their lifetime, but not all do (Golombok & Tasker, 1996). Beyond examining stability, in terms of other dimensions of gender identification, one study found that elementary school-aged children (Grades 4–8) who were questioning their heterosexuality tended to be less satisfied with their assigned gender and perceived themselves as more different from same-gender peers (Carver, Egan, & Perry, 2004). However, other studies have found no relationship between self-perceived gender nonconformity and one's sexual orientation questioning (Savin-Williams, 1998).

Overall, these mixed results may reflect the complexity involved in gender identification development for gender-variant children. For example, gender-variant children's trajectories of gender identification may not be known until later in life (Leibowitz & Telingator, 2012). Typologies of gender dysphoria have been influenced by age of onset. Although considerable literature has suggested that gender dysphoria can be traced to early childhood and prepubescent times, there are subgroups of gender dysphoric individuals who are described as late-onset (for review, see Lawrence, 2010). Further, some key developmental periods, such as puberty, may alter childhood experiences. Not all gender nonconforming children will follow trajectories similar to their nonconforming peers. More research is needed to better understand the developmental trajectories of gender identification for gender-variant children using prospective, longitudinal designs, while accounting for the diversity found among this population.

10.2.2.2 Gender-Typing

Just as with examining the trajectories of gender identification, most research on gender-variant populations has not observed changes in gender-typing from year to year. Instead, researchers have investigated whether gender-variant adults tended to show less gender-typing as children compared to gender-normative adults. There is some evidence that this is the case for appearance and play preferences. In one study of transgender youth, the majority of the youth (both female-to-male and male-to-female individuals) reported always wishing to wear clothes associated with the other gender (Grossman et al., 2005). Some retrospective studies of homosexual men and women also support a similar pattern (Bailey & Zucker, 1995). Homosexual men recalled being more feminine in their play and appearance preferences compared to childhood male peers, while homosexual women recalled being more masculine compared to childhood female peers. To minimize recall bias, Reiger, Linsenmeier, Gygax, and Bailey (2008) used childhood home videos to investigate the difference in childhood gender nonconformity and self-reports. Using both homosexual and heterosexual populations, this study found that self-reported gender nonconformity as children was confirmed by observer ratings of the childhood home videos. Additionally, gender nonconformity was significantly correlated with sexual orientation, suggesting that those who identified as homosexual as an adult were more gender nonconforming as children compared to those who identified as heterosexual adults. Thus, there is some evidence that gender-variant adults show less gender-typing as children compared to non-gender-variant adults, and sometimes even engage in other-gender-typed activities and dress.

Overall, this research suggests that for some gender-variant children, their developmental trajectories of gender identification and gender-typing diverge from the normative population. These children might identify more with the other gender from an early age, they might feel atypical of their assigned gender group, and they might show less gender-typing in activities and dress. However, more research is needed to understand whether there is change or stability in gender identification and gender-typing from early to middle childhood among gender-variant children.

10.3 Gender Identity and Gender-Typing in Relation to Health Outcomes: Theory

Thus far, we have discussed the typical developmental trajectories, from early to middle childhood, of gender identification and gender-typing. Yet, some gender-normative children do not follow these typical patterns of development. Are these children at risk for poorer health? Gender-variant populations may face many challenges across development. As a social identity, gender powerfully colors our experience of the world and is relatively permanent across situations. For example, children who feel different from their gender group may experience teasing or disapproval, not only in one instance, but across time, and possibly across situations and groups (Zucker & Bradley, 1995). Even without external teasing or disapproval, internally, children may ruminate about their gender identity or about feeling different. There is also the possibility that children may accept themselves the way they are, families may accept them as well, but children may continuously encounter others in their environments who impose their own gender stereotypes and expectations onto them. Thus, gender identity and gender-typing have the potential to have a high impact on children's health and well-being. How might gender identity and gender-typing relate to mental health and well-being? We propose that two aspects of gender identity and gender-typing are key—feeling different from others and feeling devalued by others (Fig. 10.1).

10.3.1 Mental Health and Well-Being

10.3.1.1 Feeling Different

Historically, literature on gender identity/typing and adjustment has focused on *being* different from others based on gender norms and whether *being* different from others leads to poor psychological adjustment. Controversy surrounded this question. Kagan (1964) proposed that being a typical girl or boy would lead to positive psychological adjustment, as it would minimize feelings of difference from others and would instill a healthy sense of self as a male or female. In contrast, Bem (1974) proposed that being a typical girl or boy was limiting and might lead to negative psychological adjustment. Bem was a proponent of minimizing gender distinctions and maximizing equality between the sexes (see also Woodhill & Samuels, 2003). Bem (1974, 1981) believed that androgyny—possessing both masculine and feminine traits—was ideal for girls and boys, men and women. With androgyny, individuals could acquire diverse skills, traits, and experiences that would aid them in a broader array of contexts. Although Bem's theories have been critiqued (Lippa, 2005), there has been some support for Bem's theories. For example, Woodhill and Samuels extended Bem's work and proposed that *positive* androgyny, a balance of positive masculine and positive feminine qualities, resulted in higher psychological health and well-being.

More recently, psychologists have focused on children's sense of *feeling* different from others based on gender. Similar to Kagan's (1964) arguments, researchers proposed that both feeling typical of one's gender (*felt typicality*) and feeling content with one's gender (*felt contentedness*) are beneficial for psychological adjustment (Carver et al., 2003; Egan & Perry, 2001). These two components—felt typicality and felt contentedness—have often been conceptualized as a broader concept of *gender compatibility* (Egan & Perry, 2001). Researchers hypothesized that children who feel incompatible with their gender will tend to exhibit poorer well-being. In particular, it is the combination of feeling atypical *and* feeling pressure from one's self and/or others to conform to gender norms that can likely be harmful to children's adjustment (Egan & Perry, 2001). How might feelings of atypicality and feeling pressure to conform to gender norms lead to poor adjustment? One potential mechanism that researchers have investigated is acceptance from others (Smith & Leaper, 2006). Children who feel that they are different from other children might be more likely to be teased or excluded by peers. This teasing or exclusion could, in turn, lead to anxiety, depression, and other maladaptive outcomes.

10.3.1.2 Feeling Devalued

Another pathway by which gender identity and gender-typing can affect the mental health of children is through perceiving devaluation. For example, girls may start to become aware that males have higher status than females in society and may internalize this devaluation. Children who are different from other same-gender children may also perceive devaluation, as they tend to be less popular and have lower social status among their peers compared to their gender-typical peers (Jewell & Brown, 2014). Nontraditional Children may be sensitive to this hierarchy between gender-traditional and nontraditional children, leading to distress. Children who are questioning heterosexuality may also pick up on cues that society often discriminates against lesbian, gay, bisexual, transgender, and intersex populations. Finally, children with gender dysphoria may also be sensitive to the stigma associated with gender dysphoria (Zucker & Bradley, 1995). Thus, it is possible that children might implicitly understand who is valued and who is not, whether based on gender, gender typicality, sexual orientation, or general gender variance. They might receive these messages from multiple sources, such as the media (Halim et al., 2013), language (e.g., using "gay" as a derogatory term) (Hall & LaFrance, 2012), from observing social dynamics around them, or from direct experience.

Few studies have directly examined children's perceptions of gender hierarchies. The most relevant studies conducted have mainly examined children's perceptions of men's group status compared to women's. These studies have found that awareness of male prestige and of discrimination against women is greater in older children (ages 10–15) compared to younger children (ages 5–6) (Brown & Bigler, 2004; Neff, Cooper, & Woodruff, 2007). However, even as young as age 4 there is variability in this awareness, with some children being more aware than others due to greater exposure to messages a conveying a gender hierarchy (Halim et al., 2013).

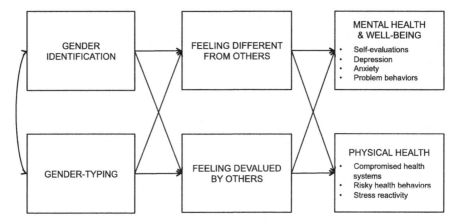

Fig. 10.1 Conceptual model of gender development and links with health

To date, to our knowledge, no studies have been conducted examining children's awareness of hierarchies based on gender typicality, sexual orientation, or gender variance.

Although there is little research on perceived devaluation based on gender and links with mental health, we can look to the racial/ethnic literature as a possible parallel. A growing body of research has shown that youth and adults who perceive devaluation based on their race or ethnicity tend to exhibit psychological distress (Ho & Sidanius, 2009; Sellers, Copeland-Linder, Martin, & Lewis, 2006). If processes involving perceived devaluation's effects on mental health generalize across both race/ethnicity and gender, then there is potential for perceived devaluation based on gender to show similar links to poorer mental health (Fig. 10.1).

10.3.2 Physical Health

How might feeling different or devalued based on gender relate to physical health? In the past few decades, health psychologists have made gains to show that our psychology can affect our bodies and our physical health. The large majority of this research has investigated links between psychology and health in adults. Thus, caution is needed in generalizing models of psychology and health from adults to children, as developmental health psychology is an emerging field. However, these models based on adults may be useful in generating ideas for future research on the effects of one's gender identity and gender-typing on physical health in children.

Feeling different and feeling devalued can potentially cause a child stress. Further, if children chronically feel different or devalued from others due to gender, they may experience a chronically stressful environment. Theories of health psychology have modeled how this chronic stress might lead to poorer physical health outcomes. One useful model that we can apply here specifically theorizes on how perceived discrimination affects physical health (Pascoe & Richman, 2009). Although perceived discrimination and feelings of difference due to gender are distinct, the same processes may apply as both share commonalities and both may induce stress. One pathway describes a direct link between feeling different or devalued and physical health. The second describes a pathway whereby feeling different can lead to a heightened physiological stress response, which can cause sustained demand on the stress response system resulting in allostatic load (McEwen & Wingfield, 2003). This load, in turn, can lead to illness and worse physical health generally. Some mechanisms whereby stress can lead to worse health include elevated ambulatory and systolic blood pressure (Brady & Matthews, 2006; Matthews, Saloman, Kenyon, & Zhou, 2005), elevated cytokines related to unhealthy inflammation profiles (Ratner, Halim, & Amodio, 2013), and possibly sleep difficulties (El-Sheikh, Buckhalt, Mize, & Acebo, 2006; Gross & Borkovec, 1982). The third describes how feeling different can lead to more risky health behaviors, which in turn leads to worse physical health. For children, unhealthy behaviors could possibly be captured in sedentary behavior, eating disturbances (eating too much or too little), or eating high caloric and fatty foods (Bennett & Cooper, 1999; Gluck, 2006). In turn, one might hypothesize, then, that these unhealthy behaviors could promote obesity and childhood diabetes. Overall, the model of perceived discrimination affecting physical health through direct and indirect means can possibly serve well in making predictions for children's health in the face of feeling different based on gender (Fig. 10.1).

Beyond current physical health, early exposure to psychosocial stress in development can have negative implications later on in development. There have been several proposed mechanisms for how early stress can affect later development, through both biological and social mechanisms, which likely interact to affect outcomes. The strongest empirical evidence for the link between early stress and poor developmental outcomes comes from literature on poverty and physical maltreatment (Miller, Chen, & Parker, 2011). It remains to be seen if stress due to feeling different based on gender is as powerful as stress from poverty or physical maltreatment. Nevertheless, the processes involved may be similar. For example, stress may cause sleeping difficulties (Sadeh, 1996), which interrupts healthy growth and development. Also, children who are rejected by others may also feel more anger and hostility, risk factors for physical attributes that, in adulthood, may put them at risk for coronary heart disease (Woodall & Matthews, 1989). Additionally, early stress during the prenatal or neonatal period can influence the brain to experience more exposure to glucocorticoids, stress-related hormones, and catecholamines. The brain's exposure to these hormones and momoamines, in turn, can interfere with executive functioning and self-regulation, which can possibly lead to developmental delays (Blair, 2010; Evans & Kim, 2013). Very recent work is beginning to suggest that early life stress (poverty, physical maltreatment) can even alter gene expression having to do with stress reactivity and inflammation, making children biologically vulnerable to behavioral and health problems (Miller et al., 2011; Romens, McDonald, Svaren, & Pollak, 2014). Hence, stressors caused by feeling different or devalued based on gender cannot only affect the concurrent physical health of children, but also potentially affect their health and development in years to come.

The literature on early childhood adversity also suggests that the early years are critical as these early negative experiences might rewire the biological system (Fagundes & Way, 2014). For example, children who had early childhood adversity, but were later educated, upward socially mobile professionals still experienced worse physical health compared to their peers who had not experienced this adversity (Kittleson et al., 2006). Again, caution is needed in comparing models of stress due to poverty and physical maltreatment to models of stress due to gender. However, we speculate that in certain cases, if a child early on feels extreme levels of stress due to feeling different or devalued based on gender, this child could potentially experience worse physical health as an adult, even if they no longer felt different from others or devalued as an adult.

10.4 Gender Identity and Gender-Typing in Relation to Health Outcomes: Empirical Evidence

We first outlined theory on how variation in gender identity and gender-typing could be related to health outcomes. We now discuss what empirical evidence exists that addresses this issue. Below we separate mental and physical health outcomes below for ease of organization. However, it is important to note that mental health and physical health are interrelated (Cohen & Herbert, 1996). For example, somatic symptoms (headaches, stomachaches, fatigue) in children are common complaints for those experiencing anxiety (Ginsburg, Riddle, & Davies, 2006).

10.4.1 Mental Health and Well-Being

10.4.1.1 Normative Population

A robust body of research has addressed the question of whether children who feel incompatible with their gender (low feelings of typicality and dissatisfaction with one's gender) might be at risk for poor adjustment. It is worth noting that perceptions of feeling and actually being different from same-gender children have been found to be positively correlated in children (Lurye, 2011). Yet, *feeling* different from same-gender children has emerged as a stronger and more consistent predictor of psychological adjustment (Lurye, 2011). The majority of this research has focused on elementary school-aged to preadolescent children and suggests that, across diverse ethnic groups, children who feel more incompatible with their gender do tend to exhibit more negative psychological adjustment (e.g., lower feelings of global self-worth and self-esteem) (Carver et al., 2003; Egan & Perry, 2001; Martin, Fabes, & Hanish, 2014). Furthermore, there has been support for the idea that the combination of felt atypicality with feelings of pressure to conform to gender norms is particularly harmful for children (Egan & Perry, 2001). Interestingly, research has found that across ethnic groups, boys, in particular, receive more pressure to conform to gender norms compared to girls, as well as receive harsher consequences for failing to do so (Carver et al., 2003; Jewell & Brown, 2014; Smith & Leaper, 2006). Thus, boys may be at particular risk for maladjustment in the face of feeling different from other boys.

Another group who might possess a particular risk for poor adjustment are girls who self-identify as tomboys. Several studies have shown that girls who either self-identify as tomboys or show tomboy-like patterns (male-typed traits, behaviors, and interests) are more likely to report feeling different from other girls and feeling discontent with being a girl compared to traditional girls (Ahlqvist et al., 2013; Martin & Dinella, 2012). Further, researchers have found that tomboys tend to have lower social self-esteem (Lobel et al., 1997) and global self-esteem when not buffered by high athleticism (Halim et al., 2011). Future research still needs to directly examine whether the lower self-esteem of tomboys is due to some feeling of gender incompatibility. Nevertheless, as a substantial number of girls today self-identify as tomboys, the risk for lower self-esteem is relevant to many.

As for the hypothesized mechanism of how gender typicality might predict adjustment, there has been some support for acceptance from peers as a key variable. A study of fourth to eighth grade children found that children who felt less gender-typical tended to have more negative peer relations (Egan & Perry, 2001). Also, one study of adolescents found that the relation between self-perceived gender typicality and self-worth was partially explained by peer acceptance (Smith & Leaper, 2006). Hence, overall, there is support for the prediction that feeling different from others, based on gender, can lead to poorer adjustment. In contrast to this robust body of work, there are few studies investigating whether feelings of devaluation based on gender also lead to poorer mental health and well-being. Future studies should address this research gap.

10.4.1.2   Gender-Variant Population

A body of research suggests that gender variance in childhood is a risk factor for poorer mental health and well-being across several indicators. First, gender-variant children are at risk for poor self-evaluations. Rijn, Steensma, Kreukels, and Cohen-Kettenis (2013) found that gender-variant girls tended to have lower global self-worth, lower self-evaluations of physical appearance, and poorer behavioral conduct compared to gender-normative girls. Gender-variant boys also reported lower global self-worth, as well as lower scholastic competence, athletic competence, and self-evaluations of physical appearance compared to gender-normative boys. Overall, gender variant compared to gender-normative children possessed more negative self-perceptions globally and across multiple domains.

Second, gender non-normative children have shown more problem behaviors compared to their normative peers (Egan & Perry, 2001; Martin et al., 2014; Zucker, Wood, & VanderLaan, 2014). Children who perceived themselves to be more similar to other- versus same-gender children, in particular, have reported more social anxiety than children who perceive themselves to be similar to same-gender children (Martin et al., 2014). Children with gender dysphoria have also been found to have more attention problems, delinquent behaviors, and aggressive behaviors compared to their gender-normative peers (Wallien, van Goozen, & Cohen-Kettenis, 2007).

Third, on top of poor self-evaluations and problem behaviors, when children experience gender dysphoria, they are also likely to experience other psychological disorders, especially anxiety and depression (Coolidge, Thede, & Young, 2002; Wallien et al., 2007; Zucker & Bradley, 1995). Most studies find that gender dysphoria is commonly comorbid with other psychiatric disorders in general, although there have been inconsistent findings (de Vries, Doreleijers, Steensma, & Cohen-Kettenis, 2011). Overall, however, several studies generally indicate that gender-variant children reported stronger negative feelings and emotional disturbances (for a review see Zucker et al., 2014).

Furthermore, the high rates of psychiatric comorbidity associated with gender variance can have serious consequences. For example, compared to non-transsexual adults, transsexual patients had higher perceived stress and reported insecure attachment patterns (Colizzi, Costa, Pace, & Todarello, 2013). Gender-variant individuals also often experience heightened anxiety and depression, which can, in turn, increase suicidal behavior (Plöderl & Fartacek, 2009; Terada et al., 2011; for a review, see Lawrence & Zucker, 2014). Terada et al. (2011) sampled Japanese patients that were diagnosed with gender dysphoria without psychiatric comorbidity and found that 72 % of the sample exhibited suicidal ideation at some point in their lifetime. Similarly, McDuffie and Brown (2010) conducted a descriptive study on US veterans with gender identity disturbances. Results indicated that 61 % had one or more suicide attempts. Compared to the rate of about 4 % in the general population (Substance Abuse and Mental Health Services Administration, 2015), these high rates of suicidal behavior or ideation are disturbing and underscore the graveness of the matter. These negative consequences may stem from the stigma related to being gender variant (Zucker & Bradley, 1995) as well as, from the distress associated with gender dysphoria (Colizzi et al., 2013).

A survey of the literature, then, suggests that gender-variant children are at risk for poorer mental health and well-being compared to their gender-normative peers. It is important to also note, however, that gender-variant children show rates of behavioral and emotional problems that are similar to children referred for other clinical issues. Gender variant compared to gender-normative children tend to show more negative self-perceptions, problem behaviors, and often experience more anxiety and depression and other psychiatric disorders. Greater anxiety and depression, in turn, can lead to suicidal ideation and behavior in one's lifetime.

10.4.2   Physical Health

Does feeling different or devalued based on gender affect the physical health of children as theory suggests? In contrast to the literature on gender and mental health, this area of research is sparse, and there is little empirical evidence for a connection between gender and physical health in children. Even in the adult literature, few studies have examined whether feeling different or devalued based on gender leads to poorer physical health outcomes. These studies, however, do lend support to the predictions made above, particularly in regard to devaluation and health. For example, hearing, "That's so gay!", with its derogatory connotations, was associated with poorer physical well-being among lesbian, gay, and bisexual college students (Woodford, Howell, Silverschanz, & Yu, 2012). In our own study of 187 ethnic minority women, we found that feeling that others regarded women more negatively than men in terms of importance, worth, and respect (*comparative gender public regard*) was associated with lower overall self-reported physical health and more frequent alcohol consumption (Lindner, Bryant, & Halim, 2014). Thus in both cases, feelings of devaluation based on gender increased the risk of poorer physical health. It remains to be seen if these dynamics seen in adults generalize to children.

10.5   Future Directions and Practical Implications

Research on the developmental trajectories of gender identification and gender-typing of gender-variant children is still scarce. We also know little about whether these children are at risk for poorer mental and physical health during childhood. As we have outlined above, research on gender dysphoric youth and adults shows that they are at risk for a number of mental and physical health problems. Research on lesbian, gay, and bisexual adults (LGB) has also shown that LGB compared to non-LGB populations are indeed at greater risk for poorer mental health, including higher rates of major depression, generalized anxiety, substance use, and suicidal behavior (Hatzenbuehler, 2009; Meyer, 2003). There are also persistent physical health disparities between LGB and non-LGB adult populations as well, spanning multiple outcomes such as overall health, cardiovascular health, and incidence of chronic disease, cancer, asthma, allergies, and headaches (Lick, Durso, & Johnson, 2013). Future research should examine whether these disparities can also be seen in children who begin to question their heterosexuality and, if so, when these disparities emerge in development. Similarly, more attention is needed to investigate the health outcomes of other types of gender-variant children and children who feel different or devalued based on their gender. To test these questions, we recommend that more longitudinal studies are needed to follow the progression and development of gender-variant children in their gender-typing and gender identification. Understanding these trajectories could potentially help inform future interventions to ameliorate health risks for these children.

Practically speaking, it would be helpful for the public to become aware that teasing, exclusion, and discrimination based on gender are not innocuous rites of childhood, but can possibly have major consequences on children's health. Further, taking care of all children's health, including children who feel different or devalued based on gender, affects public health and health expenditures more generally for the nation as a whole. We encourage schools, teachers, administration, and parents to continue to make clear statements of inclusiveness based on gender, such as establishing Gay-Straight Alliance clubs. On a more macro level, it is important to work towards removing the stigma from gender variance. Societal acceptance of all kinds of children, no matter whether they are masculine or feminine or whether they identify with one gender or the other, might potentially help to ease the impact and progression of health risks for children in childhood, and later as youth and adults.

References

Ahlqvist, S., Halim, M. L., Greulich, F. K., Lurye, L. E., & Ruble, D. N. (2013). The potential benefits and risks of identifying as a tomboy: A social identity perspective. *Self and Identity, 12,* 563–581. doi:10.1080/15298868.2012.717709.
Aron, A., Aron, E. N., & Smollan, D. (1992). Inclusion of Other in the Self Scale and the structure of interpersonal closeness. Journal of Personality and Social Psychology, 63(4), 596–612.
Arredondo, M., Walsh, A., Baeg, S. A., Halim, M. L., Ruble, D. N., Ng, F. F., … Tamis-LeMonda, C. S. (2014, April). *Gender appearance rigidity in American and Asian 4-year-olds.* Poster presented at the Western Psychological Association Convention, Portland, OR.
Ashmore, R. D., Deaux, K., & McLaughlin-Volpe, T. (2004). An organizing framework for collective identity: Articulation and significance of multidimensionality. *Psychological Bulletin, 130,* 80–114. doi:10.1037/0033-2909.130.1.80.
Bailey, J. M., Bechtold, K. T., & Berenbaum, S. A. (2002). Who are tomboys and why should we study them? *Archives of Sexual Behavior, 31,* 333–341. doi:10.1023/A:1016272209463.
Bailey, J. M., & Zucker, K. J. (1995). Childhood sex-typed behavior and sexual orientation: A conceptual analysis and quantitative review. *Developmental Psychology, 31,* 43–55. doi:10.1037/0012-1649.31.1.43.
Bem, S. L. (1974). The measurement of psychological androgyny. *Journal of Consulting and Clinical Psychology, 42,* 155–162. doi:10.1037/h0036215.
Bem, S. L. (1981). Gender schema theory: A cognitive account of sex typing. *Psychological Review, 88,* 354–364. doi:10.1037/0033-295X.88.4.354.
Bennett, D. A., & Cooper, C. L. (1999). Eating disturbance as a manifestation of the stress process: A review of the literature. *Stress and Health, 15,* 167–182.
Blakemore, J. (2003). Children's beliefs about violating gender norms: Boys shouldn't look like girls, and girls shouldn't act like boys. *Sex Roles, 48,* 411–419. doi:10.1023/A:1023574427720.
Blair, C. (2010). Stress and the development of self-regulation in context. *Child Development Perspectives, 4*(3), 181–188.
Brady, S. S., & Matthews, K. A. (2006). Chronic stress influences ambulatory blood pressure in adolescents. *Annals of Behavioral Medicine, 31,* 80–88.
Brown, C., & Bigler, R. S. (2004). Children's perceptions of gender discrimination. *Developmental Psychology, 40,* 714–726. doi:10.1037/0012-1649.40.5.714.
Campbell, A., Shirley, L., & Caygill, L. (2002). Sex-typed preferences in three domains: Do two-year-olds need cognitive variables? *British Journal of Psychology, 93,* 203–217. doi:10.1348/000712602162544.
Carver, P. R., Egan, S. K., & Perry, D. G. (2004). Children who question their heterosexuality. *Developmental Psychology, 40,* 43–53. doi:10.1037/0012-1649.40.1.43.
Carver, P., Yunger, J., & Perry, D. (2003). Gender identity and adjustment in middle childhood. *Sex Roles, 49,* 95–109.
Cohen, S., & Herbert, T. B. (1996). Health psychology: Psychological factors and physical disease from the perspective of human psychoneuroimmunology. *Annual Review of Psychology, 47,* 113–142.
Colizzi, M., Costa, R., Pace, V., & Todarello, O. (2013). Hormonal treatment reduces psychobiological distress in gender identity disorder, independently of the attachment style. *Journal of Sexual Medicine, 10,* 3049–3058. doi:10.1111/jsm.12155.

Coolidge, F., Thede, L., & Young, S. (2002). The heritability of gender identity disorder in a child and adolescent twin sample. *Behavior Genetics, 32*, 251–257.

Corby, B. C., Hodges, E. V. E., & Perry, D. G. (2007). Gender identity and adjustment in Black, Hispanic, and White preadolescents. *Developmental Psychology, 43*, 261–266. doi:10.1037/0012-1649.43.1.261.

de Vries, A. L. C., Doreleijers, T. A. H., Steensma, T. D., & Cohen-Kettenis, P. T. (2011). Psychiatric comorbidity in gender dysphoric adolescents. *Journal of Child Psychology and Psychiatry, 52*, 1195–1202. doi:10.1111/j.1469-7610.2011.02426.x.

Drummond, K. D., Bradley, S. J., Badali-Peterson, M., & Zucker, K. J. (2008). A follow-up study of girls with gender identity disorder. *Developmental Psychology, 44*, 34–45.

Egan, S. K., & Perry, D. G. (2001). Gender identity: A multidimensional analysis with implications for psychosocial adjustment. *Developmental Psychology, 37*, 451–463. doi:10.1037/0012-1649.37.4.451.

El-Sheikh, M., Buckhalt, J. A., Mize, J., & Acebo, C. (2006). Marital conflict and disruption of children's sleep. *Child Development, 77*, 31–43.

Evans, G. W., & Kim, P. (2013). Childhood poverty, chronic stress, self-regulation, and coping. *Child Development Perspectives, 7*(1), 43–48.

Fagundes, C. P., & Way, B. (2014). Early-life stress and adult inflammation. *Current Directions in Psychological Science, 23*, 277–283.

Ginsburg, G. S., Riddle, M. A., & Davies, M. (2006). Somatic symptoms in children and adolescents with anxiety disorders. *Journal of the American Academy of Child and Adolescent Psychiatry, 45*, 1179–1187. doi:10.1097/01.chi.0000231974.43966.6e.

Gluck, M. E. (2006). Stress response and binge eating disorder. *Appetite, 46*, 26–30.

Golombok, S., & Tasker, F. (1996). Do parents influence the sexual orientation of their children? Findings from a longitudinal study of lesbian families. *Developmental Psychology, 32*, 3–11. doi:10.1037/0012-1649.32.1.3.

Green, R. (1987). *The "sissy boy syndrome" and the development of homosexuality*. New Haven, CT: Yale University Press.

Gross, R. T., & Borkovec, T. D. (1982). Effects of a cognitive intrusion manipulation on the sleep-onset latency of good sleepers. *Behavior Therapy, 13*, 112–116.

Grossman, A. H., D'Augelli, A. R., Howell, T. J., & Hubbard, S. (2005). Parent' reactions to transgender youth' gender nonconforming expression and identity. *Journal of Gay & Lesbian Social Services, 18*, 3–16. doi:10.1300/J041v18n01_02.

Halim, M. D., Ruble, D. N., Tamis-LeMonda, C. S., Shrout, P. E., & Amodio, D. A. (in press). Gender attitudes among ethnic minority children: Consequences for intergroup behavior and social cognitive antecedents. *Child Development*.

Halim, M. L. (2012). *Gender rigidity and flexibility in young children's gender-typed behaviors, identity, and attitudes: A cognitive theories of gender development perspective* (Unpublished doctoral dissertation). New York University, New York, NY.

Halim, M. L., Dalmut, E., Greulich, F., Ahlqvist, S., Lurye, L. E., & Ruble, D. N. (2011). The self-esteem of tomboys and the role of athletics. *Child Development Research*. http://www.hindawi.com/journals/cdr/2011/830345/

Halim, M. L., & Lindner, N. (2013). Gender self-socialization in early childhood. In R. E. Tremblay, M. Boivin, & R. D. Peters (Eds.), *Encyclopedia on early childhood development [online]* (pp. 1–6). Montreal, Quebec: Centre of Excellence for Early Childhood Development and Strategic Knowledge Cluster on Early Childhood Development. Retrieved from http://www.child-encyclopedia.com/documents/Halim-LindnerANGxp1.pdf.

Halim, M. L., & Ruble, D. N. (2010). Gender identity and stereotyping in early and middle childhood. In J. Chrisler & D. McCreary (Eds.), *Handbook of gender research in psychology* (pp. 495–525). New York: Springer.

Halim, M. L., Ruble, D. N., Tamis-LeMonda, C., Zosuls, K. M., Lurye, L. E., & Greulich, F. K. (2014). Pink frilly dresses and the avoidance of all things "girly": Children's appearance rigidity and cognitive theories of gender development. *Developmental Psychology, 50*, 1091–1101. doi:10.1037/a0034906; 10.1037/a0034906.supp (Supplemental).

Halim, M. L., Ruble, D. N., Tamis-LeMonda, C. S., Shrout, P. E., & Amodio, D. A. (2016). Gender attitudes among ethnic minority children: Consequences for intergroup behavior and social cognitive antecedents.

Halim, M. L., Ruble, D. N., & Amodio, D. M. (2011). From pink frilly dresses to 'one of the boys': A social-cognitive analysis of gender identity development and gender bias. *Social and Personality Psychology Compass, 5*, 933–949. doi:10.1111/j.1751-9004.2011.00399.x.

Halim, M. L., Ruble, D. N., & Tamis-Lemonda, C. (2013). Four-year-olds' beliefs about how others regard males and females. *British Journal of Developmental Psychology, 31*, 128–135. doi:10.1111/j.2044-835X.2012.02084.x.

Halim, M. L., Zosuls, K. M., Ruble, D. N., Tamis-LeMonda, C. S., Baeg, A. S., Walsh, A. S., & Moy, K. H. (in press). Children's dynamic gender identities across development and the influence of cognition, context, and culture. In C. S. Tamis-LeMonda & L. Balter (Eds.), *Child Psychology: A Handbook of Contemporary Issues* (3rd ed.). New York, NY: Psychology Press/Taylor & Francis.

Hall, J., & LaFrance, B. (2012). "That's gay": Sexual prejudice, gender identity, norms, and homophobic communication. *Communication Quarterly, 60*, 35–58.

Hatzenbuehler, M. L. (2009). How does sexual minority stigma "get under the skin"? A psychological mediation framework. *Psychological Bulletin, 135*, 707–730. doi:10.1037/a0016441.

Ho, A. K., & Sidanius, J. (2009). Preserving positive identities: Public and private regard for one's ingroup and susceptibility to stereotype threat. *Group Processes & Intergroup Relations, 13*, 55–67.

Huston, A. C. (1983). Sex-typing. In E. M. Hetherington (Ed.), & P. H. Mussen (Series Ed.), *Handbook of child psychology: Vol. 4. Socialization, personality, and social development* (pp. 387–467). New York: Wiley.

Jewell, J. A., & Brown, C. S. (2014). Relations among gender typicality, peer relations, and mental health during early adolescence. *Social Development, 23*, 137–156. doi:10.1111/sode.12042.

Kagan, J. (1964). A cognitive-developmental analysis of children's sex-role concepts and attitudes. *Review of Child Development Research, 1*, 137–167.

Kittleson, M. M., Meoni, L. A., Wang, N. Y., Chu, A. Y., Ford, D. E., & Klag, M. J. (2006). Association of childhood socioeconomic status with subsequent coronary heart disease in physicians. *Archives of Internal Medicine, 166*, 2356–2361.

Kohlberg, L. (1966). A cognitive-developmental analysis of children's sex-role concepts and attitudes. In E. E. Maccoby (Ed.), *The development of sex differences* (pp. 82–172). Stanford, CA: Stanford University Press.

Lawrence, A. A. (2010). Sexual orientation versus age of onset as bases for typologies (subtypes) for gender identity disorder in adolescents and adults. *Archives of Sexual Behavior, 39*(2), 514–545. doi:10.1007/s10508-009-9594-3.

Lawrence, A. A., & Zucker, K. J. (2014). Gender dysphoria. In D. C. Beidel, B. C. Frueh, & M. Hersen (Eds.), *Adult psychopathology and diagnosis* (7th ed., pp. 603–639). Hoboken, NJ: Wiley.

Leibowitz, S., & Telingator, C. (2012). Assessing gender identity concerns in children and adolescents: Evaluation, treatments, and outcomes. *Current Psychiatry Reports, 14*, 111–120.

Leroux, A. (2008). *Do children with gender identity disorder have an in-group or an out-group gender-based bias?* Unpublished Master's thesis, University of Toronto.

Lick, D. J., Durso, L. E., & Johnson, K. L. (2013). Minority stress and physical health among sexual minorities. *Perspectives on Psychological Science, 8*, 521–548. doi:10.1177/1745691613497965.

Lindner, N., Bryant, D., & Halim, M. L. (2014, April). *Gender discrimination predicts worse health through gender public regard.* Poster presented at the Western Psychological Association Convention, Portland, OR.

Lippa, R. A. (2005). *Gender, nature, and nurture.* New York, NY: Taylor & Francis.

Lobel, T. E., Slone, M., & Winch, G. (1997). Masculinity, popularity, and self-esteem among Israeli preadolescent girls. *Sex Roles, 36*(5-6), 395–408.

Lurye, L. E. (2011). *Felt gender typicality and sex-typing: Examining felt gender typicality, sex-typing, and their relation to adjustment* (Unpublished doctoral dissertation). New York University, New York, NY.

Maccoby, E. E., & Jacklin, C. N. (1987). Gender segregation in childhood. In H. W. Reese (Ed.), *Advances in child development and behavior* (Vol. 20, pp. 239–288). New York: Academic Press.

Martin, C. L. (1990). Attitudes and expectations about children with nontraditional and traditional gender roles. *Sex Roles, 22*, 151–165. doi:10.1007/BF00288188.

Martin, C. L., Andrews, N., England, D., Ruble, D. N., & Zosuls, K. M. (in press). A dual identity approach for conceptualizing and measuring children's gender identity. Child Development.

Martin, C., & Dinella, L. (2012). Congruence between gender stereotypes and activity preference in self-identified tomboys and non-tomboys. *Archives of Sexual Behavior, 41*, 599–610. doi:10.1007/s10508-011-9786-5.

Martin, C. L., Fabes, R. A., Evans, S. M., & Wyman, H. (1999). Social cognition on the playground: Children's beliefs about playing with girls versus boys and their relations to sex segregated play. *Journal of Social and Personal Relationships, 16*, 751–771. doi:10.1177/0265407599166005.

Martin, C. L., Fabes, R. A., & Hanish, L. D. (2014). Gendered-peer relationships in educational contexts. In L. Liben & R. Bigler (Eds.), *Advances in Child Development and Behavior, 47*, 151–187. Burlington: Academic Press.

Martin, C. L., & Ruble, D. N. (2010). Patterns of gender development. *Annual Review of Psychology, 61*, 353–381. doi:10.1146/annurev.psych.093008.100511.

Martin, C. L., Ruble, D. N., & Szkrybalo, J. (2002). Cognitive theories of early gender development. *Psychological Bulletin, 128*, 903–933. doi:10.1037/0033-2909.128.6.903.

Matthews, K. A., Salomon, K., Kenyon, K., & Zhou, F. (2005). Unfair treatment, discrimination, and ambulatory blood pressure in black and white adolescents. *Health Psychology, 24*(3), 258–265. doi:10.1037/0278-6133.24.3.258.

McDuffie, E., & Brown, G. R. (2010). 70 U.S. veterans with gender identity disturbances: A descriptive study. *International Journal of Transgenderism, 12*, 21–30. doi:10.1080/15532731003688962.

McEwen, B. S., & Wingfield, J. C. (2003). The concept of allostasis in biology and biomedicine. *Hormones and Behavior, 43*, 2–15.

Meyer, I. H. (2003). Prejudice, social stress, and mental health in lesbian, gay, and bisexual populations: Conceptual issues and research evidence. *Psychological Bulletin, 129*, 674–697. doi:10.1037/0033-2909.129.5.674.

Miller, G. E., Chen, E., & Parker, K. J. (2011). Psychological stress in childhood and susceptibility to the chronic diseases of aging: Moving toward a model of behavioral and biological mechanisms. *Psychological Bulletin, 137*, 959.

Neff, K. D., Cooper, C. E., & Woodruff, A. L. (2007). Children's and adolescents' developing perceptions of gender inequality. *Social Development, 16*, 682–699.

Pascoe, E. A., & Richman, L. (2009). Perceived discrimination and health: A meta-analytic review. *Psychological Bulletin, 135*, 531–554. doi:10.1037/a0016059.

Plöderl, M., & Fartacek, R. (2009). Childhood gender nonconformity and harassment as predictors of suicidality among gay, lesbian, bisexual, and heterosexual Austrians. *Archives of Sexual Behavior, 38*, 400–410. doi:10.1007/s10508-007-9244-6.

Rankin, S., & Beemyn, G. (2012). Beyond a binary: The lives of gender-nonconforming youth. *About Campus, 17*, 2–10. doi:10.1002/abc.21086.

Ratner, K. G., Halim, M. L., & Amodio, D. M. (2013). Perceived stigmatization, ingroup pride, and immune and endocrine activity evidence from a community sample of Black and Latina women. *Social Psychological and Personality Science, 4*, 82–91.

Rieger, G., Linsenmeier, J. A., Gygax, L., & Bailey, J. M. (2008). Sexual orientation and childhood gender nonconformity: evidence from home videos. *Developmental psychology, 44*(1), 46.

Rijn, A. B., Steensma, T. D., Kreukels, B. P., & Cohen-Kettenis, P. T. (2013). Self-perception in a clinical sample of gender variant children. *Clinical Child Psychology and Psychiatry, 18*, 464–474. doi:10.1177/1359104512460621.

Romens, S. E., McDonald, J., Svaren, J., & Pollak, S. D. (2014). Associations between early life stress and gene methylation in children. *Child Development, 86*, 303–309. doi:10.1111/cdev.12270.

Ruble, D. N., Lurye, L. E., & Zosuls, K. M. (2007). Pink frilly dresses (PFD) and early gender identity. *Princeton Report on Knowledge (P–ROK), 2*. Retrieved from http://www.princeton.edu/prok/issues/2-2/pink_frilly.xml

Ruble, D. N., Martin, C. L., & Berenbaum, S. A. (2006). Gender development. In N. Eisenberg (Ed.), *Handbook of child psychology: Vol. 3. Personality and social development* (6th ed., pp. 858–932). New York: Wiley.

Ruble, D. N., Taylor, L. J., Cyphers, L., Greulich, F. K., Lurye, L. E., & Shrout, P. E. (2007). The role of gender constancy in early gender development. *Child Development, 78*, 1121–1136.

Sadeh, A. (1996). Stress, trauma, and sleep in children. *Child and Adolescent Psychiatric Clinics of North America, 5*, 685–700.

Savin-Williams, R. C. (1998). *...And then I became gay: Young men's stories*. New York: Routledge.

Sellers, R. M., Copeland-Linder, N., Martin, P. P., & Lewis, R. L. (2006). Racial identity matters: The relationship between racial discrimination and psychological functioning in African American adolescents. *Journal of Research on Adolescence, 16*, 187–216. doi:10.1111/j.1532-7795.2006.00128.x.

Signorella, M. L., Bigler, R. S., & Liben, L. S. (1993). Developmental differences in children's gender schemata about others: A meta-analytic review. *Developmental Review, 13*, 147–183. doi:10.1006/drev.1993.1007.

Singh, D. (2012). *A follow-up study of boys with gender identity disorder* (Unpublished doctoral dissertation). University of Toronto, Toronto, ON, Canada.

Slaby, R. G., & Frey, K. S. (1975). Development of gender constancy and selective attention to same-sex models. *Child Development, 46*, 849–856.

Smith, T. E., & Leaper, C. (2006). Self-perceived gender typicality and the peer context during adolescence. *Journal of Research on Adolescence, 16*, 91–104. doi:10.1111/j.1532-7795.2006.00123.x.

Steensma, T., Biemond, R., de Boer, F., & Cohen-Kettenis, P. T. (2011). Desisting and persisting gender dysphoria after childhood: A qualitative follow-up study. *Clinical Child Psychology and Psychiatry, 16*, 499–516. doi:10.1177/1359104510378303.

Steensma, T. D., McGuire, J. K., Kreukels, B. P., Beekman, A. J., & Cohen-Kettenis, P. T. (2013). Factors associated with desistence and persistence of childhood gender dysphoria: A quantitative follow-up study. *Journal of the American Academy of Child and Adolescent Psychiatry, 52*, 582–590.

Substance Abuse and Mental Health Services Administration (2015). Suicidal thoughts and behavior among adults: Results from the 2014 National Survey on Drug Use and Health. NSDUH Data Review. Retrieved from http://www.samhsa.gov/data/sites/default/files/NSDUH-FRR2-2014/NSDUH-FRR2-2014.pdf.

Susskind, J. E., & Hodges, C. (2007). Decoupling children's gender-based in-group positivity from out-group negativity. *Sex Roles, 56*, 707–716.

Tajfel, H., & Turner, J. C. (2004) The social identity theory of intergroup behavior. In J. T. Jost & J. Sidanius (Eds.), Key readings in social psychology. Political psychology: Key readings (pp.276–293). New York: Psychology Press.

Terada, S., Matsumoto, Y., Sato, T., Okabe, N., Kishimoto, Y., & Uchitomi, Y. (2011). Suicidal ideation among patients with gender identity disorder. *Psychiatry Research, 190*, 159–162. doi:10.1016/j.psychres.2011.04.024.

Trautner, H. M., Ruble, D. N., Cyphers, L., Kirsten, B., Behrendt, R., & Hartmann, P. (2005). Rigidity and flexibility of gender stereotypes in childhood: Developmental or differential? *Infant and Child Development, 14*, 365–381. doi:10.1002/icd.399.

Wallien, M. S. C., & Cohen-Kettenis, P. T. (2008). Psychosexual outcome of gender-dysphoric children. *Journal of the American Academy of Child and Adolescent Psychiatry, 47*, 1413–1423. doi:10.1097/CHI.0b013e31818956b9.

Wallien, M. S., van Goozen, S. H., & Cohen-Kettenis, P. T. (2007). Physiological correlates of anxiety in children with gender identity disorder. *European child & adolescent psychiatry, 16*(5), 309–315.

Woodall, K. L., & Matthews, K. A. (1989). Familial environment associated with Type A behaviors and psychophysiological responses to stress in children. *Health Psychology, 8*, 403–426.

Woodford, M. R., Howell, M. L., Silverschanz, P., & Yu, L. (2012). "That's so gay!": Examining the covariates of hearing this expression among gay, lesbian, and bisexual college students. *Journal of American College Health, 60*(6), 429–434.

Woodhill, B., & Samuels, C. (2003). Positive and negative androgyny and their relationship with psychological health and well-being. *Sex Roles, 48*, 555–565.

Zosuls, K. M., Ruble, D. N., Tamis-LeMonda, C. S., Shrout, P. E., Bornstein, M. H., & Greulich, F. K. (2009). The acquisition of gender labels in infancy: Implications for sex-typed play. *Developmental Psychology, 45*, 688–701. doi:10.1037/a0014053.

Zucker, K. J., & Bradley, S. J. (1995). *Gender identity disorder and psychosexual problems in children and adolescents.* New York: Guilford Press.

Zucker, K. J., Bradley, S. J., & Sanikhani, M. (1997). Sex differences in referral rates of children with gender identity disorder: Some hypotheses. *Journal of Abnormal Child Psychology, 25*, 217–227.

Zucker, K. J., Wood, H., & VanderLaan, D. P. (2014). Models of psychopathology in children and adolescents with gender dysphoria. In B. P. C. Kreukels, T. D. Steensma, & A. L. C. de Vries (Eds.), *Gender dysphoria and disorders of sex development: Progress in care and knowledge* (pp. 171–192). New York: Springer.

Chapter 11
Parameters of Preventing Substance Misuse in Adolescents

Steve Sussman, Yue Liao, Jennifer Tsai, and Diana Fishbein

11.1 Introduction

Prevention of substance use disorders involves encouraging adoption of healthy behaviors and preventing initiation or escalation of drug use behavior among teens by focusing on factors that lead to its eventual development. Keys to prevention is understanding that the antecedents of drug misuse often occur or surface earlier in life and increase the likelihood of developing risky behaviors including drug misuse. Targeting these antecedent factors prior to their full emergence through effective preventive interventions has great potential to redirect the developmental trajectory towards healthy behaviors. In contrast, in the absence of intervention, the risk for negative life consequences, such as addiction, disease and death, significantly increases (Sussman & Ames, 2008). Prevention programming works to sever the connections between these antecedent factors and drug misuse by (a) redirecting or reducing antecedent behaviors (e.g., impulsivity, aggressiveness, sensation-seeking); (b) strengthening resiliency traits (e.g., self-regulation,

S. Sussman, Ph.D. (✉)
Departments of Preventive Medicine and Psychology, and School of Social Work, Institute for Health Promotion and Disease Prevention Research, University of Southern California, 2001 N. Soto Street, SSB 302A, Los Angeles, CA 90032, USA
e-mail: ssussma@usc.edu

Y. Liao, Ph.D. • J. Tsai, M.P.H.
Department of Preventive Medicine, Institute for Health Promotion and Disease Prevention Research, University of Southern California,
2001 N. Soto Street, SSB 302A, Los Angeles, CA 90032, USA
e-mail: yueliao@usc.edu; jyktsai@gmail.com

D. Fishbein, Ph.D.
Edna Bennett Pierce Prevention Research Center, College of Health and Human Development, The Pennsylvania State University,
314 Biobehavioral Health Building, University Park, PA 16802, USA
e-mail: Dvf5211@psu.edu

© Springer Science+Business Media New York 2016
M.R. Korin (ed.), *Health Promotion for Children and Adolescents*,
DOI 10.1007/978-1-4899-7711-3_11

cognitive control); and/or (c) reducing exposure to antecedent conditions (e.g., social pressure, adversity, stress, maltreatment, toxins).

Components of substance misuse prevention programming are designed to address particular antecedents relevant to the target population. Antecedents may range from molecular to molar constituents: neurobiological makeup or phenotypes, cognitive and emotional functions, psychological and behavioral orientations, microsocial environments, and macrosocial/physical environments (e.g., Sussman & Ames, 2008). Evidence-based program components, in turn, attempt to strengthen or reha- bilitate underlying processes (e.g., neurobiological integrity), improve responses to environmental hazards (e.g., cognitive and emotional functioning, coping) or, alterna- tively, reduce exposure to microsocial or large social environmental hazards (e.g., reducing maltreatment, limiting exposure to mass media advertisements). In addition, evidence-based substance misuse prevention programming may vary as a function of (a) modality of delivery (e.g., individual, school, family, other community unit), (b) age of target group (we focus on young versus older teens in this chapter, though programming could be provided throughout the life span; see Sussman, 2013), (c) risk status of target group (universal, selective, indicated), and (d) breadth of targeted outcomes of programming (single drugs, sets of drugs, or healthy lifestyles).

This chapter focuses on prevention among adolescents. In this chapter, we will pres- ent examples of prevention program contents that attempt to modify antecedents at dif- ferent levels of analysis. We will also discuss modalities of program delivery, explain how programming might vary as a function of young versus older adolescence and risk status, and query as to whether programming should focus on a single drug, all drugs, or more broadly on healthy lifestyles. In addition, we will discuss the challenges of trans- lating scientific findings to programming. Finally, we will suggest several future needs for innovations in prevention research and practice based on the scientific evidence.

11.2 Substance Misuse Prevention Program Contents for Teens

Substance misuse prevention programs for teens teach participants how to anticipate the effects of antecedents (e.g., the desire to feel good or accepted by others), and counteract potential influences with instruction of protective cognitive or emotional regulatory skills, behaviors, or access to protective social environments. This section discusses substance misuse prevention program contents from four broad perspectives: neurobiological, cognitive, microsocial, and macrosocial/physical environmental.

11.2.1 Neurobiological

Prevention programs tailored to individuals who are more susceptible to the reinforc- ing effects of drugs due to variation in neurobiological systems and their phenotypic manifestations are relatively likely to result in favorable outcomes. For example, inadequate or aberrant mesolimbic dopaminergic neurotransmission and hypothalamic pituitary axis [HPA] response (Koob & LeMoal, 2001; Sussman & Ames, 2008) have been implicated in drug abuse propensity. Increasing evidence has shown that intact neural development underlies social and emotional competence. Accordingly, there is a growing belief among transdisciplinary scientists that prevention programs targeted to neurodevelopmental benchmarks starting in early childhood, when the brain is still rapidly developing (e.g., Fishbein, 2000), are worth exploring. For example, during this period, the development of emotional perception and regulatory skills is critical to the self-regulation of behavior. These functions are supported by the brain's prefrontal and limbic system connections which, when developmentally on par, give rise to the ability to competently perceive emotional cues (e.g., facial expressions, others' intentions, internal stress adaptations), cope with stress, and regulate the behavioral response to social demands. There is evidence that appropriately targeted mindful, socio-competency, and education programs that reinforce emotional regulatory functions may strengthen neural connections and act to normalize brain activity patterns. In turn, this trend towards normalizing neurodevelopment may help facilitate acquisition of skills necessary to avoid drug use. Furthermore, brain-based neurocognitive functions involved in behavior and emotional regulation may moderate or mediate prevention program outcomes such that those with lower levels at baseline (e.g., of executive cognitive efficiency) may show fewer preventive effects (e.g., Riggs & Greenberg, 2009).

Since emotional regulation skills are not fully developed even in the teenage years, training of self-regulatory skills may be particularly impactful for increasing program effectiveness in this age group. For example, among teens, effective self-regulation protects against substance use and buffers against the impact of various risk factors, whereas poor self-regulation, involving either delays or deficits in behavioral, affective, and cognitive functioning, is strongly related to eventual drug use, escalation, abuse and eventual dependence (Sussman & Ames, 2008).

Training in coping skills and stress adaptations, which are often awry in individuals who experience adversity and severe or frequent stressors, enhance self-regulation, likely through their impact on neural connections. In *self-regulation programming* (e.g., Project Towards No Drug Abuse [TND]), youths learn to assess their self-regulation (e.g., rate their tendency to impulsively make provocative statements, to say things they "did not mean" in stressful situations, to exhibit attention-seeking behaviors), particularly in social contexts (social self-control). They learn the importance of thinking ahead and anticipating problematic situations to prepare themselves beforehand to deal with problems that may arise. They also learn the importance of context (e.g., not laughing at a funeral, not feeling disrespected when accidentally tapped by someone). Finally, they learn assertiveness and anger management to help them better control their reactions in social settings (Sussman, 2015; Sussman & Ames, 2008). Anger, in particular, is modulated by brain regions (e.g., amygdala) in the limbic system that, when developmentally delayed or damaged in some way, causes inappropriate responses to perceived social challenges. It is possible that programs which focus on anger management may exert their effects through strengthening cognitive control (prefrontal) over affective responses (limbic). Further research is needed to flesh out these potential mechanisms of program effects.

Another neurobiological target for substance abuse prevention programming is stress reactivity. Numerous studies have suggested that exposure to frequent or severe stressors acts on the same systems recruited by both actual use of abusable drugs and drug cues. In the early stages, stress can produce an increased arousal state that is similar to drug use and cues (Kreek & Koob, 1998; Piazza & Le Moal, 1998). Eventually, after repeated stress exposures, arousal of these neurobiological systems downregulates—i.e., becomes subdued—and the brain's reward/motivational centers then lack adequate stimulation. Drug use perceptibly alleviates this state and is, thus, inherently reinforcing. Importantly, stress increases vulnerability to drug use initiation, escalation, relapse, and intractability to intervention (Briand & Blendy, 2010; Sinha, 2012). Instruction in *coping strategies*, which may include life skills, stress reduction, and mindfulness, may provide a preventive effect throughout childhood and adolescence (e.g., Botvin et al., 2000; Sussman, Sun, Rohrbach, & Spruijt-Metz, 2012). Further, there is some evidence that the effect of these techniques on improvements in brain development and function may underlie that positive outcome (Riggs & Greenberg, 2009; Wetherill & Tapert, 2013).

11.2.2 Cognitive

The influence of cognitive processes on behavior involves both rational and nonrational motivations. Substance misuse prevention strategies could focus on strategies directed at both explicit cognitive processes (e.g., rational decision-making, problem solving, goal-directedness) and relatively nonreflective (e.g., more automatic) cognitive processes (such as working memory, focus of attention, spontaneous inner speech; Thush et al., 2008). Instruction in *decision-making skills*, practice of *implementation intentions* (i.e., self-statements to engage certain behaviors during at-risk situations ["When I drive near the liquor store, I will turn right the block prior to it to avoid temptation"]), and *self-monitoring* of behavior are all examples of rational, deliberate preventive strategies. These strategies generally involve harnessing already established motivation to not misuse drugs, directing them through the strengthening of higher order executive functions (Sussman & Ames, 2008).

Relatively automatic cognitions may be reflected in tendencies to engage in certain errors during information processing, largely involving ingrained beliefs and perceptions. Three examples include prevalence overestimates, misperceptions about the dangers of drug use, and attitude–behavior discrepancies. As a first example, teens (as well as adults) may tend to overestimate the prevalence of substance use. Prevalence overestimates may promote drug use if it is considered to be a normatively acceptable or popular activity. This is particularly the case when adolescents report that "most of the friends use." Substance use prevalence overestimates may be counteracted through an *overestimates reduction* prevention activity which helps youth become aware that they tend to overestimate their perceptions of their peers' substance use and that actually it is normatively unpopular to misuse drugs. For example, teens may provide subjective ratings of the prevalence of cigarette smoking among peers (e.g., they may believe that 10 of 30 youth in their class have smoked cigarettes in the last 7 days), which are contrasted with an anonymous survey of their classmates (e.g., revealing that only 1 of their 30 classmates actually smoked a cigarette in the last 7 days). Youth learn that relatively few are using and thus they do not need to use drugs to "fit in."

As a second example, teens at risk for drug misuse often hold inaccurate relatively automatic beliefs about drug use consequences. Such inaccurate drug use beliefs can be counteracted through use of *elaborative processing*. One example of elaborative processing is a "kernel of truth" activity used in the Project TND curriculum (Sussman, 2015; Sussman et al., 2012). In this activity, youth discuss prevalent drug use myths (e.g., drug use is a means of being emotionally protected from life stressors). They discuss the kernel of truth in the myth (one may feel bemused while using some drugs), then discuss why the myth is, in fact, a myth (e.g., an individual thinks less clearly when under the influence of drugs, and is more likely to be victimized or otherwise experience greater stress). For prevention programs, it is essential to elaborate on the difference between the more immediate subjective satisfaction and the longer term negative consequences of drug use so that meaningful memories are established.

Finally, *attitude–behavior discrepancies* often occur when youth do not deliberately examine the compatibility of certain beliefs with their behavior. As a specific example, most youth prefer to consider themselves as being "moderate" (or reasonable people) and not prone to extremes. However, an individual may exhibit behaviors that are contradictory with this person's general view about himself or herself as a moderate person (e.g., escalating drug use frequency). If confronted with this discrepancy, by having the individual recognize his/her general self-attitude and then examine his/her specific drug use behavior, an individual may decrease his/her frequency of drug use (Sussman, 2015).

11.2.3   Microsocial

There are several microsocial-level strategies that can help prevent youth from misusing substances. *Communication skills instruction* may be essential, assuming that persons who have difficulty interacting with others may gravitate towards using drugs as a less demanding solution. One can improve communication skills by learning how to ask open-ended questions, using appropriate eye contact and body language, checking for a mutual understanding between speaker and listener by asking questions, and making sure that one's nonverbal behavior matches one's verbal behavior to exchange a consistent message. In general, social skills instruction involves demonstration of appropriate behavior, modeling of appropriate behavior, behavioral rehearsal, and feedback components. There may be one exception to the idea that communication skills serve a preventive function. For young and older teens, improving conversation initiation skills may increase their ability to acquire drugs from new sources. Thus, using *motivational enhancement* methods (which are cognitive-level approaches) before teaching specific communication skills may be needed to promote non-drug use-seeking behavior.

Refusal assertion is a social skill that involves how one might best refuse an offer or request from someone to use or purchase drugs. An assertive refusal is generally a simple and direct response (e.g., "No") that is not too passive (e.g., "Not today") or too aggressive (e.g., "No, you idiot!"). Assertive refusal training emphasizes acknowledging the positive intent of requester (e.g., "I know you are trying to be nice by offering me a cigarette"), stating one's own position (e.g., "I don't smoke"), and possibly offering an alternative (e.g., "I'll see you later in the gym"). One drawback of refusal assertion education is that if the focus is on how to say no to drug offers, they may come to believe that everyone "out there" uses drugs. Then, the individual may feel less certain that he/she would be able to refuse drug offers or may even become more interested in drug use. Thus, refusal assertion training is useful to those who need such skills only if closely linked to instruction of *normative education* material (e.g., prevalence overestimates reduction, described above in the cognitive subsection; and normative restructuring, described below in this subsection).

Normative restructuring involves creating a peer group (e.g., a classroom) norm of unacceptability of drug use. A class poll could be taken regarding whether peers approve of getting drunk on alcohol, using tobacco, or getting high on marijuana regularly. Youth tend to believe that they, but not their peers, are the only ones who view drug use as unacceptable behavior. By taking this group poll, youth learn that most of their peers also disapprove of regular drug use (Sussman & Ames, 2008).

Public commitment is an activity that requires writing and group action. Youth engage in a writing activity (i.e., stating a commitment to do something regarding drug use behavior) that is then stated publicly to the group. This commitment may involve thinking about not misusing drugs, discussing drug misuse with others, or cutting down or quitting one's own use of drugs. Youth may sign a written commitment regarding their stance towards drug misuse, and this commitment may be shared among the other peers in the group (generally in a classroom context).

11.2.4   Macrosocial/Physical Environmental

Substance use prevention programs at the macrosocial/environmental level can have wide-ranging effects since it has wide reach. *Prosocial resources* such as drug-free recreation alternatives, hobbies, and jobs could be an effective community-level strategy for substance use preventive interventions. Youth may increase their knowledge and self-efficacy on how to obtain prosocial resources through instruction, modeling, and structured practice in resource acquisition skills. This skill training could also help them to readily access these resources when needed. Furthermore, perception of availability of these resources in one's community could be enhanced among older teens by receiving such information through a telephone education program or mass media communication. If this strategy is used following delivery of drug misuse prevention education in school as a booster programming, it could help increase hope for lifestyle stability (Sussman & Ames, 2008).

Media literacy education involves instruction of adult advertising influences so that youth are less likely to yield to these subtle informational social influences. Often provided through school-based programming, this type of education serves to counteract macrosocial influences. Through media literacy education, teens may learn various advertisement "pitches" (e.g., one decides to smoke cigarettes to appear more sexy or sophisticated), and learn that these pitches serve to sell products and may not be correct. Youth may act on media influences through creating corrective advertisements (e.g., new tobacco ads that provide the opposite message of that portrayed in the tobacco advertisement, such as making a smoker appear unattractive or naive), or through activism activities (e.g., writing letters to the tobacco or alcohol industries requesting accurate portrayals of their advertisements).

Drug use policies involve either prohibitory mechanisms (e.g., raising the minimum drinking age), regulatory mechanisms (e.g., alcohol taxation, setting blood alcohol level limits; e.g., Holder, 2009), and/or large social climate influence (e.g., a norm that drug use is good or bad because it is legal or illegal). For example, five main categories of alcohol prevention policies have been identified in the research literature: drinking and driving sanctions, alcohol outlet density and hours of operation regulations, minimum age and access laws and enforcement, taxation, and responsible service (Holder, 2009). Each of these types of policies has been shown to reduce hazards associated with heavy or careless drinking including prevention of deaths and hospitalization.

Other environmental manipulations may also reduce demand and limit exposure to alcohol, tobacco, and other drugs, such as use of warning labels and provision of alternative youth activities outside of school. The use of warning labels also makes drug use less socially desirable (e.g., large pictorial depictions of negative use consequences on cigarette packs). It is theorized that by increasing the costs (e.g., financial, time, or social) of drug use, potential or recent drug users will consider engaging in alternative behaviors that do not involve using drugs. Some policy mechanisms, such as raising the price of cigarettes, may be particularly effective at preventing uptake among youth (Sussman et al., 2013).

11.3 Modalities of Prevention Programming Delivery

Modality of delivery refers to the channels or contexts through which prevention program content is offered. Numerous modalities have been utilized for preventive interventions including individual health care providers, families, schools, policy enforcement agencies, community organizations, and mass media channels.

Individual-level prevention programming are commonly applied by various behavioral health care providers and could impart a variety of contents, including instruction in emotional and behavioral self-regulation, decision-making and problem-solving skills, and stress reduction techniques. One popular type of programming delivered at the individual level is *Motivational Interviewing*. Motivational Interviewing involves a series of procedures for therapist (i.e., program staff) to help clients (i.e., adolescents) clarify goals and follow through with their efforts to change behavior (Barnett, Sussman, Smith, Rohrbach, & Spruijt-Metz, 2012). Motivation refers to the probability that a person will enter into, continue, or adhere to a specific change. Since motivation for change can vary over time, addressing this fluctuation is considered key for facilitating behavioral change. Intervention programming could attempt to increase a youth's motivation to desist (change intentions, for those curious about starting drug use), not escalate drug use, or to quit drug use. Contents provided through individual-level programming will likely be acting at the level of neurobiological or cognitive antecedents.

Family-based programming often attempts to promote a more positive parent–child relationship within the family. Instruction in a parenting style that fosters warm, closer, more nurturing relationships, and open communication between the child and the parent may elicit more positive childhood social behaviors. Also, parents who actively monitor their children's activity and set consequences for acceptable and unacceptable behaviors are less likely to rear drug-misusing children. Strategies that have been used to enhance family cohesiveness and improve family roles (parents as parents, children as children) include family skills training, brief family therapy, cognitive/behavioral parent training, and family group support. Most family-based programs target younger teens (Sussman, 2013). However, parents remain as a significant social influence on adolescent drug use behavior at least until the end of high school (Liao, Huh, Huang, Pentz, & Chou, 2013); although peer influences become increasing more influential with the onset of adolescence (much of microsocial-level programming is peer group focused). Family-based programming likely provides material that addresses neurobiological and cognitive antecedents, but also microsocial antecedents such as communication skills and normative restructuring.

School-based prevention programming has been the most widely implemented and assessed among modalities (Sussman & Ames, 2008). Indeed, most social influence-based substance use prevention programs occur in the school classroom setting by virtue of the ability to reach large numbers of children in several age groups. School-based programming addresses various neurobiological, cognitive, and microsocial antecedents including building self-esteem, decision-making, and other executive functions (neurobiological or cognitive-oriented strategies provided within a social group context), active listening, communicating effectively, refusal assertion learning and practice, counteracting advertising images and social activism to change norms, and public commitment. Distal program effects have been found an average of 5 years after implementation of school-based programming (Sussman et al., 2013; Sussman & Ames, 2008).

Enforcement agencies, broadly defined, attempt to arrange the social environment so that drugs are more difficult to obtain or use through increasing prices (e.g., taxation of cigarettes and alcohol), restricting access to drugs (removing cigarette vending machines, limiting hours of operation of liquor stores), or penalizing possession or use (e.g., arrests and fines for hard drug and paraphernalia possession). Enforcement agencies operate on the macrosocial and physical environment. Enforcement of restrictions on locations or hours of alcohol consumption, or on who can drink alcohol (minimum drinking age laws), or how they can be used, may serve an important impact on prevention of substance use (alcohol) disorders. As for illicit drug use or possession, enforcement operates in terms of arrests, fines, drug court diversion, or jail time. According to the Bureau of Justice Statistics in 2011, approximately 48 % of prison inmates have entered prison due to drug-related offenses (Retrieved August 29, 2013, from http://www.bjs.gov/content/pub/pdf/p11.pdf). It is not clear that such enforcement is cost-effective relative to treatment (Sussman & Ames, 2008).

Mass Media or other technology-based programming may exert preventive effects depending on the adequacy of the reach of programming, the opportunity facilitated for interaction about programming, and supplementation with other types of programming. Mass media campaigns may or may not be effective depending on their successful modification of antecedent variables such as social influences, and campaigns tend to be rather expensive with limited shelf lives (Sussman & Ames, 2008; Sussman et al., 2013). Computer or internet-based programming could provide a very pragmatic means of both surveying and intervening with various populations. Use of the Internet is inexpensive and convenient and can process information quickly (i.e., the collected data can be analyzed instantaneously). Such programming can find effects on tobacco or other drug use, and provide a macrosocial reach (e.g., Prokhorov et al., 2008, ASPIRE, effects on smoking; Chiauzzi, Green, Lord, Ma, & Ba, 2005, MyStudentBody.com, effects on alcohol use). For example, MyStudentBody.com targets 18-to-24-year-old college students, and is an online, subscription-based program that provides motivational feedback and wellness education about alcohol use and abuse. After logging in, assessment on alcohol use and consequences is conducted, followed by immediate tailored feedback based on the assessment. Coping strategies are instructed and participants are informed about available resources. Effects on alcohol use have been found among older teens and emerging adults (mean age = 19.9 year old; Chiauzzi et al., 2005). These types of programs are likely to have a macrosocial impact due to their potentially wide reach.

The use of *multiple prevention modalities* is likely to maximize prevention effects in the long term, though the efficacy of such programming depends on how well integrated the multiple modalities are. Sussman et al. (2013) found that in a majority of trials, community-wide tobacco use prevention programming, which includes multiple modalities, has not been found to achieve impacts greater than single modality programming possibly due to the lack of adequate integration. The most effective means of prevention involves a careful selection of program type combinations. Also, it is likely that a mechanism for coordinating maximally across program types (e.g., staging of programming) is needed to encourage a synergistic impact.

The Midwest Prevention Project (MPP) is among the best-known community-based interventions, which combined various modalities for intervention delivery. MPP targeted avoidance and reduction of drug use in middle/junior high school through five program components: (1) mass media coverage, promotional video-tapes, and commercials about the program, (2) an 11- to 13-session social influence-based school curriculum involving parents, (3) a parent organization program involving parent–principal meetings and parent–child communications training, (4) a community organization program to organize and train community leaders to develop action groups, and (5) drug use policy change. This program showed a 20-to-40% net program effect for the first 3 years. MPP also sustained effects on heavy drug use rate for longer than 5 years post-implementation. Overall, to have an effective multicomponent community-based program targeting youth, extensive school programming should be included to initiate behavior change, together with a community organization structure and process that promotes supplemental mass media programming and coverage, parent and adult education, and informal or formal policy change (Pentz, 1995). However, one needs to keep in mind of the relative cost-effectiveness of multicomponent community-based programs as compared to the single-channel ones. Additional components provide little or no added value if these components simply duplicate or overlap the causal mechanisms (e.g., improving social skills, establishing behavioral norms) of single-channel programs (Foxcroft & Tsertsvadze, 2011). A careful needs assessment may be helpful to determine how to appropriately map which program components at which time point within a localized target population should be implemented.

11.4   Age of Target Group

The "charge" of this chapter is a focus on adolescence although programming could be delivered throughout the life span (see Sussman, 2013). Certainly, most evidence-based programming has been developed for adolescents. Tobacco and other drug misuse prevention researchers found intriguing the critical period of young adolescence, in which tobacco and alcohol trial and experimentation increases dramatically; high-risk teens by virtue of associated antecedent conditions are particularly likely to initiate early in adolescence. Several researchers have felt that prevention programming should be delivered at this point in child development, during the trial phase of use. Young teens who are curious about experiential solutions at the beginning of their search for identity, and who are approached by other teens who share a similar curiosity, may seek out or yield to offers to try drugs or engage in other risky behaviors. Young teens are ideal candidates for the provision of comprehensive social influences/life skills program material. Drug prevalence overestimate reduction, improvement in difficulties in decision-making, media literacy, and refusal assertion may be strategies that can assist with prevention (initial trial or early use) efforts. A meta-analysis of 94 controlled trials of school-based substance abuse prevention programs with varying follow-up (most studies ranged from 6 months to 2 years follow-up) suggested that programming for middle school youth might be slightly more likely to achieve a significant effect on alcohol or other drug use than programming for elementary or senior high school youth (Gottfredson & Wilson, 2003).

Dynamic social changes occur between early adolescence (junior high school) and later adolescence (high school), including a new and growing emphasis on social interactions, autonomy, and opportunities for risky situations and behaviors. In tandem, there is tremendous growth in brain plasticity which does not conclude until the mid to late 20s (Sussman, 2013). During this period, connections are being made between neural systems responsible for goal setting, impulse control, emotion regulation, and decision-making. The combination of neurological immaturity and increasing social demands is unfortunate in that it presents the adolescent with potentially dangerous opportunities to engage in risk-taking behaviors with greater potential for negative consequences, but with reduced capacity to resist these impulses. In addition, reinforcing behaviors (including risky behaviors) may be experienced with a greater affective valence than during other developmental periods. Thus, on the one hand, adolescence is a period of heightened vulnerability to risky behaviors from neurobiological and normative perspectives, while on the other hand, this amplified period of development provides a unique window of opportunity to effectively intervene and have a lasting positive impact on future behaviors and successes. At this period of life, drug use onset and subsequent escalation is most common.

Older teens are in the process of solidifying a sense of self and tend to become more resistant to direct influence, e.g., regarding peer influence on smoking. Older teens also tend to socialize in contexts of heterosexual crowds, less mutually dependent on small groups of same-sex peers, and they tend to begin dating and engage in other preparation for an adult lifestyle. Intrapersonal motivations become more important. Yet, older teens exhibit rapid neurobiological changes. Older teens may be more sensitive and react negatively to social pressures that contradict their attempts to achieve a sense of self. Thus, instruction in such tobacco and other drug use prevention strategies as refusal assertion training may be received rather negatively by older teens compared to younger or older age groups. Tobacco and other drug use may come to serve more as a stress-coping (intrapersonal) function as the substance use acquisition process enters a more advanced phase (regular use). Some researchers suggest that drug abuse prevention programming would be relatively effective if it was implemented when drug use is truly beginning to escalate or become problematic, among older teens for most people (Sussman & Ames, 2008). Drug misuse prevention material among older teens should be provided so that youth will recall and put into practice relevant key prevention strategies that are relatively likely to involve (a) motivation enhancement, (b) stress-coping skills, and (c) decision-making, as opposed to social influences-type material.

There are several types of motivation-skills-decision-making prevention material that might be effectively utilized at this stage. Motivation enhancement material is designed to make a youth aware of a discrepancy between his or her behavior and self-perception, leading the youth to desire to bring relatively deviant behavior in line with a generally more favorable self-perception. For example, a youth may view himself or herself as a "moderate" type of person, but become aware that smoking or other drug misuse is not moderate behavior ("attitudinal perspectives" activity). Skills instruction includes listening, communication, and self-regulation skills (particularly in social situations). Decision-making skills instruction may help bolster motivation enhancement and life skills instruction (Sussman, 2013, 2015).

11.5   Risk Status

Substance use prevention programming is often directed towards groups at varying levels of risk for drug abuse. These types of programming have been labeled as "universal," "selective," or "indicated" (Gordon, 1987). *Universal* prevention programming targets the general population regardless of each individual's risk status and aims to deter or delay the onset of an undesirable behavior. Most school-based substance abuse prevention programs are universal interventions that target all students in particular schools or classrooms. From a population level, there is a general pattern of substance use initiation and escalation that occurs from early adolescence to young adulthood. This general developmental progression is typically characterized by onset of use during early adolescence, a peak in use in late adolescence, and a gradual reduction during young adulthood. Therefore, in the tween years, elementary school programs mostly aim to change attitudes and beliefs about drug use to help young teens develop strong antidrug attitudes and establish antidrug use norms prior to the years of experimentation, whereas junior high school programs delivered in young adolescence tend to address the specific contexts in which drug use occurs and provide refusal skills training (Botvin & Griffin, 2007). Programming that attempts a macrosocial impact, in general, also is intended for a universal target (e.g., mass media drug abuse prevention messages). In other words, universal prevention strategies tend to involve microsocial and macrosocial/physical environmental contents and scope of application (i.e., schools, mass media, policy).

Selective prevention programming targets subgroups of the population that are believed to be at high psychosocial risk (e.g., children of drug abusers). In addition to taking into consideration of age-appropriate programming materials as in the universal prevention programming, selective prevention programs might also focus on addressing cognition relevant to being at elevated psychosocial risk and to family roles. The Strengthening Families Program (SFP), a family skills-training program designed to increase resilience and decrease risk factors for problem behaviors in high-risk children is one example of a selective prevention program. SFP emphasizes improving family relationships, parenting skills, and children's social and life skills. Emphasis on creating a positive future orientation, age-appropriate expectations and roles, mutual empathy, making house rules, and listening to each other are essential to this program. Effects of SFP have been found on tobacco and other substance use (Sussman, 2013). In other words, selective prevention strategies tend to involve at-risk cognitive and microsocial contents and scope of application (e.g., decision-making and family counseling).

Indicated prevention programming targets high-risk individuals that already show signs of engaging in problematic drug use behaviors. Since these adolescents are at risk of continued drug use behavior as well as later treatment resistance and relapse, program strategies may be needed to focus on underlying problems (e.g., psychiatric disorders, stress, family dysfunction, impulsivity) to alleviate or treat the issues and alter behavioral patterns. For example, strategies that utilize motivation enhancement components to attempt to redirect behavior, such as Motivational Interviewing, hold promise (Barnett et al., 2012). As discussed earlier, motivational enhancement emphasizes techniques to elucidate desire for change and reduce ambivalence towards change (e.g., "attitudinal perspectives" activity, Motivational Interviewing). Cessation strategies may also be utilized. Additional strategies include cognitive rehabilitation, socio-emotional skills training, mindfulness techniques, and cognitive–behavioral therapies. Thus, indicated programming target either the individual level (e.g., strengthening executive cognitive processes) or the group level (e.g., motivation enhancement, support groups).

11.6   Targeted Outcomes of Programming

Drug abuse prevention or cessation could involve addressing use of a single drug, use of any of several drugs, or behavior that pertains to drugs and healthy lifestyles. Arguments that favor focusing on a single drug or on drug abuse include being able to provide a sufficient amount of drug-focused information, the possibility that different drugs might be used for different reasons, and the need to keep programming to a reasonable length. One main argument that favors the concurrent prevention of multiple drugs, and possibly process (behavioral) addictions (e.g., pathological gambling), and sedentary lifestyle (e.g., eating fried food, not exercising) is that different drugs and unhealthy behaviors stem from similar underlying functions (e.g., neurobiological: mesolimbic dopamine activity, anhedonia, problem proneness; cognitive: associative learning processes; microsocial: peer group social influences; macrosocial/physical environmental: large social–cultural group solidarity and environmental access). Information can be efficiently provided that counteracts use of any one of several drugs or unhealthy lifestyles in general by focusing on common underlying functions. For example, conscientiousness (industriousness and thinking of others, having a positive attitude) appears to be one such underlying remedial factor in human behavior (Sussman & Ames, 2008). Instruction in conscientiousness might counteract antecedents at multiple levels of influence.

Based on a review of a handful of studies completed at the time, Johnson, MacKinnon, and Pentz (1996) found that multipurpose programs (combining tobacco, alcohol, other drug, and diet and exercise objectives) and single-purpose programs were about equally effective for smoking prevention; however, broadly focused programs were not as effective for alcohol and other drug abuse prevention. Recently, more intervention efforts have been invested in the idea of targeting multiple health behavior change due to the fact that multiple unhealthy behaviors often co-occur (Prochaska, Spring, & Nigg, 2008). Tobacco smokers, in particular, tend to have poor behavioral health profiles. Overweightness and obesity are found to be significantly associated with smoking, drinking, and other substance use among young girls (Farhat, Iannotti, & Simons-Morton, 2010). It is believed that success in changing one or more lifestyle behavior may also increase confidence to improve risk behaviors among individuals that have low motivation to change. Therefore, a more specified health behavior change may lead to an overall healthful lifestyle change, and a healthy lifestyle may also counteract a tendency to engage in drug misuse.

Much more research is needed to discern the most appropriate outcomes of programming, which may also interface with program contents, modalities, and risk status.

11.7   Phases of Translational Prevention Research

Prevention of drug misuse among adolescents transcends the difficult task of understanding the etiological underpinnings of drug use and translating that information to the development of programs that will be effective in various populations and settings. Once that task is accomplished and an evidence-base for the ongoing use of those programs has been established, the ultimate goal is to "institutionalize" the practices for long-term sustainability (Sussman, Valente, Rohrbach, Skara, & Pentz, 2006). To capture the essence of this process of systematic information transfer from the basic sciences to practice, the terms Type 1, Type 2, and Type 3 translational research have been coined. Type I translational drug abuse research refers to the study of etiological factors in the development of drug use and escalation to abuse and dependence in both humans and animals and transfer of evidence from the basic sciences to individual applications (Pentz, Jasuja, Rohrbach, Sussman, & Bardo, 2006). That is, Type I translation considers etiologic phenomena and guides the design and preliminary testing of programs that target and, in effect, counteract factors known to increase propensity to drug misuse. For example, one important replicated etiologic finding is that people tend to overestimate drug use prevalence, and those who overestimate drug use prevalence relatively more are those who are at greater risk for later drug misuse. This knowledge has been used to create activities that counteract (decrease) prevalence overestimates and, hence, exert a preventive effect. Similarly but from a basic science standpoint, insensitivity of dopaminergic systems has been repeatedly implicated in sensation-seeking behaviors that, in turn, increase the risk for drug misuse. Based on this information, drug abuse prevention messaging content has been designed to appeal to individuals who are sensation-seekers.

Type II translation is the adoption, implementation, and sustainability of evidence-based or scientifically validated interventions by service systems (Spoth et al., 2013). Type II translation encompasses multi-level organizations and an intricate web of stakeholders that will (or will not) implement, evaluate and refine drug prevention programs in real-world settings (Rohrbach, Grana, Sussman, & Valente, 2006). Staff training of promising implementers who work in "ready" social environments (i.e., containing the labor force, resources, and motivation to implement and sustain programming) is a key element in the early detection and screening of antecedents and related problem behaviors, and the implementation of successful prevention programs in the community (Rohrbach et al., 2006). Community mobilization and evaluation are fundamental to Type II translation as communities become invested in the adoption of evidence-based approaches.

Type III translation is the actual delivery of science-based interventions to all recipients in all settings (Dougherty & Conway, 2008). Thus, Type III involves widespread dissemination and communication regarding programs being offered, and subsequently influences educational systems, practical settings, policy-making, and environmental reform. It is during this stage that there is potential to affect both supply and demand features of drug abuse in any given community. Furthermore, it is during this stage that sustainability can involve institutionalization of proven practices via longstanding alterations to public opinion, program availability, and laws/policies that have a direct impact on the way a society deals with drug abuse. Adaptations to programming and delivery systems must be made throughout this process to accommodate different and changing social environments, and to determine how the best programs can be combined to provide comprehensive services and exert the greatest impact on the greatest number.

Back translation is the feedback loop between all three types of translation. At the point of implementation and evaluation, there will invariably be a need to further investigate program components that do not work as well for some as they do for others. Additional basic research is needed at that stage to characterize unresponsive subgroups or individuals and tailor program components to their special needs.

11.8 Future Directions of Prevention Programming

Researchers and practitioners need to continuously study newly amassed evidence from the basic sciences, as well as shifting trends and perceptions associated with drug use, drug misuse, and drug prevention among adolescents. Clarification of what exactly we want to prevent (e.g., antecedents, related problem behaviors) needs to be openly discussed between researchers and health promoters. Pinpointing the differences between relatively innocuous experimentation and dangerous escalation of use may discern perhaps the most teachable moments.

11.8.1 Contents of Programming

While we know a great deal about contents of programming, there are many aspects that need additional consideration. For example, to the extent that drug misuse is an extension or expression of aberrant neurobiological functions, it is unclear what sorts of strategies would serve to redirect the behavioral pathway in a productive and healthy direction. Studies suggest that interventions designed to strengthen cognitive inhibitory controls and its connections to affect limbic structures have potential to measurably alter brain development and functioning (Davidson et al., 2003; Tang, Lu, Fan, Yang, & Posner, 2012). For antecedents that involve perceptions or normative attitudes and behaviors, perhaps positive psychology tools might be brought into prevention programming to address existing deficits or delays in neurodevelopment. These strategies include recognizing and harnessing personal strengths, listing positive daily events, writing a gratitude list, writing a gratitude letter to someone who has been helpful, savoring pleasant moments in the day, listening to others' good news, or doing and savoring one's own act of kindness to another. This approach is promising as a means of psychotherapy (Seligman, Rashid, & Parks, 2006) and might be adapted to the substance misuse prevention or treatment context.

11.8.2 Modalities of Programming

New inventions in mobile and other technology can provide innovative approaches for prevention and become cost-effective modes of prevention delivery in a prevailing technology-dependent age group. Newer modalities are being considered for implementation among youth a la high technology, including virtual reality simulations, interactive computer, and other communication devices (e.g., use of computer-based telephone conference calls and written interaction chat rooms, such as Skype), and portable computer devises (more recently, the use of smartphones). The use of social networking websites is, in particular, rising among youth and thus can be used as a great platform for assessing their social networks and delivering drug abuse preventive interventions. According to the newest Pew Internet report (Madden et al., 2013), 80 % of online American teens now use some kind of social media (compared to 55 % in 2006). Adolescents are increasingly involved with microblogging through applications such as Facebook or Twitter. In fact, one in four online teens is now using Twitter (versus 16 % in 2011). A typical teen Facebook user has 300 friends. In addition, video sharing via YouTube also could be a potentially effective way to reach adolescents. Any or all of these modalities may need exploration in the future as potential media of drug misuse prevention message contents.

11.8.3 Targets of Programming

We still don't know if the best targets of prevention are specific drugs, groups of drugs, possibly process addictions as well as drug addiction phenomena (e.g., gambling, binge eating, workaholism), or healthy lifestyles in general (i.e., wellness). Drugs such as cigarettes, alcohol, and marijuana may act as "gateway" or introductory drugs to more addictive drugs like cocaine, amphetamines, and prescribed drugs (Kandel, Yamaguchi, & Chen, 1992; Sussman & Ames, 2008). This progression from introductory to harder drugs can result in abuse and dependencies on multiple drugs (co-addictions) due to similar drug-seeking behaviors; that is, using drugs that produce similar or higher levels of stimulation from the original drug (Sussman et al., 2011). As such, drug use is oftentimes associated with other problematic behaviors, including risky sexual behaviors and violence both prior to and as a result of the drug use. The association between drug use and related problem behaviors such as risky sexual behavior and violence need to be explored and possibly incorporated into holistic prevention programs that will address and view these issues as interrelated behaviors (e.g., Sussman et al., 2012).

Understanding the implications of co-addictions can help bolster the impact of drug misuse prevention programs to encompass correlated drug addictions and behaviors and prevent substitute addictions from occurring (Sussman & Ames, 2008). Also, special attention needs to be given towards individuals who have been diagnosed with psychiatric disorders that frequently precede and then co-occur with drug- or alcohol-related problems, leading to "dual diagnoses." Individuals with various psychiatric diagnoses, especially Attention Deficit Hyperactivity Disorder, Conduct Disorder, Depression, Anxiety Disorders, Bipolar Disorder, and Borderline Personality Disorder, are predisposed to drug dependencies and a variety of other high-risk behaviors. There is evidence that psychiatric disorders and substance abuse are neurologically related—similar motivational and reward systems of the brain have been implicated—and that the presence of both increase sensitization of these systems (Post & Kalivas, 2013; Rogers, Moeller, Swann, & Clark, 2010), leading to a worsening of the disorders. Accordingly, understanding the reasons for the relationship between psychiatric disorders and substance misuse will aid in the development of early detection methods and more effective targeting of intervention components (Sussman & Ames, 2008).

11.9 Conclusions

Refinements to and improvements in prevention programs necessitate the transfer of scientific findings from the basic sciences to intervention and evaluation work to dissemination and policy, i.e., promoting the transfer of information from Type I to Type III translational approaches. Green and Glasgow (2006) have suggested that programming be developed that has a maximum likelihood of being institutionalized. Alternatively, or additionally, solid and empirically based policy changes are needed for social environments to systematically and effectively incorporate prevention programming. Evidence-based prevention curricula, for example, might become routinely and widely implemented in appropriate teaching venues, such as school health classes and community organizations. Continuous training of appropriate staff and key personnel is important to ensure fidelity of delivery as with any educational program. Finally, the success of any future substance prevention program requires a closer look at funding sources and allocations that are essential to sustain evidence-based programming as well as to explore innovative approaches to prevention.

References

Barnett, E., Sussman, S., Smith, C., Rohrbach, L. A., & Spruijt-Metz, D. (2012). Motivational interviewing for adolescent substance use: A review of the literature. *Addictive Behaviors, 37*(12), 1325–1334.

Botvin, G. J., & Griffin, K. W. (2007). School-based programmes to prevent alcohol, tobacco and other drug use. *International Review of Psychiatry, 19*(6), 607–615.

Botvin, G. J., Griffin, K. W., Diaz, T., Scheier, L. M., Williams, C., & Epstein, J. A. (2000). Preventing illicit drug use in adolescents: Long-term follow-up data from a randomized control trial of a school population. *Addictive Behaviors, 25*(5), 769–774.

Briand, L. A., & Blendy, J. A. (2010). Molecular and genetic substrates linking stress and addiction. *Brain Research, 1314*, 219–234.

Chiauzzi, E., Green, T. C., Lord, S., Ma, C. T., & Ba, M. G. (2005). My student body: A high-risk drinking prevention web site for college students. *Journal of American College Health, 53*(6), 263–274.

Davidson, R. J., Kabat-Zinn, J., Schumacher, J., Rosenkranz, M., Muller, D., Santorelli, S. F., et al. (2003). Alterations in brain and immune function produced by mindfulness meditation. *Psychosomatic Medicine, 65*(4), 564–570.

Dougherty, D., & Conway, P. H. (2008). The "3T's" road map to transform US health care: The "how" of high-quality care. *Journal of the American Medical Association, 299*(19), 2319–2321.

Farhat, T., Iannotti, R. J., & Simons-Morton, B. G. (2010). Overweight, obesity, youth, and health-risk behaviors. *American Journal of Preventive Medicine, 38*(3), 258–267.

Fishbein, D. H. (2000). The importance of neurobiological research to the prevention of psychopathology. *Prevention Science, 1*(2), 89–106.

Foxcroft, D. R., & Tsertsvadze, A. (2011). Universal multi-component prevention programs for alcohol misuse in young people. *Cochrane Database of Systematic Reviews,* doi:10.1002/14651858.CD009307.

Gordon, R. (1987). An operational classification of disease prevention. In A. Steinberg & M. M. Silverman (Eds.), *Preventing mental disorders* (pp. 20–26). Rockville, MD: Department of Health and Human Services, National Institutes of Health.

Gottfredson, D. C., & Wilson, D. B. (2003). Characteristics of effective school-based substance abuse prevention. *Prevention Science, 4*(1), 27–38.

Green, L. W., & Glasgow, R. E. (2006). Evaluating the relevance, generalization, and applicability of research: Issues in external validation and translation methodology. *Evaluation & the Health Professions, 29*(1), 126–153.

Holder, H. (2009). *Policies to prevent alcohol problems: A research agenda.* Princeton, NJ: Substance Abuse Policy Research Program (SAPRP), Robert Wood Johnson Foundation.

Johnson, C. A., MacKinnon, D. P., & Pentz, M. A. (1996). Breadth of program and outcome effectiveness in drug abuse prevention. *American Behavioral Scientist, 39*(7), 884–896.

Kandel, D. B., Yamaguchi, K., & Chen, K. (1992). Stages of progression in drug involvement from adolescence to adulthood: Further evidence for the gateway theory. *Journal of Studies on Alcohol and Drugs, 53*(5), 447–457.

Koob, G. F., & LeMoal, M. (2001). Drug addiction, dysregulation of reward, and allostasis. *Neuropsychopharmacology, 24*(2), 97–129.

Kreek, M. J., & Koob, G. F. (1998). Drug dependence: Stress and dysregulation of brain reward pathways. *Drug & Alcohol Dependence, 51*(1), 23–47.

Liao, Y., Huh, J., Huang, Z., Pentz, M. A., & Chou, C. P. (2013). Changes in friends' and parental influences on cigarette smoking from early through late adolescence. *Journal of Adolescent Health, 53*(1), 132–138.

Madden, M., Lenhart, A., Cortesi, S., Gasser, U., Duggan, M., Smith, A., & Beaton, M. (2013). Teens, social media, and privacy. Pew Research Center: Internet, Science & Technology. Retrieved August 14, 2015, from http://www.pewinternet.org/Reports/2013/Teens-Social-Media-And-Privacy.aspx

Pentz, M. A. (1995). A comprehensive strategy to prevent the abuse of alcohol and other drugs: Theory and methods. In R. Coombs & D. Ziedonis (Eds.), *Handbook on drug abuse prevention* (pp. 62–92). Englewood Cliffs, NJ: Prentice Hall.

Pentz, M. A., Jasuja, G. K., Rohrbach, L. A., Sussman, S., & Bardo, M. T. (2006). Translation in tobacco and drug abuse prevention research. *Evaluation & the Health Professions, 29*(2), 246–271.

Piazza, P. V., & Le Moal, M. (1998). The role of stress in drug self-administration. *Trends in Pharmacological Sciences, 19*(2), 67–74.

Post, R. M., & Kalivas, P. (2013). Bipolar disorder and substance misuse: Pathological and therapeutic implications of their comorbidity and cross-sensitisation. *British Journal of Psychiatry, 202*(3), 172–176.

Prochaska, J. J., Spring, B., & Nigg, C. R. (2008). Multiple health behavior change research: An introduction and overview. *Preventive Medicine, 46*(3), 181–188.

Prokhorov, A. V., Kelder, S. H., Shegog, R., Murray, N., Peters, R., Agurcia-Parker, C., et al. (2008). Impact of a smoking prevention interactive experience (ASPIRE), an interactive, multimedia smoking prevention and cessation curriculum for culturally diverse high-school students. *Nicotine & Tobacco Research, 10*(9), 1477–1485.

Riggs, N. R., & Greenberg, M. T. (2009). Neurocognition as a moderator and mediator in adolescent substance misuse prevention. *American Journal of Drug and Alcohol Abuse, 35*(4), 209–213.

Rogers, R. D., Moeller, F. G., Swann, A. C., & Clark, L. (2010). Recent research on impulsivity in individuals with drug use and mental health disorders: Implications for alcoholism. *Alcoholism: Clinical and Experimental Research, 34*(8), 1319–1333.

Rohrbach, L., Grana, R., Sussman, S., & Valente, T. W. (2006). Type II translation: Transporting prevention interventions from research to real-world settings. *Evaluation & the Health Professions, 29*(3), 302–333.

Seligman, M. E. P., Rashid, T., & Parks, A. C. (2006). Positive psychotherapy. *American Psychologist, 61*(8), 774–788.

Sinha, R. (2012). How does stress lead to risk of alcohol relapse? *Alcohol Research, 34*(4), 432–440.

Spoth, R., Rohrbach, L. A., Greenberg, M., Leaf, P., Brown, C. H., Fagan, A., et al. (2013). Addressing core challenges for the next generation of type 2 translation research and systems: The translation science to population impact (TSci Impact) framework. *Prevention Science, 14*(4), 319–351.

Sussman, S. (2013). A lifespan developmental-stage approach to tobacco and other drug abuse prevention. *ISRN Addiction, 2013*, 745783.

Sussman, S. (2015). Evaluating the efficacy of Project TND: Evidence from seven research trials. In L. M. Scheier (Ed.), *Handbook of adolescent drug use prevention: Research, intervention strategies, and practice*. Washington, DC: American Psychological Association.

Sussman, S., & Ames, S. L. (2008). *Drug abuse: Concepts, prevention, and cessation*. New York: Cambridge University Press.

Sussman, S., Leventhal, A., Bluthenthal, R. N., Freimuth, M., Forster, M., & Ames, S. L. (2011). A framework for the specificity of addictions. *International Journal of Environmental Research and Public Health, 8*(8), 3399–3415.

Sussman, S., Levy, D., Hassmiller, K., Cena, D. W., Kim, M., Rohrbach, L. A., & Chaloupka, F. (2013). Comparing effects of tobacco use prevention modalities: need for complex system models. *Tobacco Induced Diseases, 11*(2), 14.

Sussman, S., Sun, P., Rohrbach, L., & Spruijt-Metz, D. (2012). One-year outcomes of a drug abuse prevention program for older teens and emerging adults: Evaluating a motivational interviewing booster component. *Health Psychology, 31*(4), 476–485.

Sussman, S., Valente, T. W., Rohrbach, L. A., Skara, S., & Pentz, M. A. (2006). Translation in health behavior research: Converting science into action. *Evaluation & the Health Professions, 29*(1), 7–32.

Tang, Y. Y., Lu, Q., Fan, M., Yang, Y., & Posner, M. I. (2012). Mechanisms of white matter changes induced by meditation. *Proceedings of the National Academy of Sciences, 109*(26), 10570–10574.

Thush, C., Wiers, R. W., Ames, S. L., Grenard, J. L., Sussman, S., & Stacy, A. W. (2008). Interactions between implicit and explicit cognition and working memory capacity in the prediction of alcohol use in at-risk adolescents. *Drug & Alcohol Dependence, 94*, 116–124.

Wetherill, R., & Tapert, S. F. (2013). Adolescent brain development, substance use, and psychotherapeutic change. *Psychology of Addictive Behaviors, 27*(2), 393–402.

Chapter 12
Violence Affecting Youth: Pervasive and *Preventable*

Larry Cohen, Rachel Davis, and Anna Realini

12.1   Introduction

Violence is a preventable, public health crisis in the United States. We see violence all around us, and we mourn its victims. We want to know what can be done about it, but, by and large, we stand by as a society and allow a culture of violence to flourish without protest.

We are *all* affected by violence. It affects where we live, where we work, where we go to school, and *whether* our children go to school or *if* we can work. Further, these impacts are disproportionately felt by disenfranchised and under-resourced communities where residents nearly always suffer the most and bear the greatest burden of reduced health and safety, but have the fewest resources to respond to these mounting challenges.

Violence particularly affects youth. They are three times more likely than adults to be victims of violence (Arredondo et al., 1999). Reports of child abuse and neglect in the United States in 2012 totaled 678,810 (Morgan & Truman, 2014). Over the last 20 years, practitioners and researchers have revealed the impact of multiple forms of violence on children, including child abuse, sexual abuse, dating violence/sexual assault, witnessing domestic violence, and witnessing/experiencing violence in street, school, and community settings. Young people are powerfully affected by violence in the environments they grow up in.

The founder of the Los Angeles Violence Prevention Coalition, Billie Weiss, went back to school after raising her children to study maternal and child health where she thought she would focus on preventing disease. To her astonishment, she learned that after year one, injuries and trauma exceeded disease as the leading cause of death to children and adolescents (Centers for Disease Control and

L. Cohen, M.S.W. (✉) • R. Davis, M.S.W. • A. Realini
Prevention Institute, Oakland, CA, USA
e-mail: larry@preventioninstitute.org; rachel@preventioninstitute.org; anna@preventioninstitute.org

© Springer Science+Business Media New York 2016   235
M.R. Korin (ed.), *Health Promotion for Children and Adolescents*,
DOI 10.1007/978-1-4899-7711-3_12

Prevention, 2012a, 2012b). Homicide is the second most lethal threat for 15- to 24-year-olds, accounting for 4828 deaths in that age bracket alone in 2010 and homicide has been the leading cause of death among African-American males between the ages of 15–24 for more than 10 years (Centers for Disease Control and Prevention, 2012a, 2012b). In low-income communities and among youth of color, violence is the leading cause of injury (Centers for Disease Control and Prevention, 2012a, 2012b). On a typical day, six or seven youth are murdered in this country and youth 7- to 17-years-old are equally likely to be victims of suicide or victims of homicide (Center for the Study and Prevention of Violence). Eighty two percent of all murdered juveniles are killed with a firearm and more than a fifth of US teenagers from 14 to 17 report having witnessed a shooting (Center for the Study and Prevention of Violence). Additionally, nineteen percent of undergraduate women experience attempted or completed sexual assault (Fisher, Krebs, Lindquist, Martin, & Warner, 2009). Domestic violence, which accounted for 21 % of all violent crimes from 2003 to 2012, was most prevalent for 18- to 24-year-olds (Morgan & Truman, 2014).

It is clear that experiencing violence directly impacts children's physical and emotional health. Experiencing or fearing violence in the street, in their homes, and in their relationships also has immediate and long-term emotional and mental health consequences that can, in turn, further affect physical health, relationships, learning, and the ability to work (Anda et al., 2005). Trauma from violence and chronic adversity also become a basis for how children perceive and respond to events in their lives and communities.

Fortunately, there is a strong and growing evidence-base that confirms that violence is preventable. Preventing childhood exposure to violence before it occurs saves lives, reduces injuries and illnesses, helps communities thrive, and saves money. It is critical that prevention be included as a vital part of the solution to defend childhood. This awareness has begun to reach a tipping point, resulting in mobilized groups advocating for social and political solutions. *We know what to do to prevent violence. We need to refine that knowledge, and even more importantly, we need to develop the political will to translate that knowledge into practice in communities so we can save lives.*

12.2 Prevention Strategies: Upfront, in the Thick, but Mostly Aftermath

Prevention strategy is often categorized in public health as primary, secondary, and tertiary prevention. In a prevention planning process focused on community street violence, Philadelphia youth modified these terms to make them more user-friendly and community-relevant, renaming the categories *Upfront, In the Thick,* and *Aftermath.*

Upfront, or primary prevention, explicitly focuses on action *before* there are symptoms/risks to implement strategies that every community needs, primarily focused on changing policies, practices, and norms that underlay violence. Examples include positive social connections in neighborhoods, economic development, reducing the availability of firearms, quality early care and education, parenting skills, quality after-school programming, conflict resolution, and youth leadership.

In the Thick, or secondary prevention, focuses on the *immediate* responses *after* symptoms/risks have appeared and are aimed at those communities and individuals who may be at increased risk for violence. Examples include street outreach and violence interruption, family support services, and mentoring.

Aftermath, or tertiary prevention, focuses on *longer term* responses to deal with the consequences of violence after it has occurred to reduce the chances it will reoccur. Prevention examples include successful re-entry following incarceration, mental health services, (e.g., therapeutic foster care, functional family therapy, and multi-systemic therapy), and restorative justice, which fundamentally shifts the way we think about and do justice to invite victims, offenders, and community members to work together to repair the harm caused by incidents.

So far, the vast majority of US violence-related efforts have focused on after-the-fact programs. Historically, society has relied almost exclusively on the criminal justice system to respond to violence. This approach has been rooted in a few assumptions: (1) violence is an individual's criminal choice; (2) punishment or the threat of punishment is both warranted and a deterrent to violent acts; and (3) violence is an inevitable aspect of the behaviors of some people.

Law enforcements' goal and role, for the most part, is the identification, prosecution, and punishment of violent offenders, the result of which is an immense criminal justice and incarceration system. While few disagree that policing is an important piece of addressing violence, a prescription to treat violent crime that focuses primarily on criminal justice is not only insufficient and often ineffective and inhumane, it's expensive and often contributes to the cycle of violence. The emphasis on incarceration of youth in the United States is far greater than in any other country (Redburn, Travis, & Western, 2014). Approximately 93,000 young people are held in juvenile facilities across the country with 70% at state-funded institutions at an average cost of 240 dollars per inmate, per day (Justice Policy Institute, 2009). California spends almost $180,000 per year per inmate (Legislative Analyst's Office) in its juvenile justice system and less than $8500 per year per K-12 student (California Department of Education, 2013). By the age of 23, nearly a third of US youth have been arrested for an offense other than a minor traffic violation (Goode, 2011).

Despite the fact that the juvenile justice system was created with a fundamental belief in the potential for prevention and rehabilitation among children, its major responsibility is punishment, which has not been shown to be affective for addressing violent behavior or for preventing further violence. Many incarcerated youth are put away for nonviolent crimes and return home with fewer opportunities, increased trauma, and reduced connections to their communities (Campaign for Youth Justice, 2011). Additionally, too many states ignore the evidence of the negative long-term impacts of incarceration on children and, in fact, incorporate youth into the adult criminal process (Campaign for Youth Justice, 2011).

The realities of violence beg for strategies beyond aggressive, traditional efforts that blame and punish. This requires a more comprehensive set of prevention activities—changes in social norms, organizational practice, public education, and policy—as well as cooperation between multiple partners, including public health and criminal justice.

12.2.1   The Need for Prevention Strategy in the First Place

Initiatives to prevent violence have primarily been *in the thick* focused on individually-oriented efforts and early intervention services. Interventions, such as universal screening in health care settings and improved access to mental health services help to alleviate trauma and potentially prevent future incidents; however, early identification, while very important, comes after actual or threatened violence and seldom alters the broader community and societal environment that gave rise to the violence that caused the trauma *in the first place*. As Dr. George Albee put it, no epidemic can ever be resolved solely by attention to the affected individual (Albee, 1983).

The next step in preventing violence requires expanding the overarching dialog to emphasize approaches that prevent children and youth from experiencing and being exposed to violence before it occurs. Primary prevention includes systemic change to environmental factors—such as economic inequalities—and norms—such as privacy and silence around family violence—that shape the behaviors of a population to promote healthy and safe environments for children.

A greater emphasis on violence prevention *in the first place* complements the field's continued commitment to improving responses. This shift will require increased effort and cross-sector collaboration from multiple partners to advance promising prevention approaches—essential to achieving dramatic reductions in rates of child exposure to violence.

12.3   Violence Is a Health Equity Issue

All people and communities deserve equal opportunities to be healthy and safe, but opportunities to be healthy and safe aren't distributed evenly across our society. For example, research by the Alameda County, CA, Health Department concluded that an African-American child born in West Oakland, a low-income community, can expect to die an average of 15 years earlier than a white child born in the Oakland Hills, where there is historically higher household incomes, lower unemployment rates, and fewer Black and Latino residents than in the flatlands of Oakland (Alameda County Public Health Department, 2008). The same study showed that for every $12,500 in additional family income, one could expect an additional year of life (Alameda County Public Health Department, 2008). This pattern is repeated in cities across United States and internationally. Poverty, racism, and lack of educational and economic opportunities are among the fundamental determinants of poor health and lack of safety, and inequities in the distribution of resources perpetuate patterns of poor health. Some neighborhoods and groups are far more exposed to the conditions that give rise to violence and other health inequities. Some communities have an overwhelming number of accumulated risk factors for violence and at the same time lack adequate compensatory resilience factors to protect against violence. In many neighborhoods across the United States, entire communities experience traumatizing events and conditions. Young people in urban neighborhoods are often exposed to persistent or chronic traumatic stress and fear of violence. It is not our genetic codes, but our ZIP codes that primarily dictate our experiences, norms, and behaviors.

Further, when our communities become unsafe, the investment of financial and personal capital is diminished. Community and interpersonal violence not only jeopardize health and safety directly—causing injuries, death, and emotional trauma—witnessing, directly experiencing, and the fear of violence can also contribute to unhealthy behavior and impact people's choices, purchasing patterns, and access to resources such as safe places to play and healthy food (Cohen, Davis, Lee, & Valdovinos, 2010). In communities with pervasive violence or where residents have fear of violence, people are less likely to walk and talk on the streets, parents do not allow their children to play or bike outside or walk to school, businesses are less likely to open and invest in neighborhoods, and there is less investment in improving deteriorating parks, housing, and schools.

These neighborhood factors and reduced options for healthy eating and activity exacerbate already existing illnesses and increase the risk for onset of disease (Prevention Institute, 2011a, 2011b). Due to community risk factors, many chronic illnesses and mental health problems are more prevalent in African American, Hispanic, and Asian American groups than for white people, and these chronic health issues are made significantly worse by exposure to violence (Braveman, Egerter, & Williams, 2011; Cespedes & Stanley, 2008). Preventing violence is an important component of achieving equity in health and in all communities (Prevention Institute, 2011a, 2011b).

12.4 Norms: Commonly Held Attitudes and Beliefs that Shape Behaviors

Societal and community environments play a strong role in shaping norms and behavior. Often based in culture and tradition, norms are attitudes, beliefs, and standards that we take for granted and that pattern our behavior—they are environmental signals telling people what is okay and not okay to do. Norms label what actually occurs and also signify a standard of proper behavior.

As the Institute of Medicine puts it, "It is unreasonable to expect that people will change their behavior easily when so many forces in the social, cultural and physical environment conspire against such change" (Smedley & Syme, 2000). But that is exactly what we expect too often.

A prevention strategy must account for norms because these standards are pervasive, powerful determinants of behavior. For example, when smoking was prevalent and legal in virtually all venues, many more people smoked. At the time, prevention initiatives focused on individual smoking cessation, which didn't impact the powerful norms of smoking as sexy and universally accepted. Coalitions of health advocates worked together to pass policies that restricted smoking in public places, which proved to be the tipping factor in shifting smoking norms. As places to smoke were reduced and nonsmokers began to expect environments with cleaner air, we saw dramatic changes in behavior. In California, for example, where the first no smoking laws emerged, the number of smokers dropped by more than 50 % within one generation (U.S. Department of Health and Human Services, 2012).

This approach is equally important in the prevention of violence. For example, alcohol abuse is heavily correlated with violence. Alcohol density and marketing is far greater in low-income communities (LaVeist & Wallace, 2000) and billboards advertising malt liquor typically are only placed in low-income communities of color. Sexual depictions of women and symbols of aggression and power are often used to promote cheap products with high alcohol content and that imagery reinforces the dynamics of structural violence (Pinderhughes & Davis, 2013). These marketing practices significantly impact norms surrounding alcohol use and therefore impact behavior, compounding risk factors for violence as well as perpetuating disparities in physical and mental health (Anderson, Angus, de Bruijn, Gordon, & Hastings, 2009).

As an example of successful strategy to implement policy to change norms, Community Coalition—a nonprofit organization that works with African American and Latino residents to build a prosperous and healthy South Los Angeles—solicited input from residents who recommended reducing the number of liquor stores in the community as one way to address crime and violence. At the time, there were more than 700 liquor stories in South L.A. (population 820,000; 71.3 miles²), more than in the entire state of Pennsylvania (population 12,281,054; 44,820 miles²). Community Coalition launched a grassroots advocacy campaign to influence L.A. County's policies on conditional-use permits and ultimately succeeded in shutting down nearly 200 liquor stores. As a result of the coalition's activities, the neighborhood saw a 27 % reduction in violent and drug-related crime within a four-block radius of each closed liquor store (Aboelata, 2004).

In work on preventing violence against women, Prevention Institute identified and clustered five norms that underlay violence. Practitioners who work to prevent violence confirmed that addressing these norms is critical for preventing child abuse, violence against women, and sexual assault (Cohen, 2012).

1. *A Narrow Definition of Manhood*, where society promotes the behaviors of domination, exploitation, objectification, control, oppression, and dangerous risk-taking by men and boys, too often victimizing women and children.
2. *Limited Roles for Women*, where from a young age females are often encouraged, through subtle and overt messages, to act and be treated as objects, to be used and controlled by others.

3. *Power*, where value is placed on claiming and maintaining control over others. Traditional power expectations make children a particularly vulnerable population.
4. *Violence as the Way We Solve Problems*, where aggression is tolerated and accepted as normal behavior and can be used as a way to get what one wants.
5. *Privacy and Silence*, where norms associated with individual and family privacy are considered sacrosanct and secrecy and silence is fostered. Children who experience violence may keep it secret and those who witness violence are discouraged from intervening. Though changing, the value placed on privacy, can render victims and their families immobile in the face of fear, public shame, and stigma.

It is important to understand that these norms are not just individual traits, but are standardized cultural patterns. For example, in our society, we glamorize violence, overlook it, accept it as a private matter, and regularly encourage it through "egging" others on. While condoning children's exposure to violence is certainly not the norm, we have an overarching set of norms that insidiously contributes to the likelihood that it will happen. If violence is typical, expected, and reinforced by the media, family, community, peers, or school, it is far more likely to occur. It will occur, in fact, with greater frequency and potency. If norms discourage safe behavior and are unsupportive of healthy and safe relationships, then programs focused on change at the individual level will not produce safe behavior unless social norms are changed with them.

We must work together to change norms if we are to make major strides in preventing violence affecting youth.

12.5   Three Keys to Prevent Violence that Impacts Youth

There are many ways to characterize multifaceted strategy to reduce violence before it occurs. Perhaps the simplest is the Three Keys, a framework for understanding a comprehensive approach to preventing violence that incorporates public health, law enforcement, social service, and education perspectives.

12.5.1   *Key 1: Youth Violence Is Complex and Requires a Comprehensive Community Approach*

Since childhood and youth exposure to violence is rooted in norms and environments, no single program can address the magnitude of the issue or the diverse root factors underlying it. Violence is a complex issue and effectively preventing violence involves comprehensive and multidisciplinary efforts to address the underlying contributors and to build resilience in youth, families, and communities. This is sometimes called a public health approach to preventing violence.

THE SPECTRUM OF PREVENTION

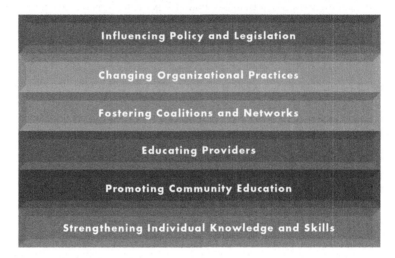

Fig. 12.1 The spectrum of prevention

Prevention of violence is often seen as unachievable because prevention is rarely approached with the level of commitment and attention required for long-term success. As with many national issues, one way to find effective solutions is to start locally, with the unit of analysis being the city. As urban successes are realized, they build momentum and serve as models for other locales, both revealing the pathways and also providing a sense of hope and opportunity. By building on the wisdom of communities, the experience of national experts, and the infrastructure built through coalitions and networks over the last 20 years, we can harness the willingness and capture the opportunity to collectively construct a national movement to prevent childhood and youth exposure to violence.

Successful prevention initiatives require comprehensive solutions for addressing community conditions at multiple levels simultaneously. The Spectrum of Prevention (as shown in Fig. 12.1, Prevention Institute, 1999) provides a systematic framework for developing effective and sustainable community prevention efforts. Prevention activities can be implemented at any of the Spectrum's six levels, but when all Spectrum levels are applied as part of a cohesive plan, the effect can be transformative (Davis, Kilburn, & Schultz, 2009). In most instances, environmental change requires efforts at the broadest levels of the Spectrum, such as by changing legislation and adopting regulations (Levels 1 and 2). Applied in concert, the other levels of the Spectrum build momentum for change and contribute to improved health and safety. For example, efforts to influence policy (Level 1) are more likely to succeed when public awareness and support are garnered through individual and community education (Levels 6 and 5), and when a variety of partners in different sectors work together to effect the desired change (Levels 3 and 4).

12.5.1.1   The Spectrum of Prevention and Recommendations for Salinas, CA

The city of Salinas, a rural, agricultural area in California, used the Spectrum of Prevention in a comprehensive plan to prevent violence that included the mayor, grass roots activists, local businesses, the faith community, and major city and county leaders from varying sectors, including law enforcement and health. During the course of a year, they developed a framework for reducing violence based upon the Spectrum of Prevention, *Cultivating Peace in Salinas* (Cohen & Erlenborn, 2001). It was used to foster community momentum and create a shared sense of strategy. Further, the City Council used it when making decisions regarding priorities and funding. With a clear, all-encompassing action framework in place, violence rates dropped and local residents noted improved perceptions of safety (Table 12.1).

Table 12.1 Spectrum of prevention and its application to preventing violence in Salinas, California

Spectrum level	Recommendations for Salinas
1. Influencing policy and legislation	• Engage with planning commission to set zoning restrictions on alcohol density • Develop public policies to address gun regulations in Salinas • Review all funding requests to the City by comparing to the violence prevention plan
2. Changing organizational practices	• Increase after-school and recreation opportunities • Prioritize economic development and job training for youth • Implement measures to promote walkability and bicycling • Promote family-friendly practices among employers
3. Fostering coalitions and networks	• Develop collaboration between City, County, and School Districts to implement this plan • Establish an intergovernmental youth services board
4. Educating providers	• Collaborate to produce annual report card and share data • Promulgate a shared strategy to reduce gang violence • Support practitioners who work in violence prevention
5. Promoting community education	• Develop initiatives that promote positive community values • Enhance positive media messages and reduce the impact of negative messages • Encourage more positive role models and mentors for youth • Convene community-wide dialog on inequitable use of discipline practices
6. Strengthening individual knowledge and skills	• Invest in early childhood and parent support initiatives • Improve literacy rates for children and adults

12.5.2 Key 2: A Focus on Reducing Risk and Enhancing Resilience Is Needed

Risk factors are *community, family, or individual* characteristics or circumstances that increase the likelihood that violence will occur; resilience factors support the healthy development of individuals, families, schools, and communities, and build capacity for positive relationships and interactions, thereby reducing the long-term impact from exposure to violence. Removing a specific exposure to risk is not enough without complementary development of resilience factors. As Jordan Simmons, Executive Director of the East Bay Center for the Performing Arts in Richmond, CA, said, "what's critical in terms of the continuum is that it's not a direct relationship in terms of opposites—it's that resilience factors are protective against risk factors. So it's not enough to take the gun or the knife from a gang member's hand, you have to replace it with something—a paint brush, a computer keyboard" (Simmons, 2009). We also have to consider the critical impact of *community* risk and resilience factors in addition to *individual* factors.

On an individual and family level, risk factors include high levels of family disruption and family violence; poor discipline practices, including authoritarian child-rearing attitudes and harsh, lax, or inconsistent disciplinary practices; low parental involvement; and parental substance abuse or mental illness, criminality, and/or incarceration.

Alternately, resilience factors for children include caring relationships, connection to family, a sense of connection to school, high academic expectations, and opportunities for participation in school and community networks (Byrne, Pattavina, & Taxman, 2005).

The ACE (Adverse Childhood Experience) Studies are longitudinal studies that assess the extent of adverse experiences as a child and compare them to the child's health and social outcomes more than a generation later. The ACE studies reveal that the experiences of violence and trauma in childhood accumulate. As Jim Garbarino, who studies children's well-being, summarizes, "No one risk factor accounts for much by itself. It is the overwhelming accumulation without compensatory protective factors that puts kids at risk" (Prevention Institute, 2005). The ACE studies also reveal that violence and trauma are major risk factors for further violence and also for the leading causes of illness and death as well as poor quality of life in the United States (Anda et al., 2005). The ACE framework demonstrates a link between (1) specific violence-related stressors in childhood, including child abuse, neglect, and repeated exposure to intimate partner violence, and (2) resulting risky behaviors and health problems in adulthood including alcoholism and alcohol abuse; depression; illicit drug use; and chronic diseases. In addition, ACEs also strongly correlate with health-related behaviors and outcomes during childhood and adolescence including early initiation of smoking, sexual activity, and illicit drug use; adolescent pregnancies; social rejection and antisocial attitudes; lack of involvement in conventional activities and school problems, including poor academic performance; and suicide attempts.

Research shows that, like risk, the effects of resilience factors accumulate; children with more assets are less likely to engage in violence and other high-risk behaviors. Having more resilience factors also increases the chances that young people will have positive attitudes and behaviors such as good health, success in school, and self-control. Reducing the impact of adverse childhood experience requires advancing greater resilience; indeed, building community resilience factors can counteract the risks. Research shows that developing relationships with caring adults protects "at-risk" youth against becoming involved in violence (Prevention Institute, 2001). The National Longitudinal Study of Adolescent Health found that young people's sense of connection to their parents and other family members was the most consistently protective factor across all the health outcomes. Teens with parents who are physically present in the home are less likely to engage in violent behavior (Prevention Institute, 2001).

Schools are, of course, a critical venue for youth that shapes their learning, norms, environmental exposures, and risk and resilience factors. School risk factors include school system failure, illiteracy, truancy, and bullying. These factors are more prevalent in under-resourced schools in low-income communities and in communities of color (see textbox below). Violence and fear of violence in schools permeates how children experience their daily lives as well as if they succeed academically—those who are scared at school prioritize safety over learning (Prevention Institute, 2011a, 2011b).

High-quality education that fosters positive social–emotional development in young people protects against violence, whereas lack of resources for academic success increases the risk of future violence (Brewer et al., 2000; Dahlberg, 1998; Maguin & Loeber, 1996). Young people living in more affluent communities report greater access to education and employment opportunities, which are associated with higher expectations for success and better grades (Chung, Mulvey, & Steinberg, 2011). Students whose parents express high expectations for school performance are also less likely to engage in violent behavior.

Students who feel they are a part of their school and are treated fairly by teachers are more emotionally healthy and less inclined toward drug and alcohol abuse, suicidal thoughts and attempts, and involvement in violence (Prevention Institute, 2001). Involving students in decisions about school policies and programs is key to helping create a school climate of inclusion, respect, and safety (Cohen, McCabe, Michelli & Pickeral, 2009). Research has found that when students are offered opportunities to acquire skills and engage in social activities, their problem-solving, communication, and analytical skills improve (Prevention Institute, 2001). In addition, they demonstrate enhanced leadership and autonomous decision-making and are more likely to reach academic goals such as graduating from school. Such factors are all protective against involvement in violent activities (Prevention Institute, 2001).

The community is a critical focal point for promoting resilience and reducing risk. Examples of *Community* risk factors are diminished economic opportunities and high concentrations of poverty; low levels of community participation; lack of safe streets and parks; discrimination and oppression; availability of firearms; availability of alcohol and other drugs; community deterioration (blight, graffiti, vacant buildings, high levels of transiency); and high levels of incarceration/re-entry. The textbox below describes many contributing factors to community risk exacerbated by inequity.

On a community level, resilience factors include economic capital, including living wage opportunities; the ability to access social capital, including strong social networks and trust, meaningful opportunities for participation, and willingness of the community to act on its own behalf; positive ethnic, racial, and intergroup relations; good lighting and community design and upkeep that fosters physical activity, interaction, and artistic and creative opportunities.

Strong neighborhood connections protect against violence (Dahlberg, 1998; Earls, Raudenbush, & Sampson, 1997) and correspond with significantly lower rates of homicide and alcohol and drug abuse (Nation & Wandersman, 1998). Social cohesion of neighborhoods combined with intergenerational connections and neighbors' willingness to intervene on behalf of the common good account for more than 70 % of the variation between neighborhoods in levels of violence (Earls et al., 1997). Economically disadvantaged communities foster lower levels of trust and social cohesion than wealthier communities, which benefit from lower rates of violence (Dahlberg, 1998). Participation in community networks, neighborhood associations, and religious and school organizations helps students to develop strong formal and informal ties with adults and increases their sense of connection and self-efficacy.

It is unreasonable to blame certain individuals, families, communities, or schools for the exposures and behaviors that lead to risk or resilience, which we know result from the environmental and social factors within communities and neighborhoods. It is also unreasonable to continue to focus on treatment of individual risks and outcomes of violence. The burden of trauma and the drain of limited community resources make prevention a priority. As Dr. Vincent Felitti, the co-founder of the ACE's framework, stated to a large conference of health clinicians, "If we don't prevent violence there are huge health costs not just criminal justice costs. We know, you know, there will never be enough resources to address the impacts. Primary prevention is the only option we have to pay attention to the breadth of the problem. The cost of this exposure to the individual, family, community, and society is staggering."

Due to the frequency of violence, the high cost of medical and social services, and the lack of dedicated funding for interventions, after-the-fact approaches, while important, are unlikely to ever meet the demand. More importantly, after-the-fact strategies will never prevent childhood exposure to violence from occurring in the first place. Our children and youth deserve an investment in prevention.

Community Risk Factors Emerging from or Exacerbated by Inequity
Poverty
Areas of concentrated poverty that have low housing values and schools with low high school graduation rates put residents at increased risk of death from homicide (Robert Wood Johnson Foundation, 2009), and low-income neighborhoods suffer disproportionately high rates of street violence (Prevention Institute, 2011b). Low-income neighborhoods are more likely to have higher

(continued)

unemployment and poverty rates, and lower homeownership and educational attainment rates than middle- and high-income neighborhoods (Acevedo-Garcia, Krimgold, Lefkowitz, McArdle, & Osypuk, 2007; Arnett et al., 2001).

In high-poverty urban areas, four out of five residents are non-white (Collins & Williams, 2001; Geronimus, 2000). African American, American Indian, and Latino children are six to nine times more likely than white children to live in areas of concentrated poverty, as are children with parents born outside the United States (The Annie E. Casey Foundation, 2012).

While economic opportunity protects against violence (Dahlberg, 1998), neighborhoods without employment opportunities deny residents the means to earn a living wage as part of the mainstream economy. People without access to job training, support services, and loans and investment capital are more likely to suffer from chronic stress and may be engaged in alternative economies and means of earning income, including the drug economy and other illegal activities (Dahlberg, 1998).

Residential Segregation

Concentrating poverty and social problems in segregated neighborhoods creates the physical and social conditions that increase the likelihood of violence (Allard & Greene, 2011). Discriminatory housing and mortgage practices persist today to restrict the housing options of low-income populations and people of color to the least desirable residential areas (Kubrin & Squires, 2005). Sub-standard housing is more common in poor communities, and homes with severe physical problems are more likely to be occupied by Black people (1.7 times more likely than the general population) and those with low incomes (2.2 times) (Collins & Williams, 2001; Higgins & Krieger, 2002).

Residential segregation affects the quality of neighborhoods by increasing poverty, poor housing conditions, overcrowding, and social disorganization in some areas, while limiting access to quality healthcare and other services and institutions in others (Collins & Williams, 2001; Corral & Landrine, 2009). This creates inequitable conditions and clear patterns of poor health.

Community Deterioration and the Built Environment

Community deterioration and how communities are designed affects the likelihood of violence. Appearances shape perceptions of safety, and neighborhoods with higher levels of litter, graffiti, abandoned cars, dilapidated housing, and other signs of disorder are associated with increased violence (Beyers, Hipwell, Loeber, Pardini, & Wei, 2005). Well-designed and safe streets help develop active, healthy neighborhoods with greater economic development; zoning policies can help create vital community centers and increase the presence of businesses, thus increasing neighborhood foot traffic and improving safety. Public transportation should be placed where it is equitably responsive to community needs and encourages links to vibrant centers, but unfortunately, needs of local residents in low-income communities and communities of color are often not included in transportation planning processes.

(continued)

The presence of quality schools, health and mental health facilities, libraries, recreational centers, and parks buffer against the likelihood of violence, but neighborhoods that are predominantly low-income and African American have higher numbers of abandoned buildings and grounds, and inadequate city services and amenities (Collins & Williams, 2001). Cuts in government spending affect these neighborhoods more than affluent neighborhoods. The disinvestment of economic resources has contributed to a decline in the urban infrastructure and physical environment in these communities (Collins & Williams, 2001).

Alcohol and Other Drugs
Alcohol is involved in two-thirds of all homicides and the presence of illegal drug markets contribute to higher levels of violence (Cohen & Swift, 1991; Dahlberg, 1998). Low-income census tracts and predominantly Black census tracts have significantly more liquor stores per capita than more affluent communities and predominantly white neighborhoods (LaVeist & Wallace, 2000). Predominantly white neighborhoods also have less outdoor advertising for alcohol and tobacco than predominantly non-white neighborhoods (LaVeist & Wallace, 2000). Alcohol advertising contributes to higher consumption and heavier drinking, which increases the risk for violence (Anderson et al., 2009). Alcohol and other drugs have a multiplier effect that heightens aggression and violence, and neighborhoods with a concentration of liquor stores often suffer higher incidence of alcohol-related problems (United Nations Office for Drug Control and Crime Prevention, 2002).

Academic Failure and Quality Schools
Students who do not have the opportunity to develop their learning and cognitive skills, or who do not graduate have less access to economic opportunities, and these young people may not enjoy stable employment that pays a living wage (Robert Wood Johnson Foundation, 2009). Urban schools with higher concentrations of Black and Latino students offer fewer advanced courses and have lower levels of achievement than schools attended by predominately white students in adjacent suburban school districts (Collins & Williams, 2001). The student body of schools in high-poverty areas is 43 % Black and Hispanic, but only 4 % white (Acevedo-Garcia et al., 2007), whereas white children primarily attend schools where 80 % of the student body is white (Chungmei, Frankenberg, & Orfield, 2003). Affluent communities offer greater access to support systems for parents and young people, and these resources reduce the risk of truancy (Teasley, 2004).

School systems subject their students of color to harsher discipline than their white counterparts for the same infractions, which affects school achievement and graduation rates for students of color (Office of Civil Rights, 2012). Only 17 % of students in US public schools are Black, yet Black students represented more than one-third of all students suspended and expelled in 2006 (Children's Defense Fund, 2012). Dropping out of school is twice as

(continued)

likely to occur among Black, Latino, and American Indian children as white children (Children's Defense Fund, 2007). The average high school graduation rate in the nation's 50 largest cities is 53 %, compared with 71 % in the suburbs (Swanson, 2008).

Weapons
Access to firearms and other weapons greatly increases the risk of violence (Prothrow-Stith & Spivak, 2004) and the availability of guns and ammunition greatly increases the likelihood of severe injury and death (Clark, Ruback, & Shaffer, 2011; The Graduate Institute, 2009). There are 270 to 310 million guns in the United States (Desilver, 2013) and two-thirds of all murders in the United States are gun related (Wilkinson & Pickett, 2009). Homicide rates due to firearms are higher in cities (Clark et al., 2011) and residents of large cities are more likely to carry a weapon on their person than residents of suburbs, small cities, or rural areas (Klec & Gertz, 1998). As a result of community conditions, most gun violence associated with young people is concentrated in urban neighborhoods.

Incarceration and Re-entry
The persistent removal of people from communities and into prisons diminishes community members' economic, social, and political standing, and contributes to an increase in recidivism and future criminality. Mass imprisonment damages social networks, distorts social norms, destroys social citizenship, and increases child poverty (King, Mauer, & Young, 2005).

People of color are more likely to serve time and serve more time than whites charged with similar offenses. African-Americans are imprisoned at nearly six times the rate of whites, and Latinos at nearly double the rates of whites (Policy Link). Even though illicit drug use is about the same for African Americans and whites, for example, African Americans are sentenced to prison for drug offenses at a rate of 34 times that of whites, and time served in federal prison for drug offenses committed by African Americans is almost as long (58.7 months) as time served for violent offenses committed by whites (61.7 months) (Beyers et al., 2008). More than 1.7 million children in the United States have a parent in prison. Having an incarcerated parent is an "Adverse Childhood Experience" that puts young people at risk for poorer health outcomes (Anda et al., 1998).

For white children, the estimated risk that their mother or father will be imprisoned by the time they turn 14-years-old is one in 25. For Black children, the risk is one in four (Wildeman, 2009). At large, African-American children are nine times more likely than white children to have a parent in prison, and a Latino child is three times more likely than a white peer to have a parent in prison (Davis, Kilburn, & Schultz, 2009).

Urban neighborhoods that are under-resourced have higher concentrations of formerly incarcerated people or those on probation or parole (Lynch & Sabol, 2001). Prisoners are more likely to come out of poor communities (and

(continued)

to return to them). This means that communities with the least capacity to absorb former prisoners are home to the largest share of them. This also means that economic, social and political problems that result from incarceration tend to fall on communities that have the fewest resources and opportunities (National Research Council of the National Academies, 2014). A lack of neighborhood resources makes successful re-entry less likely, which increases the likelihood of further violence (Re-Entry Policy Council, 2003).

Air of Inevitability
Even when individual news stories are accurate, the cumulative picture presented by the media as a whole is distorted, conflating youth, race, crime, and violence. Positive stories about young people are rare, and the public harbors a skewed view of who commits crime and who suffers from violence (Dorfman & Wallack, 2009). The news is more likely to cover a story if the victim is white than if a victim is Black, and people of color tend to be overrepresented as perpetrators of violence in stories (Dorfman & Schiraldi, 2001). This contributes to a view of violence as inevitable rather than preventable.

According to Lori Dorfman and Larry Wallack, who study the impact of media coverage of violence, "The result is a misinformed public motivated by fear to be more accepting of punishment-oriented public policies that are often discriminatory." The public overlooks the larger social and economic forces that shape violence, and are thus less likely to support policies that effectively prevent violence.

12.5.3   Key 3: Preventing Violence Requires an Integrated Strategy for Action

The multifaceted efforts described in Key 1 and the focus on risk and resiliency in Key 2 provide the framework for a vision for keeping our children safe. It is essential to put this vision into action and develop and implement effective initiatives to prevent violence. While traditional views of and responses to violence have relied on individual programs and services, it is time to reflect the complexity of violence by incorporating a perspective that moves toward an integrated, community-centered approach to prevention.

Large US cities have increasingly incorporated a multifaceted approach to improving community environment in order to prevent violence. Since 2005, UNITY (Urban Networks to Increase Thriving Youth Through Violence Prevention), a national initiative initially funded by the CDC, has built support for effective, sustainable efforts in cities to prevent violence before it occurs, so urban youth can thrive in safe environments with ample opportunities and supportive relationships. As violence rates have generally dropped in cities across the United States, the 8-year UNITY evaluation demonstrated that cities are relying more on comprehensive prevention strategies to address the issue of violence, including increased public health involvement in efforts to address violence affecting youth; improved collaboration and engagement across sectors and with communities most impacted by violence; enhanced city-wide strategic planning to address violence; and more attention to preventing violence before it occurs, i.e., not relying solely on intervention, suppression, or enforcement (Prevention Institute, 2010).

12.5.3.1 The UNITY Roadmap

In 2006, UNITY conducted the *Assessment of Youth Violence Prevention Activities in US Cities* (Weiss, 2008). Researchers conducted interviews with mayors, police chiefs, school superintendents, and public health directors in one-third of the largest US cities. The assessment revealed that violence was a major concern; law enforcement and criminal justice were the most prevalent strategy used to address it; responses were not perceived to be highly effective or adequate; most cities lacked a comprehensive strategy; few cities reported using primary prevention to stop violence before it occurs; and informants lacked a shared knowledge of existing youth violence prevention resources available in their cities. The cities with the greatest coordinated approach also had the lowest rates of youth violence.

In response to these findings, UNITY developed The *UNITY RoadMap: A Framework for Effectiveness and Sustainability* (Prevention Institute, 2008). It was developed by UNITY staff in partnership with city representatives and advisors from across the United States as a framework for understanding the key elements needed to prevent violence before it occurs and to sustain these efforts in cities. The *UNITY RoadMap,* (1) helps cities understand the current status of their efforts (starting point); (2) describes the core elements necessary to prevent violence before it occurs (milestones); and (3) provides information, resources, and examples to support cities in planning, implementation, and evaluation. As a framework, the *UNITY RoadMap* is most effective when tailored to the needs of a particular city.

UNITY RoadMap
Who? Partnerships

1. *High-level leadership*: Mayors, agency and department heads, police chiefs, and public health directors, superintendents, and other local leaders insist that the violence stops, lead policy change, provide necessary supports and resources to ensure efficacy and long-term sustainability, and engage broader support by eliciting multiple partnerships between the public and private sector, and hold people accountable.
2. *Collaboration and staffing*: A formal structure is in place for multidisciplinary collaboration to coordinate priorities and actions across multiple jurisdictions and there is dedicated staffing in place to support collaboration and implement priorities.
3. *Community engagement*: Members of the community—youth and adults, community-based organizations, the faith community, the business sector,

and survivors—are actively engaged in setting priorities and planning ongoing activities.

What? Prevention

4. *Programs, organizational practices, and policies*: There are effective and far-reaching efforts in place to prevent violence, particularly in highly impacted neighborhoods.
5. *Training and capacity building*: Participants, practitioners, and policy makers have the skills and capacities necessary to work across multiple disciplines and in partnership with community to implement effective prevention programs, policies, and practices.
6. *Communication*: The case has been made for preventing violence before it occurs to foster buy-in for prevention strategies and priorities and people are aware of what's being done effectively to prevent it.

How? Strategy

7. *Strategic plan*: There is a plan in place that prioritizes prevention, is well-known, and informs priorities and actions for multiple departments, agencies, jurisdictions, and community groups.
8. *Data and evaluation*: Efforts are informed by data and continuously improved through ongoing evaluation.
9. *Funding*: Adequate resources support collaboration and staffing; community engagement; the implementation of programs, policies, and practices; skills development and capacity building; communications; strategic planning; and data and evaluation.

12.5.3.2 Interdisciplinary Collaboration: Convening Community Partners

"Violence is not the problem of one neighborhood or group and the response and solution are not the responsibility of one agency or one sector," said Deborah Prothrow-Stith, co-chair of UNITY.

Research, practitioners' experience, and community wisdom all confirm that efforts to prevent violence will be more effective when multiple private, public, and community players come together in a strategic and coordinated way. No one sector can prevent violence on its own and almost every department in city government can contribute to safety, including social services, public health, parks and recreation, housing, schools (including school boards and superintendents), law enforcement and probation, public works, transportation, workforce development, and others. Private sectors such as business, healthcare, the faith community, and news media can also contribute in important ways. Sectors, agencies, and departments that align their strategies and approaches are better equipped to achieve goals in common. When practitioners understand the solutions to violence and how their activities align with those of other sectors, they can more readily carry out their work in ways that also reduce community violence. UNITY's *Assessment of Youth Violence Prevention Activities in US Cities* (Weiss, 2008) revealed that cities with the greatest coordination and communication across sectors also had the lowest rates of youth violence. Multi-sector collaboration is essential for preventing youth violence. It can dramatically reduce violence by multiplying the effectiveness of individual efforts, (Weiss, 2008). Both by aggregating the activities and investments of diverse sectors in one coherent approach, and by leveraging the efforts of different sectors so that they build on one another to achieve broader outcomes than could be accomplished by any single sector alone. Assessing and prioritizing key risk and resilience factors can inform which partners should be engaged further in planning and implementation.

Benefits of Multi-Sector Collaboration:

- *Capacity to define a problem and shape a solution*: Achieves collective outcomes; leverages diverse expertise; cultivates innovation and creativity; fosters a unified approach with shared buy-in
- *Enhanced resources to achieve success*: Leverages investments; supports access to resources and fosters resource-sharing; allows for more flexible use of existing resources and decreases duplication of efforts
- *Credibility and advocacy*: Strengthens authority and influence; maximizes advocacy power
- *Staying power*: Promotes broader reach and impact; supports sustainability

Securing *community* involvement is critical, including community-based organizations and youth development organizations; families, such as caregivers, family members, and parents; and individuals, including community members, former gang members, formerly incarcerated individuals, and survivors of violence and youth. Engaging community members as leaders and encouraging collaboration among community partners early in planning builds a common understanding and language; helps identify key local priorities, needs, and assets; forges a shared vision; and enhances buy-in for selected strategies.

Developing a truly collaborative way of addressing the problem of violence requires authentic engagement of community leadership, sharing decision-making power with community members, and creating a role for residents in the development of city and county strategies that address violence as well as ordinances related to parks, school reform, social services, employment, and economic development. It is critical that any approach to preventing violence provides the mechanisms and resources for community members to play a consistent, positive, and significant role in shaping the solutions, leading initiatives, and working to change policies that lead to violence. Community engagement and leadership increases the effectiveness and sustainability of the initiatives and helps to ensure that strategies continue to be funded despite changes in agency leadership or political administration.

The principles below, adapted (Cohen, 2012) from "Life and Death from Unnatural Causes in Alameda County" (Beyers et al., 2008), served as a foundation for bringing together diverse agencies and community members concerned with preventing violence:

- Our overall approach should shift toward changing community conditions and away from blaming individuals or groups for their disadvantaged status.
- Acknowledging the cumulative impact of stressful experiences and of multiple risk factors in the environment is crucial, especially since these sources of chronic stress and risk factors tend to occur in areas of concentrated poverty. For some families, poverty lasts a lifetime and is perpetuated to next generations, leaving its family members with few opportunities to make healthful decisions.
- Meaningful public participation is needed with attention to outreach, follow-through, language, inclusion, and cultural understanding. Government and private funding agencies should actively support efforts to build resident capacity to be engaged.
- Preventing violence is an opportunity to invest in community. The social fabric of neighborhoods needs to be strengthened. Residents need to be connected and supported and feel that they hold power to improve the safety and well-being of their families. All residents need to have a sense of belonging, dignity and hope.
- The developmental needs and transitions of all age groups should be addressed.
- Working across multiple sectors of government and society is key to making the structural changes necessary. Such work should be in partnership with community advocacy groups that continue to pursue a more equitable society.
- Groups that are the most impacted by violence must have a voice in identifying policies that will make a difference and must be empowered to hold government accountable for implementing these policies.
- Setting a Policy Agenda: Faced with fragmented and inadequate funding streams, a lack of coordination across supporting agencies, and hit hard by the nation's economic downturn, local efforts, more than ever, need federal support to achieve and sustain their efforts. Through UNITY (Urban Networks to Increase Thriving Youth), the UNITY City Network, including representatives from the largest US cities, identified and prioritized strategies that, if adopted at the federal level, will enhance the ability of local leaders to prevent violence and thereby prevent childhood exposure to violence. The UNITY Urban Agenda for Preventing Violence was endorsed by 13 US cities and serves as a guiding document for national and local systems change (Prevention Institute and the UNITY City Network, 2010).

12.6 Preventing Violence: Four Models in Practice

Diverse communities have come together and mobilized their resources to prevent childhood and youth exposure to violence.

12.6.1 Minneapolis

Minneapolis serves as an example of a successfully implemented, coordinated, multi-sector approach to preventing violence that affects youth. As Mayor *R.T. Rybak* of Minneapolis said, "The public health approach means backing up from the emergency room where you bandage the wound and starting at the beginning, understanding why that person is there in the ER at all" (Rybak, 2014).

The city's strategic plan, *Minneapolis Blueprint for Action to Prevent Youth Violence*, included specific goals: Foster violence-free social environments; Promote positive opportunities and connections to trusted adults for all youth; Intervene with youth and families at the first sign of risk; Restore youth who have gone down the wrong path; Protect children and youth from violence in the community; facilitate everyone to unlearn the culture of violence (Rybak, 2014).

Within 2 years of developing the strategic plan in 2006, Minneapolis saw a 43 % drop in juvenile crime in its most violent neighborhoods (Minneapolis Police Department, 2008). Following this success, in 2009 the city expanded from a focus on five neighborhoods to the 22 neighborhoods most impacted by violence. From 2006 to 2012, violent crime among youth decreased 57 %, incidents with guns among youth decreased 67 %, youth gunshot victims decreased 39 %, youth homicides decreased 60 %, and youth gun-related assault injuries decreased 62 % (City of Minneapolis, 2013).

12.6.2 Cure Violence

The CeaseFire Chicago model, created by the Cure Violence initiative, implements trained violence interrupters and outreach workers and community mobilization to connect with at-risk children and youth to prevent violence and shootings by identifying and mediating potentially lethal conflicts, making referrals to social services, following up to ensure that the conflict does not reignite, and changing beliefs about the acceptability and inevitability of violence. The model has been replicated 16 times and has been validated by a three-year US Department of Justice study conducted by four universities, showing 41–73 % drops in shootings and killings, and 100 % drops in retaliation murders (Bump, Dubois, Hartnett, & Skogan, 2008). The first year of impact regularly shows 25–45 % drops in shootings and killings. Additionally, businesses have returned to neighborhoods following the reduction in violence (Bump et al., 2008). The US Office of Juvenile Justice and Delinquency Prevention and the National Forum on Youth Violence Prevention have identified Cure Violence as promising for significantly reducing youth violence.

12.6.3   Boston

Boston, Massachusetts, which has seen dramatic and sustained decline in youth violence, also serves as a model of multilevel programmatic activity with exemplary integration between public health and policing strategies (Prothrow-Stith & Spivak, 2004). The Boston Public Health Commission's Violence Intervention and Prevention Initiative (VIP) is a community-organizing approach to violence prevention that focuses on building coalitions and engaging residents to address the issue of community gun violence and to change norms and expectations around the issue. The program is public led, organized by residents who bring in other community members to develop strategies that build community resilience, such as reclaiming public spaces, enhancing social connections, and promoting positive activity. Two decades of activities within public health and criminal justice, and most importantly within the broader community of parents, teens, and survivors of violence, resulted in the creation of an extensive set of programs for youth throughout the city. The Boston Public Health Commission also employs neighborhood residents to organize, lead, and implement community-based solutions that prevent violence (Boston Public Health Commission, 2010). Boston's efforts reflect the range needed both to reduce the extent of violent behavior and to respond to the violence that does occur. It is not only an example for elected officials and community activists; it is also a model for professionals within public health and criminal justice.

12.6.4   Colorado

Colorado's Department of Public Health and Environment developed a Violence Prevention Advisory group to complete a statewide analysis of violence impacting children and adolescents and build a violence prevention strategic plan for the state. The plan promotes integrated policies and programs that impact multiple forms of violence by addressing shared risk and resilience factors. Through collaborative partnerships, universal and selected prevention strategies, and research-based approaches, the plan presents steps to most effectively reduce the rates of child and adolescent violence throughout Colorado (Colorado Department of Public Health and Environment, 2014).

Peer Solutions' Stand and Serve program targets the underlying conditions that foster violence through youth-led trainings, community and coalition meetings, school-based activities, and service projects. This peer leadership initiative promotes positive norms that reduce the likelihood that violence will occur and disrupts systems of oppression in which such norms are often rooted (Peer Solutions).

Included in this set of initiatives are efforts to advance changes in the built environment—the ways communities are designed—that can have a significant effect on making communities look and feel safer. The *built environment* refers to everything that we design and construct—including homes, schools, offices, places of worship, theaters, parks, and restaurants, as well as the streets and open spaces that connect these places. Just as the quality of air and water impacts our health and safety, so do our decisions about community design, which can significantly increase or decrease the likelihood of violence or injury.

12.7 Conclusion: We Know What To Do

The most effective and sustainable strategies for preventing violence are community- or population-based, addressing the complex interplay of social, behavioral, and environmental contributors to violence. Preventing violence, particularly in communities that have been inequitably exposed to these factors requires addressing the multiple risk factors associated with violence; building resilience in individuals, families, and communities; and implementing approaches that are distinct, though complementary at times, from violence containment or suppression. Efforts must shift policies and realign institutions to be more inclusive and receptive to responding to community needs. Preventing violence contributes to empowerment and educational and economic progress while fostering healthy communities in which people can live with dignity and safety.

There is growing attention to preventing violence nationally and internationally. As Nelson Mandela said in the World Health Organization's World Report on Violence and Health:

> The twentieth century will be remembered as a century marked by violence. It burdens us with the legacy of mass destruction... Less visible, but even more widespread, is the legacy of day-to-day, individual suffering. It is the pain of children who are abused by people who should protect them, women injured or humiliated by violent partners, elderly persons maltreated by their caregivers, youths who are bullied by other youths, and people of all ages who inflict violence on themselves. This suffering—and there are many more examples that I could give—is a legacy that reproduces itself, as new generations learn from the violence of generations past, as victims learn from victimizers, and as the social conditions that nurture violence are allowed to continue. No country, no city, no community is immune. But neither are we powerless against it ... Many who live with violence day in and day out assume that it is an intrinsic part of the human condition. But this is not so. Violence can be prevented. Violent cultures can be turned around. We owe our children—the most vulnerable citizens in any society—a life free from violence and fear. In order to ensure this, we must be tireless in our efforts not only to attain peace, justice and prosperity for countries, but also for communities and members of the same family. We must address the roots of violence (Dahlberg, Krug, Lozano, Mercy, & Zwi, 2002).

Violence is preventable if it is approached with commitment and sustained attention. Any one group, organization or field cannot prevent violence in isolation. It requires coordinated and comprehensive efforts and resources, and the active cooperation of sectors and fields that might not typically work together. There is far more to learn but we know what to do to save lives, improve community conditions and reduce trauma and fear right now. It is past time to seize the opportunity to work together collaboratively, building on what we know works to prevent violence. The current generation's learnings about prevention of violence lead to a critical opportunity for the next generation of leaders. Take what we know and put it to use. Build further political will so successful efforts become common practice. Build enhanced understanding, ties and shared strategy between advocates of different types of violence. The upcoming generation—the readers of this book—can make our neighborhoods, our country, and the world safer.

References

Aboelata, M. (2004, July). *The built environment and health: 11 profiles of neighborhood transformation.* Retrieved from http://www.preventioninstitute.org/index.php?option=com_jlibrary&view=article&id=114&Itemid=127

Acevedo-Garcia, D., Krimgold, B. K., Lefkowitz, B., McArdle, N., & Osypuk, T. L. (2007, January). *Children left behind: How metropolitan areas are failing America's children.* Retrieved from http://diversitydata-archive.org/Downloads/children_left_behind_final_report.pdf

Alameda County Public Health Department. (2008). *Life and death from unnatural causes: Health and social inequity in Alameda County.* Retrieved from http://www.acphd.org/media/53628/unnatcs2008.pdf

Albee, G. W. (1983). Psychopathology, prevention, and the just society. *Journal of Primary Prevention, 4*, 5–40.

Allard, P., & Greene, P. (2011). *Children on the outside: Voicing the pain and human costs of parental incarceration* (pp. 1–54). Brooklyn, NY: Justice Strategies.

Anda, R. F., Chapman, D. F., Dong, M., Dube, S. R., Edwards, V. J., & Felitti, V. J. (2005). The wide-ranging health consequences of adverse childhood experiences. In K. Kendall-Tackett & S. Giacomoni (Eds.), *Victimization of children and youth: Patterns of abuse, response strategies.* Kingston, NJ: Civic Research Institute.

Anda, R. F., Edwards, V., Felitti, V. J., Koss, M. P., Marks, J. S., Nordenberg, D.,...& Williamson, D. F. (1998). Relationship of childhood abuse and household dysfunction to many of the leading causes of death in adults. The Adverse Childhood Experiences (ACE) Study. *American Journal of Prevention Medicine, 14*(4), 245–258.

Anderson, P., Angus, K., de Bruijn, A., Gordon, R., & Hastings, G. (2009). Impact of alcohol advertising and media exposure on adolescent alcohol use: A systematic review of longitudinal studies. *Alcohol and Alcoholism, 44*(3), 229–243.

Arnett, D., Chambless, L., Diez Roux, A. V., Massing, M., Merkin, S. S., Nieto, J.,... & Watson, R. L. (2001). Neighborhood of residence and incidence of coronary heart disease. *New England Journal of Medicine, 345*(2), 99–106.

Arredondo, S., Aultman-Bettridge, T., Johnson, T. P., Williams, K. R., Ninneman, L., & Torp, K. (1999). *Preventing youth handgun violence: A national study with trends and patterns for the State of Colorado (CSPV-014).* Boulder, CO: Center for the Study and Prevention of Violence, Institute of Behavioral Science, University of Colorado.

Beyers, M., Brown, J., Cho, S., Desautels, A., Gaska, K., Horsley, K., ... Witt, S. (2008). *Life and death from unnatural causes: Health and social inequity in Alameda County.* Retrieved from http://www.acphd.org/media/53628/unnatcs2008.pdf

Beyers, J. M., Hipwell, A., Loeber, R., Pardini, D., & Wei, E. (2005). Block observations of neighbourhood physical disorder are associated with neighbourhood crime, firearm injuries and deaths, and teen births. *Journal of Epidemiology and Community Health, 59*(10), 904–908.

Boston Public Health Commission. (2010). *Violence intervention and prevention initiative (VIP) executive summary.* Boston: Division of Violence Prevention, Boston Public Health Commission.

Braveman, P., Egerter, S., & Williams, D. (2011, April). *Race, socioeconomic factors and health.* Retrieved from http://www.rwjf.org/en/research-publications/find-rwjf-research/2011/04/race-and-socioeconomic-factors-affect-opportunities-for-better-h.html

Brewer, J. D., Catalano, R. F., Cothern, L., Farrington, D. P., Hawkins, D., Harachi, T. W., & Herrenkohl, T. I. (2000, April). *Predictors of youth violence*. Retrieved from https://www.ncjrs. gov/pdffiles1/ojjdp/179065.pdf

Bump, N., Dubois, J., Hartnett, S., & Skogan, W. (2008). *Executive summary: Evaluation of cease fire-Chicago*. Chicago, IL: Northwestern University.

Byrne, J., Pattavina, A., & Taxman, F. (2005). Racial disparity and the legitimacy of the criminal justice system: Exploring consequences for deterrence. *Journal of Health Care for the Poor and Underserved, 16*(4b), 57–77.

California Department of Education. (2013). *Current expense of education & per-pupil spending*. Retrieved from http://www.cde.ca.gov/ds/fd/ec/currentexpense.asp

Campaign for Youth Justice. (2011). *Legislative victories from 2005 to 2010 removing youth from the adult criminal justice system*. Retrieved from http://www.campaignforyouthjustice.org/documents/CFYJ_State_Trends_Report.pdf

Center for the Study and Prevention of Violence. *Facts*. Retrieved from http://www.colorado.edu/cspv/

Centers for Disease Control. (2012a). *Youth violence: Facts at a glance*. Retrieved from http://www.cdc.gov/violenceprevention/pdf/yv-datasheet-a.pdf

Centers for Disease Control. (2012b, April 19). *Protect the ones you love: Child injuries are preventable*. Retrieved from http://www.cdc.gov/safechild/NAP/background.html

Cespedes, Y. M., & Stanley, J. H. (2008). Depression in Latino adolescents: A cultural discrepancy perspective. *Cultural Diversity & Ethnic Minority Psychology, 14*(2), 168–172.

Children's Defense Fund. (2007). *America's cradle to prison pipeline*. Retrieved from http://www.childrensdefense.org/child-research-data-publications/data/cradle-prison-pipeline-report-2007-full-highres.html

Children's Defense Fund. (2012). *Portrait of inequality 2012—Black children in America*. Retrieved from http://www.childrensdefense.org/child-research-data-publications/data/portrait-of-inequality-2011.html

Chung, H. L., Mulvey, E. P., & Steinberg, L. (2011). Understanding the school outcomes of juvenile offenders: An exploration of neighborhood influences and motivational resources. *Journal of Youth and Adolescence, 40*(8), 1025–1038.

Chungmei, L., Frankenberg, E., & Orfield, G. (2003). *A multiracial society with segregated schools: Are we losing the dream?* Retrieved from http://civilrightsproject.ucla.edu/research/k-12-education/integration-and-diversity/a-multiracial-society-with-segregated-schools-are-we-losing-the-dream/frankenberg-multiracial-society-losing-the-dream.pdf

City of Minneapolis. (2013, August). *Minneapolis blueprint for action to prevent violence*. Retrieved from http://www.minneapolismn.gov/www/groups/public/@health/documents/web-content/wcms1p-114466.pdf

Clark, V., Ruback, B., & Shaffer, J. (2011). Easy access to firearms: Juveniles' risks for violent offending and violent victimization. *Journal of Interpersonal Violence, 26*(10), 2111–2138.

Cohen, J., McCabe, L., Michelli, N.M & Pickeral, T. (2009). School Climate: Research, Policy, Teacher Education and Practice. Teachers College Record, 111(1), 180–213. Retrieved from http://www.ijvs.org/files/Publications/School-Climate.pdf

Cohen, L. (2012). *Larry Cohen's written testimony for the task force for defending childhood*. Retrieved from http://www.preventioninstitute.org/about-us/lp/856-lc-testimony.html

Cohen, L., Davis, R., Lee, V., & Valdovinos, E. (2010, May). *Addressing the intersection: Preventing violence and promoting healthy eating and active living*. Retrieved from http://www.preventioninstitute.org/component/jlibrary/article/id-267/127.html

Cohen, L., & Erlenborn, J. (2001, June). *Cultivating peace in Salinas: A framework for violence prevention*. Retrieved from http://www.preventioninstitute.org/index.php?option=com_jlibrary&view=article&id=51&Itemid=127

Cohen, L., & Swift, S. (1991). *Beyond brochures: Preventing alcohol-related violence and injuries*. Retrieved from http://thrive.preventioninstitute.org/alcohol.html

Collins, C., & Williams, D. (2001). Racial residential segregation: A fundamental cause of racial disparities in health. *Public Health Reports, 116*(5), 404–416.

Colorado Department of Public Health and Environment. (2014). *Bold steps toward child and adolescent health: A plan for youth violence prevention in Colorado peer solutions. About peer solutions* Retrieved from http://www.peersolutions.org/about-us/; http://www.ccasa.org/wp-content/uploads/2014/10/Bold-Steps.pdf

Corral, I., & Landrine, H. (2009). Separate and unequal: Residential segregation and black health disparities. *Ethnicity and Disease, 19*(2), 179–184.

Dahlberg, L. (1998). Youth violence in the United States. Major trends, risk factors, and prevention approaches. *American Journal of Preventative Medicine, 14*(4), 259–272.

Dahlberg, L. L., Krug, E. G., Lozano, R., Mercy, J. A., & Zwi, A. B. (2002). *World report on violence and health. World Health Organization.* Retrieved from http://www.who.int/violence_injury_prevention/violence/world_report/en/introduction.pdf

Davis, L., Kilburn, R., & Schultz, D. (2009). *Reparable harm: Assessing and addressing disparities faced by boys and men of color in California.* Retrieved from http://www.rand.org/content/dam/rand/pubs/monographs/2009/RAND_MG745.pdf

Desilver, D. (2013, June 4). *A minority of Americans own guns, but just how many is unclear.* Retrieved from http://www.pewresearch.org/fact-tank/2013/06/04/a-minority-of-americans-own-guns-but-just-how-many-is-unclear/

Dorfman, L., & Schiraldi, V. (2001). *Off balance: Youth, race & crime in the news. Building blocks for youth.* Retrieved from http://www.cclp.org/documents/BBY/offbalance.pdf

Dorfman, L., & Wallack, L. (2009). *Moving from them to us: Challenges in reframing violence among youth.* Retrieved from http://www.bmsg.org/pdfs/BMSGReframingViolenceRev.pdf

Earls, F., Raudenbush, S. W., & Sampson, R. J. (1997). Neighborhoods and violent crime: A multilevel study of collective efficacy. *Science, 277*(5328), 918–924.

Fisher, B. S., Krebs, C. P., Lindquist, C. H., Martin, S. L., & Warner, T. D. (2009). College women's experiences with physically forced, alcohol- or other drug-enabled, and drug-facilitated sexual assault before and since entering college. *Journal of American College Health, 57*(6), 639–647.

Geronimus, A. (2000). To mitigate, resist, or undo: Addressing structural influences on the health of urban populations. *American Journal of Public Health, 90*(6), 867–872.

Goode, E. (2011, December 19). Many in U.S. are arrested by age 23, study finds. *The New York Times*, p. A16.

Higgins, D. L., & Krieger, J. (2002). Housing and health: Time again for public health action. *American Journal of Public Health, 92*(5), 758–768.

Justice Policy Institute. (2009). *The costs of confinement: Why good juvenile justice policies make good fiscal sense.*

King, R. S., Mauer, M., & Young, M. C. (2005). *Incarceration and crime: A complex relationship.* Retrieved from http://www.sentencingproject.org/doc/publications/inc_iandc_complex.pdf

Klec, G., & Gertz, M. (1998). Carrying guns for protection: Results from the National Self-Defense survey. *Journal of Research in Crime and Delinquency, 35*(2), 193–224.

Kubrin, C. E., & Squires, G. D. (2005). Privileged places: Race, uneven development and the geography of opportunity in urban America. *Urban Studies, 42*(1), 47–68.

LaVeist, T. A., & Wallace, J. M., Jr. (2000). Health risk and inequitable distribution of liquor stores in African American neighborhoods. *Social Science & Medicine, 51*(4), 613–617.

Legislative Analyst's Office. (2012, February 15). *The 2012–13 budget: Completing juvenile justice realignment.* Retrieved from http://www.lao.ca.gov/analysis/2012/crim_justice/juvenile-justice-021512.aspx

Lynch, J. P., & Sabol, W. J. (2001). Prisoner reentry in perspective. *The Urban Institute.* Retrieved from http://www.urbaninstitute.org/UploadedPDF/410213_reentry.PDF

Maguin, E., & Loeber, R. (1996). Academic performance and delinquency. *Crime and Justice, 20*, 145–264.

Minneapolis Police Department. (2008). *2008 Fourth precinct juvenile crime suspect & arrest statistics.*

Morgan, R. E., & Truman, J. L. (2014, April 16). *Nonfatal domestic violence 2003–2012.* Retrieved from http://www.bjs.gov/index.cfm?ty=pbdetail&iid=4985

Nation, M., & Wandersman, A. (1998). Urban neighborhoods and mental health: Psychological contributions to understanding toxicity, resilience, and interventions. *American Psychologist, 53*(6), 647–656.

National Research Council of the National Academies. (2014). *The growth of incarceration in the United States: Exploring causes and consequences.* Retrieved from http://www.nap.edu/openbook.php?record_id=18613&page=R1

Office of Civil Rights. (2012). *Civil rights data collection.* Retrieved from http://ocrdata.ed.gov/

Peer Solutions. *About Peer Solutions.* Retrieved from http://www.peersolutions.org/about-us/

Pinderhughes, H., & Davis, R. (2013, November). *Addressing and preventing trauma and the community level.* Retrieved from http://www.preventioninstitute.org/component/jlibrary/article/id-347/127.html

Policy Link. (n.d.). *Why place and race matter: Impacting health through a focus of place and race.* Retrieved from http://www.policylink.org/sites/default/files/WHY_PLACE_AND_RACE%20MATTER_FULL%20REPORT_WEB.PDF

Prevention Institute. (1999). *The Spectrum of Prevention: Developing a comprehensive approach to injury prevention.* Retrieved from http://preventioninstitute.org/component/jlibrary/article/id-105/127.html

Prevention Institute. (2001, September). *Preventing and reducing school violence fact sheets: What factors foster resiliency against violence?* Retrieved from http://www.preventioninstitute.org/component/jlibrary/article/id-50/288.html

Prevention Institute. (2005, July). *A lifetime commitment to violence prevention: The Alameda County blueprint.* Retrieved from http://www.preventioninstitute.org/component/jlibrary/article/id-38/127.html

Prevention Institute. (2008, November). *UNITY roadmap: A framework for effectiveness and sustainability.* Retrieved from http://www.preventioninstitute.org/index.php?option=com_jlibrary&view=article&id=30&Itemid=127

Prevention Institute. (2010). *A public health approach to preventing violence. Prevention is primary: Strategies for community well-being.* San Francisco: Jossey-Bass, 2, 323–350.

Prevention Institute. (2011a). *Fact Sheets: Links between violence and chronic diseases, mental illness and poor learning.* Retrieved from http://www.preventioninstitute.org/component/jlibrary/article/id-301/127.html

Prevention Institute. (2011b). *Links between violence and health equity.* Retrieved from http://www.preventioninstitute.org/component/jlibrary/article/id-311/127.html

Prevention Institute and the UNITY City Network. (2010). *Unity policy platform.* Retrieved from http://www.preventioninstitute.org/component/jlibrary/article/id-290/127.html

Prothrow-Stith, D., & Spivak, H. (2004). *Murder is no accident: Understanding and preventing youth violence in America.* San Francisco: Jossey-Bass.

Redburn, S., Travis, J., & Western, B. (2014). *The growth of incarceration in the United States: Exploring causes and consequences.* Washington, DC: The National Academies Press.

Re-Entry Policy Council. (2003). *Report of the re-entry council: Charting the safe and successful return of prisoners to the community.* Retrieved from http://reentrypolicy.org/jc_publications/rpc_report_full/RPC_Report_Full.pdf

Robert Wood Johnson Foundation. (2009). *Education matters for health. Exploring the social determinants of health: Education and health.* Retrieved from http://www.rwjf.org/files/research/commission2009eduhealth.pdf

Rybak, R. T. (2014). *City voices and perspectives.* Retrieved from http://www.minneapolismn.gov/www/groups/public/@health/documents/webcontent/wcms1p-088219.pdf

Simmons, J. (2009). Personal communication, June 6, 2009.

Smedley, B. D., & Syme, S. L. (2000). *Promoting health: Intervention strategies from social and behavioral research.* Washington, DC: National Academy Press.

Swanson, C. (2008). *Cities in crisis: A special analytic report on high school graduation.* Retrieved from http://www.edweek.org/media/citiesincrisis040108.pdf

Teasley, M. (2004). Absenteeism and truancy: Risk, protection, and best practice implications for school social workers. *Children & Schools, 26*(2), 117.

The Annie E. Casey Foundation. (2012). *Data snapshot on high-poverty communities.* Retrieved from http://www.aecf.org/resources/data-snapshot-on-high-poverty-communities/

The Graduate Institute. (2009). *Small arms survey 2009: Shadows of war.* Retrieved from http://www.smallarmssurvey.org/fileadmin/docs/A-Yearbook/2009/en/Small-Arms-Survey-2009-Prelims-Intro-EN.pdf

U.S. Department of Health and Human Services. (2012, August). *Ending the tobacco epidemic: Progress towards a healthier nation.* Retrieved from http://www.hhs.gov/ash/initiatives/tobacco/tobaccoprogress2012.pdf

United Nations Office for Drug Control and Crime Prevention. (2002). *Lessons learned in drug abuse prevention: A global review.* Retrieved from http://www.mentorfoundation.org/uploads/Lessons_Learned_in_Drug_Prevention.pdf

Weiss, B. (2008). *An assessment of youth violence prevention activities in U.S.A. cities.* Retrieved from http://www.preventioninstitute.org/component/jlibrary/article/id-137/127.html

Wildeman, C. (2009). Parental imprisonment, the prison boom, and the concentration of childhood disadvantage. *Demography, 46*(2), 265–280.

Wilkinson, R., & Pickett, K. (2009). *The spirit level: Why greater equality makes societies stronger.* New York: Bloomsbury Press.

Chapter 13
Pediatric and Adolescent Obesity

Stephenie Wallace and Bonnie A. Spear

13.1 Introduction

The campaign against obesity has been the latest battle in health promotion in pediatrics. In the last several generations, the number of US children with obesity has increased epidemically. Excess weight is correlated with a host of medical conditions—diabetes, heart disease, and cancer—particularly when obesity starts in childhood (Reilly et al., 2003). Fortunately, reduction of excess weight can lower the risk of these diseases, thus helping children and their families make the necessary changes is crucial for those working in child health.

13.1.1 Epidemiology

The number of overweight or obese infants and young children (aged 0–5 years) increased globally from 31 million in 1990 to 44 million in 2012, with the highest prevalence is in middle and high income countries such as the USA, but rapidly rising in low income countries (WHO, 2015). In the USA, 32 % of children 2–19 years old were considered to be overweight or obese (Ogden, Carroll, Kit, & Flegal, 2014), and of this group, 17 % of youth were considered obese, or at highest risk for health concerns due to weight. While the prevalence of youth obesity has been stable for the USA since 2003, health disparities continue, with Hispanic and African American children in the USA disproportionately affected.

S. Wallace, M.D., M.S.P.H. (✉) • B.A. Spear, Ph.D., R.D.N.
Department of Pediatrics, University of Alabama School of Medicine,
1600 5th Ave South, CPP1 310, Birmingham, AL 35216, USA
e-mail: swallace@peds.uab.edu; bspear@peds.uab.edu

© Springer Science+Business Media New York 2016
M.R. Korin (ed.), *Health Promotion for Children and Adolescents*,
DOI 10.1007/978-1-4899-7711-3_13

Table 13.1 BMI categories in children

BMI percentiles	Category
<5th percentile	Underweight
5th–84th percentile	Healthy weight
85th–94th percentile	Overweight
>95th percentile	Obese
>97th percentile	Has not been named, but children at this level have significant increases for comorbidities (Kelly et al., 2013)

13.1.2 Definition and Assessment of Childhood Obesity

The most commonly used assessment tool in screening for childhood obesity is the body mass index (BMI). The BMI is a calculation that adjusts weight for height. It is defined as weight (in kilograms) divided by height (in meters) squared. For BMI, age and gender standards are reported as percentiles for which the calculation for a given child is compared. A child's BMI will change with age as their height and weight distribution changes as they grow, and thus percentiles have to be used to better track BMI changes. Age and gender BMI percentiles for children above 2 years old allow clinicians to determine which children are at the highest risk in the population (Centers for Disease Control and Prevention, 2010).

In 2007, an Expert Committee, comprised of representatives from 15 national health organizations, described how to use the BMI and the classifications of weight status for children and adolescents (Barlow, 2007). The Expert Committee Recommendations for the screening, assessment and treatment of childhood overweight and obesity recommended classifications for the assessment of BMI found in Table 13.1.

The recommendations states that higher BMIs are accompanied with greater health and social risk (Kelly et al., 2013), and there is a need to identify those young people in the highest percentiles of pediatric standards. This is in contrast to adult care, where there is a 3-staged definition for the highest obesity category in order to better in characterize patients with the greatest health risk. However, in pediatrics, there has not been agreement on a set of definitions for this highest group. The CDC pediatric BMI charts for age only displayed up to the 97th percentile, which may not fully capture the population at risk. Leading health organizations have identified a need to better define severe obesity in children given many already have significant health problems related to their weight (Kelly et al., 2013).

13.1.3 Alternative Measurements to BMI

The use of weight class definitions based on BMI percentiles in children has some limitations, as outlined by the Expert Recommendations (Barlow, 2007). While BMI correlates well with excess body fat and health conditions, it does not measure body fat directly as it only examines body weight in proportion to height. Body weight can be a factor of water weight, lean body mass, and adipose tissue, which is not distinguished in the BMI calculation. It is higher adipose tissue that is of concern, as it is correlated with premature death and comorbidities (Pischon et al., 2008). There are children, such as student athletes, with an elevated BMI and possible classified in the overweight category class due to a higher proportion of lean muscle mass instead of adipose tissue. Classifying these children as overweight may inaccurately convey health risk concerns. However, children with BMI ≥95th percentile, or obese, have higher levels of adipose and health concerns (Freedman, Khan, Dietz, Srinivasan, & Berenson, 2001; Mei et al., 2002; Pietrobelli et al., 1998). Given the ease at determining the BMI and percentiles for each child, it is a useful screening tool for identifying obese patients, but additional evaluations are needed to determine if the elevated BMI indicates a riskier health assessment.

There are several other tools that can be utilized to assess body composition in children and adolescents, as outlined in Table 13.2. These tools can be used in conjunction with BMI calculation for assessing patients at higher risk for obesity-related illness.

Table 13.2 Assessment tools beyond BMI and their use in pediatrics

Assessment tools	What measures	Use in pediatrics	References
Skinfolds	Uses specific sites to measure body fat	• Accuracy and precision can be a concern,	Krebs et al. (2007), Wells and Fewtrell (2006)
		• Limited formulas available for children under 16 years of age,	
		• Does not provide additional information beyond BMI in children	
Waist circumference	Measures central obesity	• Corresponds with risk for morbidity in adults	Fernandez et al. (2004), Katzmarzyk et al. (2004), Krebs et al. (2007), Wells and Fewtrell (2006)
		• Studies in children have been inconsistent with MRI and abdominal obesity	
		• Emerging evidence of use in identifying children at high risk for cardiovascular disease	
		• Utility in clinical setting has not been fully determined	
		• No national standards exist	
		• Not recommended by the 2007 Expert Committee	

(continued)

Table 13.2 (continued)

Assessment tools	What measures	Use in pediatrics	References
Bioelectrical Impedance (BIA)	Measures total body fat using resistance based on body fat, water, and muscle	• Since children have higher body water and lower bone density BIA is not accurate in children • Accuracy concerns for obese and children from different racial and ethnic populations	Talma et al. (2013)
Dual energy X-ray absorptiometry (DEXA)	Use to measure bone density but can determine total body fat	• Percentile references exist • Primarily used in research settings • Exposes children to small doses of X-rays	Ogden, Li, Freedman, Borrud, and Flegal (2011)

13.2 Obesity Prevention Strategies

13.2.1 The Role of Clinicians

The Expert Recommendations stress primary preventions as well as secondary prevention of obesity throughout all ages and stages of development in childhood (Barlow, 2007). Primary prevention is focused on preventing normal weight children from gaining weight and excess fat. Secondary prevention is for children who are already overweight and obese, and aims at preventing the development of weight-related diseases such as diabetes, hypertension, stroke, and hypercholesterolemia (Reilly et al., 2003).

In pediatric medicine, the well child/health supervision visits serve as the most commonly used encounter to provide early screening, diagnosing, and treating of medical conditions in children. These visits include medical history interview, vital signs assessments, physical examinations, and anticipatory guidance to promote optimal health and development. The Expert Committee recommends individual growth assessments of children and adolescents as a regular part of well-visits, and BMI to be calculated for children above 2 years old (WORKGROUP, 2015). These visits serve a great opportunity to review of current symptoms, family history, dietary, and activity behaviors with the child's weight status in mind.

The review of this medical information will distinguish those children whose BMI is classified as overweight without other health concerns. In these cases, the individual evaluation will reveal healthy eating and adequate physical activity without any additional risk factors. While these children should have their BMI monitored on an annual basis, they should also be praised for their healthy lifestyle choices. For those children found to be at risk during their medical review or have an elevated BMI status, productive conversations are needed on how to have a healthy lifestyle in order to prevent excessive weight gain.

13.2.2   Conversations with Patients and Families

Health care providers are encouraged to discuss weight status with patients and families during their clinical encounters. This subject should be approached with sensitivity, where clinicians are supportive and nonjudgmental. Adult patients prefer more neutral terms during counseling than "obese," "fat," and "excess fat" (Wadden & Didie, 2003). With children, there is even greater concern about the language used because of their developing self-esteem and risk of promoting eating disorders. As discussed above, clinician should keep in mind that the goal of the conversation is guided by the child's symptoms and their medical and family history with regard weight-related health problems. It should be a three-way conversation between the health care professional, child, and parent such that all sides are heard and a course of action is agreed upon mutually.

Patient-centered communication styles and counseling methods are the recommended to facilitate a discussion about weight and health concerns (Krebs et al., 2007). The commonly used strategies are the Transtheoretical Model and Motivational Interviewing. The Transtheoretical Model of Change (Prochaska & DiClemente, 1982) can serve as a basis for behavioral counseling as it describes how a person or family moves toward changing behaviors to improve health. There are five stages that describe the patient's readiness to make a change: (1) pre-contemplative (not concern or interested in making the change), (2) contemplative (considering making the change), (3) preparation (making arrangements to accept the change), (4) action (made stated change), and (5) maintenance (the change is incorporated into their lifestyle). In a discussion regarding a child's weight, health professionals would determine which stage the parent or child are in regarding the child's health and weight. Motivational interviewing (Rollnick, Mason, & Butler, 1999) is a counseling technique recommended to guide this discussion (Daniels & Hassink, 2015). By engaging the conversation through the tenants of motivational interviewing, health care professionals can simultaneously determine families' readiness for change and help patients move forward from one stage to another. By using a nondirective judgmental tone, open-ended questions, and reflective listening throughout the conversation, patients and families would share with their thoughts on weight-related health through their own words. This conversation hopefully guides patients and families in ways they can improve their unhealthy weight-related behaviors.

13.3   Social Ecology Model

Obesity in adults and children is a multifactorial disease. However, promoting health and preventing disease in children presents different challenges. The social ecological model (SEM) was first presented by Bronfenbrenner and is often used as a guide to examine the influences at multiple levels on pediatric obesity (Bronfenbrenner, 1979). In Fig. 13.1, these influences are represented as five concentric circles or spheres. This model has identified multiple influences that can be

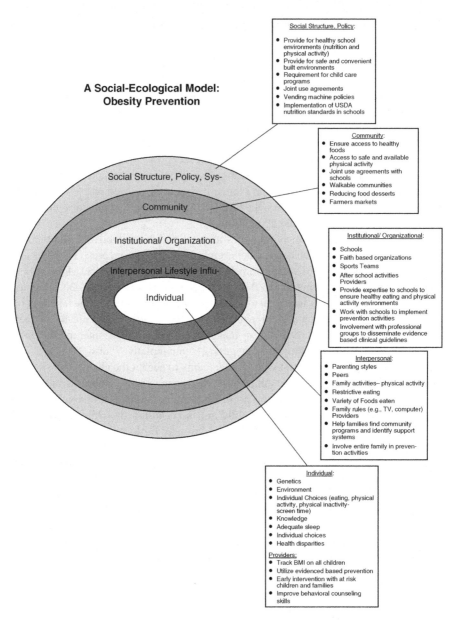

Fig. 13.1 Illustrates the social ecology model and childhood obesity. *Adapted from McLeroy KR, Bibeau D, Steckler A. Glanz K (1988). A Perspective on Health Promotion Programs. Health Education Quarterly 15:351–377, 1988*

targeted in the prevention of pediatric obesity. These influences are: (1) individual factors, (2) interpersonal relationships, (3) institutions and organizations, (4) communities, and (5) policies. The following sections will highlight ways in which obesity prevention efforts take place at each level of influence.

13.3.1 Individual Sphere

The first level in the social ecological model represents individual factors. Research aims to provide a better understanding of individual characteristics through genetics and how this interplays with people's choices and environment. The Human Genome project has been able to identify several genetic mutations associated with obesity and excess weight gain (Loos, 2009; Rankinen et al., 2006). However, the mechanisms for which these genetic mutations and how much of they contribute to obesity is not yet determined. Thus far, we know this process starts at a young age where in an obesogenic environment responsive genes are activated promoting obesity (Maes, Neale, & Eaves, 1997). Since the genetics of obesity are not fully understood, this factor is not amendable to modification and plays minimal role in obesity prevention.

Of the all contributions to individual weight gain, it is individual choices around diet and exercise that are modifiable. Thus, helping children make healthy choices has been the cornerstone in the prevention of pediatric obesity. This is the basis for several evidence-based recommendations for children and is highlighted in the 2007 guidelines for obesity prevention (Davis et al., 2007). Meta-analyses have shown that increased sugar intake, often from sugar sweetened beverages, is associated with weight gain in children (Bruening et al., 2014; Morgan, 2013). In addition, several eating habits have also been studied regarding its impact on the development of pediatric obesity. Meal skipping, especially breakfast, in older children and adolescents is associated with increased adiposity accruement (Rampersaud, Pereira, Girard, Adams, & Metzl, 2005), and youth who eat more meals out of the house, especially in fast food restaurants have higher caloric intakes and weight gain (Bruening et al., 2014). Conversely, the more often family meals together is inversely associated with overweight in youth (Lee et al., 2011).

Individual choices around activity are also emphasized in the Expert Committee Recommendations. Sixty minutes of daily moderate to vigorous activity is recommended for children and adolescents (Committee, 2008), as it has been shown to lower the odds of being overweight (Patrick et al., 2004). Unfortunately, most youth do not meet this activity goal (Fakhouri et al., 2014). Surveys indicate that the percentage of US adolescents in daily physical education classes has decreased in the last 20 years, while, sedentary activities have been increasing (Lowry, Lee, Fulton, & Kann, 2009; Lowry, Wechsler, Kann, & Collins, 2001; Rideout, Foehr, & Roberts, 2010). Thus, more attention should be given to the amount of free play children are given in addition to time with organized sports or physical educational classes.

13.3.2 Interpersonal Factors

The second sphere in the social ecological model is interpersonal factors, which includes one's social network of parents, family, and friends. Particularly, parents and families often serve as the most important influences in their children's choices and behaviors (Whitaker, Wright, Pepe, Seidel, & Dietz, 1997). However, peers and other social network connections have a large impact on children behaviors, especially as they become adolescents and young adults.

13.3.2.1 Families

The importance of parents and families as an influence of healthy behaviors is well understood. Their role of obesity prevention is paramount. Parents and adult caregivers are key in the dietary choices children make and have a strong influence on their physical activity practices. In the past 20 years, parental influences on dietary and activity behaviors have been the focus of research and interventions in obesity prevention for children. There are three levels of parents' influences: specific parental practices regarding food and activity for the child, parent's behaviors for themselves, and general parenting decisions that shape the development of habits in the children (Rhee, 2008).

Parents and caretakers set rules and practices that often set the stage for a child's eating and activity habits. For example, children are often told to eat all the food given or rewarding a "clean plate" with a treat. As children get older, they are less responsive to their natural cue to satiety, and prompting them to eat more. (Birch & Fisher, 1998; Cecil et al., 2005; Johnson & Taylor-Holloway, 2006). Additionally, parents can also set rules regarding activity and inactivity. Setting limits on sedentary activities like television watching encourages children to increase their level of activity (Nowicka & Flodmark, 2008) while having a TV in the child's bedroom will promote fewer calories to be expended by children throughout the day.

There are general parental behaviors that are not targeted toward the child but influence the development of child behaviors. As Bandura (1977) explains through social modeling, parents serve as role models for their children, and children often base their own health behaviors on the actions of their parents. Parents decide what food comes into the house, the portion sizes served, and how food is distributed (Ritchie et al., 2005). For example, parents who eat more fruits and vegetables encourage their children to do the same (Pearson, Biddle, & Gorely, 2009). Unhealthy habits also have a negative influence as well, as studies have shown that families with mothers who drank sweetened beverages pass this habit to their daughters (Fisher, Mitchell, Smiciklas-Wright, & Birch, 2001), and prolonged sedentary TV watching by parents is associated with the same in children (Jago, Fox, Page, Brockman, & Thompson, 2010).

Parenting style and family functioning impact children's food choices and eating behaviors by providing a certain social and emotional environment in which to make decisions. Parents who have authoritarian style (e.g., high parental decision-making with less child input) is associated with high weight gain in children (Davis et al., 2007), and children who are neglected and have other adverse life events have higher BMI (Pretty, O'Leary, Cairney, & Wade, 2013).

13.3.2.2 Friends and Social Networks

As children become older, friends and social networks have increasing influence on dietary and activity choices (Zimmer-Gembeck & Collins, 2003). As with parents, Bandura's social modeling theory can also describe the influence of friends on children's health behaviors (Bandura, 1977). Children often choose friends that have similar activity levels to themselves (de la Haye, Robins, Mohr, & Wilson, 2011). Studies have shown that having friends to play with facilitates physical activity, and conversely being alone appears to deter youth from being physically active. Peers also play a role in modeling eating habits, and studies have consistently found that children not only eat more when around their peers, but overweight children were especially susceptible to modeling poor eating behaviors of their peers (Salvy, de la Haye, Bowker, & Hermans, 2012). Thus, obesity prevention efforts need to involve children's social networks in order to be effective.

13.3.3 Third Sphere: Institutions and Organizations

13.3.3.1 Schools

Schools are the most prominent institution in the lives of most children given it is where they spend most of their day and year (Guinhouya et al., 2009). There has been a great deal of focus and research on the role of schools in the prevention of obesity in children.

There are several roles that schools play in prevention of obesity in children. First, through the classroom curricula, educators can teach children the recommended dietary and activity habits discussed above. Educational programs can focus on nutritional habits, physical/inability habits or a combination of both. Although curricula focused on only healthier activity alone has not shown to change BMI, a meta-analysis demonstrated that programs with instructions on healthier activity and dietary choices together did show improvements in BMI (Harris, Kuramoto, Schulzer, & Retallack, 2009; Shaya, Flores, Gbarayor, & Wang, 2008).

The second strategy used in school settings to promote healthier lives in children has been to change the school environment. For example, schools can provide healthier food choices in the cafeteria for breakfast and lunch, as well as at school stores and vending machines. Recent policies with the United States Department of Agriculture (USDA) have provided guidance to increase students' intake of dairy, fruits, and vegetables consumption while decreasing sodium, fats, and sugars ("National School Lunch Program Fact Sheet," 2013). Their policies have targeted the availability of sugar sweetened beverages, high-calorie snacks, food available at classroom events, and as competitive goods in vending machine on campus. These policies have demonstrated improvement in fruit consumption (Schwartz, Henderson, Read, Danna, & Ickovics, 2015) which is a great factor in preventing obesity.

To promote physical activity, providing recess time and physical education classes in schools are effective ways to help children reach the recommended goal of 60 min of physical activity each day (Committee, 2008). The organization, Active Living Research, reports that requiring physical education and in-class activity breaks can contribute 23 min and 19 min to that goal, respectively (Ward, 2011). Their report emphasizes that schools should consider a physical education (PE) curriculum yearly for grades K-12 as well increase physical activity outside of PE with recess and after school programs.

Research has shown that increasing physical activity levels improves academic performance. Studies have found that the odds of passing both standardized math and English increased as the number of fitness test passed increases (Chomitz et al., 2009), physically fit children perform better on test of memory (Chaddock et al., 2010), and children who perform better cardiovascular fitness tests have high academic achievements (Torrijos-Nino et al., 2014). Similarly, children who participate in school breakfast programs do better with achievement (Frisvold, 2015). As there are financial challenges to implementing these changes in schools, collaborating with school administrators, educators, health professionals, and community leaders to overcome these barriers is crucial.

13.3.3.2   Early Child Care

For preschool children, the policies and curricula in their preschools and early child care centers center influence their habits related to weight gain. Since obesity has significantly increased for children entering kindergarten over a 12-year periods (Datar & Chung, 2015), making changes early is paramount. The strategy is similar as with the elementary schools: change the food offered at preschools, educate the young children, teachers, caregivers, and parents about appropriate healthy lifestyle habits, and providing more opportunities for age-appropriate physical activities. Research has shown that child care centers did not serve meals that were consistent with a healthy diet in terms of saturated fat, sodium dietary fibers, and dairy as recommended by IOM (Schwartz et al., 2015). Reviews of interventions to promote physical activity in this area have reported that significant effects were largely seen with environmental and playground changes (Temple & Robinson, 2014). While comprehensive healthy eating interventions with multiple components such as parents' education, child education, and greater exposure to fruits and vegetables increased consumptions of vegetables; changes in BMI and anthropometrics were not found consistently in preschools (Mikkelsen, Husby, Skov, & Perez-Cueto, 2014).

13.3.4   Fourth Sphere: Community

In the social ecological model for pediatric obesity prevention, the fourth sphere is the child's community. There are several ways in which the community can have an impact on the development of excess weight gain in children. In this section, we will focus on neighborhoods and churches as the focus of prevention in excess weight gain in children.

13.3.4.1 Neighborhoods

The three aspects of neighborhoods that have been the focus of obesity prevention in children: access to healthier foods, areas for active living, and neighborhood safety. Easy access to healthier foods would help parents and caregivers provide healthier food to children in the home. Typically in the neighborhoods that are void of healthy food options, more fast food and unhealthy options prevails. The USDA defines food deserts (Gallagher, 2011) as parts of the country without access to fresh fruit, vegetables, and other healthy whole foods, usually found in impoverished areas. This is largely due to a lack of grocery stores, farmers' markets, and healthy food providers. Research has shown that residents who have access to supermarkets and limited access to convenient stores tend to have healthier diets and lower levels of obesity (Larson, Story, & Nelson, 2009). In young adults, the CARDIA study has shown that more convenient stores were associated with lower diet quality, especially for participants with lower incomes (Rummo et al., 2015), and urban children that live a significant distance from the nearest grocery store had higher BMI than those that liver closer to grocery stores (Carroll-Scott et al., 2013). Community leaders can help recruit healthier eating options into affected communities once this problem has been identified.

Other aspects of neighborhoods that affect healthy lifestyles in children are options for physical activity. For example, the presences of sidewalks, bike lanes, parks, and playgrounds help families and children become more active. The availability of neighborhood parks was associated with higher participation in active sports for all adolescents, while greater green space demonstrated more wheel-based sports and exercise for female adolescents (Boone-Heinonen, Popkin, Song, & Gordon-Larsen, 2010). Increasing walkability in an urban city has been associated with low BMI scores in children and adolescents (Duncan et al., 2014). Studies have shown that people who live in near trails are 50 % more likely to be active and communities that are walkable increase the physical activity of its residents twofold (Huston, Evenson, Bors, & Gizlice, 2003). Even access to playgrounds for children can have a significant positive impact on physical activity (Carroll-Scott et al., 2013). Leaders can plan communities with these features in mind or modify older communities to accommodate more active lifestyles.

Lastly, communities leaders can help ensure neighborhood are safe for children to play without being exposed to crime and violence. Parental concern about neighborhood safety is associated with overweight and obesity in children (Lumeng, Appugliese, Cabral, Bradley, & Zuckerman, 2006). Even the perception of a high crime environment is associated with higher weight status. In a study looking at adolescents, elevated BMI was positively associated with perceived crime for boys and girls, where it was associated with reported crime in girls (Forsyth et al., 2015). One proposed solution is to allow community children to use playgrounds and gyms when schools are closed allowing youth to get more daily activity time in a safe place (Lopez, 2011). This was successful in New Orleans, LA where the number of children outside and active in participating neighborhoods increased by 84 % (Farley et al., 2007).

13.3.4.2 Churches

Churches are community institutions and for many a trusted source of information and care. Leveraging the influence churches have on neighborhoods has been studied, especially in minority populations. Involving the church in the education and health of children has been instrumental in addressing the disparate levels of obesity in certain racial/ethnic groups in the USA (Fryar, Carroll, & Ogden, 2012; Rossen & Talih, 2014). Families who report a higher level of religiosity have children with lower BMI (Limbers, Young, Bryant, & Stephen, 2015). In the African American community, churches have been the setting for obesity interventions for women and men with some success in reducing weight, increasing intake of fruits and vegetables, and increasing levels of physical activity (Lancaster, Carter-Edwards, Grilo, Shen, & Schoenthaler, 2014). There have been several faith-based interventions focused on children and adolescents, all using the community leaders input to design the program (Horton, Alvear, & Horton, 2014; Reifsnider, Hargraves, Williams, Cooks, & Hall, 2010; Resnicow, Taylor, Baskin, & McCarty, 2005). In the Latino community, church leaders suggested that the church can become the conduit for obesity prevention programs and opportunities for both children and parents (He et al., 2013). It has been suggested that religious leaders would be effective leaders in promoting critical change toward a healthier lifestyle (Anshel & Smith, 2014).

13.3.5 Fifth Sphere: Public Policy

The last sphere in the social ecological model for childhood obesity prevention is social structure policy and systems. This would include local, state and national laws that promote better health often through change discussed in the other spheres in this chapter. Additionally, policy influences how obesity is treated within medical community. By enacting public policy, more people, including children, would be impacted by implemented changes.

Local leaders and governances can enact changes within communities and local neighborhoods by enacting laws that provide access to playgrounds and safe traffic patterns. Laws can restrict unhealthy food sources which encourages healthier choices. For example, in King County, Washington, guidance was mandated to add calorie information to menus, which has shown to help certain populations make more informed decisions regarding their food choices (Chen et al., 2015). One policy specifically aimed to prevent obesity in young children was in changing the New York City Health Code in early child care centers. In 2006, the regulations required increased physical activity, limited screen time, and sugar sweetened beverages in the centers (Nonas, Silver, Kettel Khan, & Leviton, 2014).

Additionally, leaders have responded nationally to prevent childhood obesity. The USDA issues the 2010 Dietary Guidance for Americans and adopted the MyPlate (Choose My Plate, 2010) as the symbol and educational tool. This change was implemented to emphasis the importance of eating more low-fat dairy products, fruits, and vegetables. As already discussed earlier, the USDA also changed polices to the National School Lunch Program which affected 31 million children in 2012 ("National School Lunch Program Fact Sheet," 2013).

National organizations in health care, such as the American Academy of Pediatrics, Institute of Medicine, American Heart Association, Academy of Nutrition and Dietetics, and the Society of Adolescent Health and Medicine, have issued position papers and recommendations toward the prevention and treatment of pediatric obesity (Daniels and Hassink, 2015; Fitzgerald, Morgan, & Slawson, 2013; Kelly, et al., 2013; Kohn et al., 2006; Prevention & Glickman, 2012). The US Preventive Task Force provides accurate, up-to-date, and relevant recommendations about preventive services in primary care and has adopted many of the recommendations presented here (WORKGROUP, 2015). However, a big endorsement toward obesity prevention efforts occurred in 2013 from the American Medical Association (AMA). It made a strong statement to when it recognized obesity as a disease requiring a range of medical interventions to advance obesity treatment and prevention (AMA Adopts New Policies on Second Day of Voting at Annual Meeting, 2013). The classification of obesity as a disease will help health professionals receive reimbursement for their counseling and efforts with patients, including children, to identify those at risk and prevent further weight gain. It is hoped that by this action insurers will examining their provision to provide preventive care, especially with children.

In recent years, one of the biggest efforts toward obesity prevention has been through US politics. *Let's Move!* Campaign (Let's Move), promoted by Michelle Obama, was started in 2010 and brought the issues of childhood obesity to the forefront. This campaign addresses all sectors of the epidemic in youth, similar to the social ecological model. It includes tools and guidance regarding nutrition and activity and speaks to a broad audience of kids, parents, schools, and community leaders.

13.4   Conclusion

In this chapter, we reviewed the role of obesity prevention in health promotion for youth. Although the prevalence appears to be stabilizing in the USA, there is still great concern as approximately 30% of our children and youth are overweight or obese, and the health-related conditions that are triggered by excess weight, such as diabetes, heart disease, and cancers, are occurring at younger ages. BMI percentiles still remains the best screening tool available, and once at-risk youth are identified, pediatric providers are asked to engage families to make specific changes. The social–ecological model provides structure to the discussion of all factors that can contribute to weight gain in children. Both parents and schools have strong influences on the development of negative and positive habits that contrite to weight gain in youth. Community and neighborhoods factors also contribute to the activity and dietary choices children and families make. Politicians and national leaders have made several policy changes to impact many. Clinicians should support opportunities to help children, families, schools, communities, and lawmakers in their efforts to promote lifestyle changes with better diet and activity habits. To promote better health for children, assisting children in making healthier choices will be paramount.

References

AMA Adopts New Policies on Second Day of Voting at Annual Meeting. (2013). [Press release]. Retrieved from http://www.ama-assn.org/ama/pub/news/news/2013/2013-06-18-new-ama--policies-annual-meeting.page

Anshel, M. H., & Smith, M. (2014). The role of religious leaders in promoting healthy habits in religious institutions. *Journal of Religion and Health, 53*(4), 1046–1059. doi:10.1007/s10943-013-9702-5.

Bandura, A. (1977). Self-efficacy: Toward a unifying theory of behavioral change. *Psychological Review, 84*(2), 191–215. doi:10.1037/0033-295X.84.2.191.

Barlow, S. E. (2007). Expert committee recommendations regarding the prevention, assessment, and treatment of child and adolescent overweight and obesity: Summary report. *Pediatrics, 120*(Suppl 4), S164–S192. doi:10.1542/peds.2007-2329C.

Birch, L. L., & Fisher, J. O. (1998). Development of eating behaviors among children and adolescents. *Pediatrics, 101*(3 Pt 2), 539–549.

Boone-Heinonen, J., Popkin, B. M., Song, Y., & Gordon-Larsen, P. (2010). What neighborhood area captures built environment features related to adolescent physical activity? *Health & Place, 16*(6), 1280–1286. doi:10.1016/j.healthplace.2010.06.015.

Bronfenbrenner, U. (1979). *The ecology of human development: Experiments by design and nature*. Cambridge, MA: Harvard University Press.

Bruening, M., MacLehose, R., Eisenberg, M. E., Nanney, M. S., Story, M., & Neumark-Sztainer, D. (2014). Associations between sugar-sweetened beverage consumption and fast-food restaurant frequency among adolescents and their friends. *Journal of Nutrition Education and Behavior, 46*(4), 277–285. doi:http://dx.doi.org/10.1016/j.jneb.2014.02.009

Carroll-Scott, A., Gilstad-Hayden, K., Rosenthal, L., Peters, S. M., McCaslin, C., Joyce, R., & Ickovics, J. R. (2013). Disentangling neighborhood contextual associations with child body mass index, diet, and physical activity: The role of built, socioeconomic, and social environments. *Social Science and Medicine, 95*, 106–114. doi:10.1016/j.socscimed.2013.04.003

Cecil, J. E., Palmer, C. N., Wrieden, W., Murrie, I., Bolton-Smith, C., Watt, P., . . . Hetherington, M. M. (2005). Energy intakes of children after preloads: Adjustment, not compensation. *The American Journal of Clinical Nutrition, 82*(2), 302–308.

Centers for Disease Control and Prevention, N. C. f. H. S. (2010, September 9). Growth chart. Retrieved from http://www.cdc.gov/growthcharts/

Chaddock, L., Erickson, K. I., Prakash, R. S., Kim, J. S., Voss, M. W., Vanpatter, M., . . . Kramer, A. F. (2010). A neuroimaging investigation of the association between aerobic fitness, hippocampal volume, and memory performance in preadolescent children. *Brain Research, 1358*, 172–183. doi:10.1016/j.brainres.2010.08.049

Chen, R., Smyser, M., Chan, N., Ta, M., Saelens, B. E., & Krieger, J. (2015). Changes in awareness and use of calorie information after mandatory menu labeling in restaurants in King County, Washington. *American Journal of Public Health, 105*(3), 546–553. doi:10.2105/ajph.2014.302262.

Chomitz, V. R., Slining, M. M., McGowan, R. J., Mitchell, S. E., Dawson, G. F., & Hacker, K. A. (2009). Is there a relationship between physical fitness and academic achievement? Positive results from public school children in the northeastern United States. *Journal of School Health, 79*(1), 30–37. doi:10.1111/j.1746-1561.2008.00371.x.

Choose My Plate. (2010). Retrieved from http://www.choosemyplate.gov/about

Committee, P. A. G. A. (2008). *Physical activity guidelines advisory committee report, 2008* (pp. A1–H14). Washington, DC: US Department of Health and Human Services.

Daniels, S. R., & Hassink, S. G. (2015). The role of the pediatrician in primary prevention of obesity. *Pediatrics, 136*(1), e275–e292. doi:10.1542/peds.2015-1558.

Datar, A., & Chung, P. J. (2015). Changes in socioeconomic, racial/ethnic, and sex disparities in childhood obesity at school entry in the United States. *JAMA Pediatrics, 169*(7), 696–697. doi:10.1001/jamapediatrics.2015.0172.

Davis, M. M., Gance-Cleveland, B., Hassink, S., Johnson, R., Paradis, G., & Resnicow, K. (2007). Recommendations for prevention of childhood obesity. *Pediatrics, 120*(Suppl 4), S229–S253. doi:10.1542/peds.2007-2329E.

de la Haye, K., Robins, G., Mohr, P., & Wilson, C. (2011). How physical activity shapes, and is shaped by, adolescent friendships. *Social Science and Medicine, 73*(5), 719–728. doi:10.1016/j.socscimed.2011.06.023.

Duncan, D. T., Sharifi, M., Melly, S. J., Marshall, R., Sequist, T. D., Rifas-Shiman, S. L., & Taveras, E. M. (2014). Characteristics of walkable built environments and BMI z-scores in children: Evidence from a large electronic health record database. *Environmental Health Perspectives, 122*(12), 1359–1365. doi:10.1289/ehp.1307704

Fakhouri, T. H., Hughes, J. P., Burt, V. L., Song, M., Fulton, J. E., & Ogden, C. L. (2014). Physical activity in U.S. youth aged 12–15 years, 2012. *NCHS Data Brief, 141*, 1–8.

Farley, T. A., Meriwether, R. A., Baker, E. T., Watkins, L. T., Johnson, C. C., & Webber, L. S. (2007). Safe play spaces to promote physical activity in inner-city children: Results from a pilot study of an environmental intervention. *American Journal of Public Health, 97*(9), 1625–1631. doi:10.2105/ajph.2006.092692.

Fernandez, J. R., Redden, D. T., Pietrobelli, A., & Allison, D. B. (2004). Waist circumference percentiles in nationally representative samples of African–American, European–American, and Mexican–American children and adolescents. *Journal of Pediatrics, 145*(4), 439–444. doi:10.1016/j.jpeds.2004.06.044.

Fisher, J. O., Mitchell, D. C., Smiciklas-Wright, H., & Birch, L. L. (2001). Maternal milk consumption predicts the tradeoff between milk and soft drinks in young girls' diets. *The Journal of Nutrition, 131*(2), 246–250.

Fitzgerald, N., Morgan, K. T., & Slawson, D. L. (2013). Practice paper of the Academy of Nutrition and Dietetics abstract: The role of nutrition in health promotion and chronic disease prevention. *Journal of the Academy of Nutrition and Dietetics, 113*(7), 983. doi:10.1016/j.jand.2013.05.007.

Forsyth, A., Wall, M., Choo, T., Larson, N., Van Riper, D., & Neumark-Sztainer, D. (2015). Perceived and police-reported neighborhood crime: Linkages to adolescent activity behaviors and weight status. *Journal of Adolescent Health, 57*(2), 222–228. doi:10.1016/j.jadohealth.2015.05.003.

Freedman, D. S., Khan, L. K., Dietz, W. H., Srinivasan, S. R., & Berenson, G. S. (2001). Relationship of childhood obesity to coronary heart disease risk factors in adulthood: The Bogalusa Heart Study. *Pediatrics, 108*(3), 712–718.

Frisvold, D. E. (2015). Nutrition and cognitive achievement: An evaluation of the school breakfast program. *Journal of Public Economics, 124*, 91–104. doi:10.1016/j.jpubeco.2014.12.003.

Fryar, C. D., Carroll, M. D., & Ogden, C. L. (2012). Prevalence of obesity among children and adolescents: United States, trends 1963–1965 through 2009–2010. *National Center for Health Statistics, 1960*.

Gallagher, M. (2011). USDA defines food deserts. *Nutrition Digest*. Retrieved from http://americannutritionassociation.org/newsletter/usda-defines-food-deserts

Guinhouya, B. C., Lemdani, M., Vilhelm, C., Hubert, H., Apete, G. K., & Durocher, A. (2009). How school time physical activity is the "big one" for daily activity among schoolchildren: A semi-experimental approach. *Journal of Physical Activity and Health, 6*(4), 510–519.

Harris, K. C., Kuramoto, L. K., Schulzer, M., & Retallack, J. E. (2009). Effect of school-based physical activity interventions on body mass index in children: A meta-analysis. *Canadian Medical Association Journal, 180*(7), 719–726. doi:10.1503/cmaj.080966.

He, M., Wilmoth, S., Bustos, D., Jones, T., Leeds, J., & Yin, Z. (2013). Latino church leaders' perspectives on childhood obesity prevention. *American Journal of Preventive Medicine, 44*(3 Suppl 3), S232–S239. doi:10.1016/j.amepre.2012.11.014.

Horton, S. E., Alvear, E. E., & Horton, D. L. (2014). Health ministry partnerships: Creating a habit for health. *Journal of Christian Nursing, 31*(1), 28–33.

Huston, S. L., Evenson, K. R., Bors, P., & Gizlice, Z. (2003). Neighborhood environment, access to places for activity, and leisure-time physical activity in a diverse North Carolina population. *American Journal of Health Promotion, 18*(1), 58–69.

Jago, R., Fox, K. R., Page, A. S., Brockman, R., & Thompson, J. L. (2010). Parent and child physical activity and sedentary time: Do active parents foster active children? *BMC Public Health, 10*, 194. doi:10.1186/1471-2458-10-194.

Johnson, S. L., & Taylor-Holloway, L. A. (2006). Non-Hispanic white and Hispanic elementary school children's self-regulation of energy intake. *The American Journal of Clinical Nutrition, 83*(6), 1276–1282.

Katzmarzyk, P. T., Srinivasan, S. R., Chen, W., Malina, R. M., Bouchard, C., & Berenson, G. S. (2004). Body mass index, waist circumference, and clustering of cardiovascular disease risk factors in a biracial sample of children and adolescents. *Pediatrics, 114*(2), e198–e205.

Kelly, A. S., Barlow, S. E., Rao, G., Inge, T. H., Hayman, L. L., Steinberger, J., . . . Daniels, S. R. (2013). Severe obesity in children and adolescents: Identification, associated health risks, and treatment approaches: A scientific statement from the American Heart Association. *Circulation, 128*(15), 1689–1712. doi:10.1161/CIR.0b013e3182a5cfb3

Kohn, M., Rees, J. M., Brill, S., Fonseca, H., Jacobson, M., Katzman, D. K., . . . Schneider, M. (2006). Preventing and treating adolescent obesity: A position paper of the Society for Adolescent Medicine. *Journal of Adolescent Health, 38*(6), 784–787.

Krebs, N. F., Himes, J. H., Jacobson, D., Nicklas, T. A., Guilday, P., & Styne, D. (2007). Assessment of child and adolescent overweight and obesity. *Pediatrics, 120*(Suppl 4), S193–S228. doi:10.1542/peds.2007-2329D.

Lancaster, K. J., Carter-Edwards, L., Grilo, S., Shen, C., & Schoenthaler, A. M. (2014). Obesity interventions in African American faith-based organizations: A systematic review. *Obesity Reviews, 15*(Suppl 4), 159–176. doi:10.1111/obr.12207.

Larson, N. I., Story, M. T., & Nelson, M. C. (2009). Neighborhood environments: Disparities in access to healthy foods in the U.S. *American Journal of Preventive Medicine, 36*(1), 74–81. doi:10.1016/j.amepre.2008.09.025.

Lee, H. A., Lee, W. K., Kong, K. A., Chang, N., Ha, E. H., Hong, Y. S., & Park, H. (2011). The effect of eating behavior on being overweight or obese during preadolescence. *Journal of Preventive Medicine and Public Health, 44*(5), 226–233. doi:10.3961/jpmph.2011.44.5.226

Let's Move. Retrieved from http://www.letsmove.gov/

Limbers, C. A., Young, D., Bryant, W., & Stephen, M. (2015). Associations between family religious practices, internalizing/externalizing behaviors, and body mass index in obese youth. *International Journal of Psychiatry in Medicine, 49*(3), 215–226. doi:10.1177/0091217415582191.

Loos, R. J. (2009). Recent progress in the genetics of common obesity. *British Journal of Clinical Pharmacology, 68*(6), 811–829. doi:10.1111/j.1365-2125.2009.03523.x.

Lopez, R. (2011). *The potential of safe, secure and accessible playgrounds to increase children's physical activity*. Princeton, NJ. Retrieved from www.activelivingresearch.org

Lowry, R., Lee, S. M., Fulton, J. E., & Kann, L. (2009). Healthy people 2010 objectives for physical activity, physical education, and television viewing among adolescents: National trends from the Youth Risk Behavior Surveillance System, 1999–2007. *Journal of Physical Activity and Health, 6*(Suppl 1), S36–S45.

Lowry, R., Wechsler, H., Kann, L., & Collins, J. L. (2001). Recent trends in participation in physical education among US high school students. *Journal of School Health, 71*(4), 145–152.

Lumeng, J. C., Appugliese, D., Cabral, H. J., Bradley, R. H., & Zuckerman, B. (2006). Neighborhood safety and overweight status in children. *Archives of Pediatrics and Adolescent Medicine, 160*(1), 25–31. doi:10.1001/archpedi.160.1.25.

Maes, H. M., Neale, M., & Eaves, L. (1997). Genetic and environmental factors in relative body weight and human adiposity. *Behavior Genetics, 27*(4), 325–351. doi:10.1023/A:1025635913927.

Mei, Z., Grummer-Strawn, L. M., Pietrobelli, A., Goulding, A., Goran, M. I., & Dietz, W. H. (2002). Validity of body mass index compared with other body-composition screening indexes for the assessment of body fatness in children and adolescents. *The American Journal of Clinical Nutrition, 75*(6), 978–985.

Mikkelsen, M. V., Husby, S., Skov, L. R., & Perez-Cueto, F. J. (2014). A systematic review of types of healthy eating interventions in preschools. *Nutrition Journal, 13*, 56. doi:10.1186/1475-2891-13-56.

Morgan, R. E. (2013). Does consumption of high-fructose corn syrup beverages cause obesity in children? *Pediatric Obesity, 8*(4), 249–254. doi:10.1111/j.2047-6310.2013.00173.x.

National School Lunch Program Fact Sheet. (2013). In U. S. D. o. Agriculture (Ed.). Alexandria, VA.

Nonas, C., Silver, L. D., Kettel Khan, L., & Leviton, L. (2014). Rationale for New York City's regulations on nutrition, physical activity, and screen time in early child care centers. *Preventing Chronic Disease, 11*, E182. doi:10.5888/pcd11.130435.

Nowicka, P., & Flodmark, C. E. (2008). Family in pediatric obesity management: a literature review. *International Journal of Pediatric Obesity, 3*(Suppl 1), 44–50. doi:10.1080/17477160801896994.

Ogden, C. L., Carroll, M. D., Kit, B. K., & Flegal, K. M. (2014). Prevalence of childhood and adult obesity in the United States, 2011–2012. *Journal of the American Medical Association, 311*(8), 806–814. doi:10.1001/jama.2014.732.

Ogden, C. L., Li, Y., Freedman, D. S., Borrud, L. G., & Flegal, K. M. (2011). Smoothed percentage body fat percentiles for U.S. children and adolescents, 1999–2004. *National Health Statistics Reports 43*, 1–7.

Patrick, K., Norman, G. J., Calfas, K. J., Sallis, J. F., Zabinski, M. F., Rupp, J., & Cella, J. (2004). Diet, physical activity, and sedentary behaviors as risk factors for overweight in adolescence. *Archives of Pediatrics and Adolescent Medicine, 158*(4), 385–390. doi:10.1001/archpedi.158.4.385

Pearson, N., Biddle, S. J., & Gorely, T. (2009). Family correlates of fruit and vegetable consumption in children and adolescents: A systematic review. *Public Health Nutrition, 12*(2), 267–283. doi:10.1017/s1368980008002589.

Pietrobelli, A., Faith, M. S., Allison, D. B., Gallagher, D., Chiumello, G., & Heymsfield, S. B. (1998). Body mass index as a measure of adiposity among children and adolescents: A validation study. *Journal of Pediatrics, 132*(2), 204–210.

Pischon, T., Boeing, H., Hoffmann, K., Bergmann, M., Schulze, M. B., Overvad, K., . . . Riboli, E. (2008). General and abdominal adiposity and risk of death in Europe. *New England Journal of Medicine, 359*(20), 2105–2120. doi:10.1056/NEJMoa0801891

Pretty, C., O'Leary, D. D., Cairney, J., & Wade, T. J. (2013). Adverse childhood experiences and the cardiovascular health of children: A cross-sectional study. *BMC Pediatrics, 13*, 208. doi:10.1186/1471-2431-13-208.

Prevention, I. o. M. C. o. A. P. i. O., & Glickman, D. (2012). *Accelerating progress in obesity prevention: Solving the weight of the nation*. Washington, DC: National Academies Press.

Prochaska, J. O., & DiClemente, C. C. (1982). Transtheoretical therapy: Toward a more integrative model of change. *Psychotherapy: Theory, Research & Practice, 19*(3), 276.

Rampersaud, G. C., Pereira, M. A., Girard, B. L., Adams, J., & Metzl, J. D. (2005). Breakfast habits, nutritional status, body weight, and academic performance in children and adolescents. *Journal of the American Dietetic Association, 105*(5), 743–760. doi:http://dx.doi.org/10.1016/j.jada.2005.02.007

Rankinen, T., Zuberi, A., Chagnon, Y. C., Weisnagel, S. J., Argyropoulos, G., Walts, B., . . . Bouchard, C. (2006). The human obesity gene map: The 2005 update. *Obesity (Silver Spring), 14*(4), 529–644. doi:10.1038/oby.2006.71

Reifsnider, E., Hargraves, M., Williams, K. J., Cooks, J., & Hall, V. (2010). Shaking and rattling: Developing a child obesity prevention program using a faith-based community approach. *Family & Community Health, 33*(2), 144–151. doi:10.1097/FCH.0b013e3181d59487.

Reilly, J. J., Methven, E., McDowell, Z. C., Hacking, B., Alexander, D., Stewart, L., & Kelnar, C. J. (2003). Health consequences of obesity. *Archives of Disease in Childhood, 88*(9), 748–752.

Resnicow, K., Taylor, R., Baskin, M., & McCarty, F. (2005). Results of go girls: A weight control program for overweight African-American adolescent females. *Obesity Research, 13*(10), 1739–1748. doi:10.1038/oby.2005.212.

Rhee, K. (2008). Childhood overweight and the relationship between parent behaviors, parenting style, and family functioning. *The Annals of the American Academy of Political and Social Science, 615*(1), 11–37. doi:10.1177/0002716207308400.

Rideout, V. J., Foehr, U. G., & Roberts, D. F. (2010). Generation M [superscript 2]: Media in the Lives of 8-to 18-Year-Olds. *Henry J. Kaiser Family Foundation.*

Ritchie, L. D., Welk, G., Styne, D., Gerstein, D. E., & Crawford, P. B. (2005). Family environment and pediatric overweight: what is a parent to do? *Journal of the American Dietetic Association, 105*(5 Suppl 1), S70–S79. doi:10.1016/j.jada.2005.02.017.

Rollnick, S., Mason, P., & Butler, C. (1999). *Health behavior change: A guide for practitioners.* Philadelphia, PA: Elsevier Health Sciences.

Rossen, L. M., & Talih, M. (2014). Social determinants of disparities in weight among US children and adolescents. *Annals of Epidemiology, 24*(10), 705–713. e702. doi:10.1016/j. annepidem.2014.07.010

Rummo, P. E., Meyer, K. A., Boone-Heinonen, J., Jacobs, D. R., Jr., Kiefe, C. I., Lewis, C. E., .. . Gordon-Larsen, P. (2015). Neighborhood availability of convenience stores and diet quality: Findings from 20 years of follow-up in the coronary artery risk development in young adults study. *American Journal of Public Health, 105*(5), e65–73. doi:10.2105/ajph.2014.302435

Salvy, S. J., de la Haye, K., Bowker, J. C., & Hermans, R. C. (2012). Influence of peers and friends on children's and adolescents' eating and activity behaviors. *Physiology and Behavior, 106*(3), 369–378. doi:10.1016/j.physbeh.2012.03.022.

Schwartz, M. B., Henderson, K. E., Grode, G., Hyary, M., Kenney, E. L., O'Connell, M., & Middleton, A. E. (2015). Comparing current practice to recommendations for the child and adult care food program. *Child Obesity, 11*(5), 491–498. doi:10.1089/chi.2015.0041

Schwartz, M. B., Henderson, K. E., Read, M., Danna, N., & Ickovics, J. R. (2015). New school meal regulations increase fruit consumption and do not increase total plate waste. *Child Obesity, 11*(3), 242–247. doi:10.1089/chi.2015.0019

Shaya, F. T., Flores, D., Gbarayor, C. M., & Wang, J. (2008). School-based obesity interventions: A literature review. *Journal of School Health, 78*(4), 189–196. doi:10.1111/j.1746-1561.2008.00285.x.

Talma, H., Chinapaw, M. J., Bakker, B., HiraSing, R. A., Terwee, C. B., & Altenburg, T. M. (2013). Bioelectrical impedance analysis to estimate body composition in children and adolescents: A systematic review and evidence appraisal of validity, responsiveness, reliability and measurement error. *Obesity Reviews, 14*(11), 895–905. doi:10.1111/obr.12061.

Temple, M., & Robinson, J. C. (2014). A systematic review of interventions to promote physical activity in the preschool setting. *Journal for Specialists in Pediatric Nursing, 19*(4), 274–284. doi:10.1111/jspn.12081.

Torrijos-Nino, C., Martinez-Vizcaino, V., Pardo-Guijarro, M. J., Garcia-Prieto, J. C., Arias-Palencia, N. M., & Sanchez-Lopez, M. (2014). Physical fitness, obesity, and academic achievement in schoolchildren. *Journal of Pediatrics, 165*(1), 104–109. doi:10.1016/j. jpeds.2014.02.041.

Wadden, T. A., & Didie, E. (2003). What's in a name? Patients' preferred terms for describing obesity. *Obesity Research, 11*(9), 1140–1146. doi:10.1038/oby.2003.155.

Ward, D. (2011). *Policies on physical education and physical activity. A research synthesis.* Princeton, NJ. Retrieved from www.activelivingresearch.org

Wells, J. C., & Fewtrell, M. S. (2006). Measuring body composition. *Archives of Disease in Childhood, 91*(7), 612–617. doi:10.1136/adc.2005.085522.

Whitaker, R. C., Wright, J. A., Pepe, M. S., Seidel, K. D., & Dietz, W. H. (1997). Predicting obesity in young adulthood from childhood and parental obesity. *New England Journal of Medicine, 337*(13), 869–873. doi:10.1056/nejm199709253371301.

World Health Organization. (2015). Obesity and Overweight. Fact Sheet. Retrieved September 30, 2015, from http://www.who.int/mediacentre/factsheets/fs311/en/#.

WORKGROUP, B. F. P. S. (2015). 2015 Recommendations for preventive pediatric health care committee on practice and ambulatory medicine and bright futures periodicity schedule workgroup. *Pediatrics, 136*(3), e727.

Zimmer-Gembeck, M. J., & Collins, W. A. (2003). Autonomy development during adolescence. In G. R. Adams & M. Berzonsky (Eds.), *Blackwell handbook of adolescence* (pp. 175–204). Oxford: Blackwell.

Chapter 14
Preventing Eating Disorders in Adolescents

Maribel Plasencia, Salomé A. Wilfred, and Carolyn Black Becker

14.1   Overview of Eating Disorders

Eating disorders (EDs) comprise anorexia nervosa (AN), bulimia nervosa (BN), binge eating disorder (BED), and other specified feeding or eating disorder (OSFED) (American Psychiatric Association, 2013). Anorexia nervosa is characterized by excessive restriction of energy intake as well as significantly low body weight, body image disturbance, and an intense fear of gaining weight (American Psychiatric Association, 2013). The latter criteria may be fulfilled by behavior that undermines weight gain when at a significantly low weight. Bulimia nervosa involves frequent episodes of binge eating. Binge eating is defined as episodes of eating large amounts of food given the context during which individuals feel a loss of control. Individuals with BN also must engage in compensatory behaviors, such as purging, excessive dieting, exercise, or use of laxatives or diuretics, with the aim of preventing weight gain. Binge eating disorder is characterized by episodes of binge eating without a succeeding compensatory behavior. OSFED is a diagnosis used for individuals who

M. Plasencia, B. A.
Department of Psychology, Rutgers, The State University of New Jersey,
152 Frelinghuysen Road, Piscataway, NJ 08854, USA
e-mail: maribel.plasencia@rutgers.edu

S.A. Wilfred, B. A.
Department of Psychology, Assumption College,
500 Salisbury Street, Worcester, MA 01609, USA
e-mail: salome.wilfred@assumption.edu

C.B. Becker, Ph. D. (✉)
Department of Psychology, Trinity University, 1 Trinity Place, San Antonio, TX 78212, USA
e-mail: cbecker@trinity.edu

© Springer Science+Business Media New York 2016   285
M.R. Korin (ed.), *Health Promotion for Children and Adolescents*,
DOI 10.1007/978-1-4899-7711-3_14

have a clinically significant ED that does not meet criteria for one of the three listed above. Examples include atypical anorexia nervosa that does not meet the low weight requirement and purging disorder (American Psychiatric Association, 2013).

Often chronic (Beumont & Touyz, 2003), EDs are both costly (e.g., Agras, 2001) and difficult to treat (e.g., Agras et al., 2004). Together, studies support average durations of 4–11 years (Agras, Walsh, Fairburn, Wilson, & Kraemer, 2000; Beumont & Touyz, 2003; Stice, Marti, Shaw, & Jaconis, 2009). EDs additionally have the highest mortality rate out of any of the psychiatric disorders (Arcelus, Mitchell, Wales, & Nielsen, 2011; Sullivan, 1995). Research indicates that mortality rates typically result from complications arising from the disorder (e.g., cardiovascular complications; Jáuregui-Garrido & Jáuregui-Lobera, 2012), as well as suicide (Herzog et al., 2000). Unfortunately, EDs are frequently undertreated (Hudson, Hiripi, Pope, & Kessler, 2007). In addition to costs in terms of psychological and physical well-being, treatment for EDs is often financially expensive. For instance, BN and BED are as costly to treat as obsessive–compulsive disorder, and AN has treatment costs comparable to schizophrenia (Agras, 2001). Given the typical course and costs of EDs, recent efforts have targeted the prevention of their development.

Although EDs may onset at various points in the lifespan, adolescence is a particularly vulnerable time for the emergence of factors increase risk for developing an ED. Additionally, research demonstrates higher rates of EDs and/or disordered eating behaviors among this age group (e.g., Jones, Bennett, Olmsted, Lawson, and Rodin, 2001). In terms of mere prevalence, studies suggest that a high percentage of adolescent populations may present with partial or full syndromal EDs. For example, Jones et al. (2001) found that disordered eating behaviors were present in 27% of a sample of teenage girls ages 12–18. In terms of the development over the adolescent time-span, longitudinal research by Stice and colleagues (2009) suggests that between 13 and 17% of individuals with subthreshold status for an ED go on to develop threshold cases for BN and BED, respectively. Subthreshold cases were prevalent in about 17% of this sample (mean age = 13 years), providing evidence for the need for earlier prevention efforts. Research supported by the Mcknight Foundation (McKnight Investigators, 2003) additionally found that across time, 3% of a sample of adolescent girls in grades 6–9 developed at least sub-syndromal eating disordered behavior.

In addition to the finding that a subthreshold foundation for EDs may develop in early adolescence, research indicates that full criteria EDs commonly emerge in late adolescence. Anorexia nervosa, for example, has an average age of onset of 17 years (e.g., Steiner et al., 2003; Wentz, Gillberg, Anckarsäter, Gillberg, & Råstam, 2009). With regard to EDs more generally, research by Hudson et al. (2007) yielded an average age for onset for AN, BN, BED, subthreshold BED, and any binge eating of 18–21 years. Further, Stice and Agras (1998) found that an estimated 3% of adolescents engage in binge eating and purging. Given the high prevalence of risk factors and subclinical symptoms in adolescent populations, as well as the emergence of EDs in late adolescence, this particular age group is of great interest to researchers who seek to prevent the onset of an ED. The following provides a brief overview of the rationale for targeting adolescents, structural elements of prevention interventions, risk factors related to the onset of EDs, as well as a review of a selection of specific interventions that seek to reduce or eliminate these known risk factors in early to late adolescent populations.

14.2   Why Target Adolescence?

As noted above, significant evidence suggests that many EDs onset during adolescence and into young adulthood. As a result, a great deal of research has focused on the trajectory of the development of disordered eating behaviors among adolescent samples. Although the exact causes of adolescent onset are not entirely established, etiology likely involves a myriad of biological, psychological, and social–environmental factors. More specifically, adolescence is a period of time in which children undergo various changes that occur at these three levels. For instance, increases in levels of gonadal steroid hormones (e.g., testosterone, estrogen) lead to the development of external characteristics of reproductive maturation such as enlarged breast and facial hair (Sisk & Zehr, 2005). Thus, adolescents experience the development of both primary and secondary reproductive characteristics (Herpertz-Dahlmann, Bühren, & Remschmidt, 2013), which may impact body image. Importantly, body dissatisfaction has been found to be a potent risk factor for EDs (Jacobi & Fittig, 2010; see below for discussion).

Cognitively, a rewiring of cortical and limbic systems occurs, which leads to the development of adult cognitions, decision-making strategies, and social behaviors (Sisk & Zehr, 2005). Importantly, changes in the brain may differ by gender. Boys, for example, experience volume growth in the amygdala, an area involved in emotion processing and motivation, while girls experience growth in the hippocampus, an area associated with spatial navigation and memory (Herpertz-Dahlmann et al., 2013). Such changes are of significance, as they may indicate a neurological basis for gender-biased disorders among this population (e.g., depression, EDs). In addition to changes associated with puberty, the *timing* of such changes is also a factor that may influence the development of certain forms of psychopathology. Sisk and Zehr (2005) suggest that variations in the onset of puberty potentially lead to individual differences in behavior. Specifically, the development of EDs and depression has been found to be associated with early onset of puberty (Herpertz-Dahlmann et al., 2013; Stice, Presnell, & Bearman, 2001). Thus, interactions between such hormonal and cognitive changes may increase risk for developing some forms of psychopathology, particularly those that appear to be gender biased.

Research also has investigated genetic influence across this time period, demonstrating a variable influence of genetics over time. For instance, research conducted by Klump, McGue, and Iacono (2003) indicates that heritability for ED symptoms increases across puberty with genetics accounting for 0 % of variance in 11-year-old prepubertal twins and 54 % of the variance in 11- and 17-year-old *pubertal* twins. Thus, regarding heritability, 11-year-old pubertal twins appear more similar to 17-year-old pubertal twins than prepubertal twins their own age. Additional research suggests that the *influence* of genetics on disordered eating increases linearly as females advance through puberty (Klump, Burt, McGue, & Iacono, 2007). In summary, the multilevel changes experienced by this population have thus facilitated research investigating factors that adolescent populations may experience that put them at further risk for developing EDs, as well as strategies for prevention.

14.3 Eating Disorders Prevention: Overview

Prevention programs targeting adolescents generally employ a public health approach to mitigating the emergence of new ED cases by reducing associated risk factors. A risk factor is an initial condition that is associated with a later outcome (World Health Organization, 2002). ED prevention interventions seek to reduce the strength of risk factors or prevent them altogether as a means of decreasing one's likelihood for developing an ED. For example, body dissatisfaction is one of the most empirically supported risk factors for the development of an ED (e.g., Jacobi & Fittig, 2010; Neumark-Sztainer, Paxton, Hannan, Haines, & Story, 2006). An ED prevention program might then seek to reduce/eliminate body dissatisfaction as a way of decreasing onset of EDs. Public health approaches thus rely on the identification of known risk factors in the creation and implementation of prevention interventions.

True prevention is commonly taken to mean that one has prevented the emergence of the disorder. In other words, prevention happens when an intervention has reduced the actual onset of EDs that otherwise would have occurred. To demonstrate this, researchers typically utilize a randomized controlled trial (RCT) in which participants are randomly assigned to either the intervention condition or an assessment-only/wait-list control condition; the latter condition allows for observation of the natural occurrence of new cases of the disorder during the course of the trial. One challenge in ED prevention research is that the base rate of full syndrome EDs is high enough to be problematic but low enough to make finding statistical differences in onset challenging. As such, studies aimed at documenting true prevention typically need to be quite large (hundreds of participants) and have a fairly long follow-up. In other words, they are expensive to conduct.

In the absence of sufficient resources to investigate true prevention effects, many researchers measure reductions in known risk factors as a proxy for prevention effects. This is not an uncommon approach. For instance, researchers in other areas measure risk factors such as smoking cessation (a known risk factor for lung cancer and heart disease) as well as reductions in blood pressure and cholesterol as study outcomes. Yet, it is important to recognize that successfully reducing a very well-established risk factor may or may not actually prevent onset of the disorder of interest. For example, a given intervention might successfully reduce blood pressure but not sufficiently to actually impact heart attack onset. Thus, it is important to distinguish between studies that clearly demonstrate true prevention effects (e.g., a reduction in EDs) versus those that simply document a reduction in a risk factor (e.g., body dissatisfaction) and may or may not have yielded true prevention effects if such effects had been studied.

With regard to types of prevention efforts, according to the Institute of Medicine (Mrazek & Haggerty, 1994), prevention programs can be classified as universal, selective, or indicated. Universal programs seek to reach all individuals regardless of whether or not they are at a high or low risk for developing a disorder. Selective programs, alternatively, target individuals identified to be at risk for developing a disorder. Indicated programs are those designed to reach individuals who are experiencing symptoms of a disorder but do not yet meet full criteria. Thus, if an individual is provided with a prevention program due to the presentation of early symptoms, the program is considered indicated. Many ED prevention programs work at a somewhat selected level, though recent efforts have focused on universal programs. It is important to note that the Institute of Medicine's classification of programs applies categorical classification to degree of population risk, a variable which actually is more continuous in nature. As such, it can be difficult at times to accurately classify prevention efforts using the three category system. For instance, because being female is a significant risk factor for the development of EDs, one could argue that any prevention approach aimed at females is selective. Yet this obscures important differences between prevention approaches that target all females in a given community (thus reaching females who are at lower- and higher relative risk) versus those who target females with additional risk factors (e.g., elevated body dissatisfaction). For this reason, we focus more on whether or not programs clearly target high-risk samples (e.g., females with elevated body dissatisfaction) versus those that seek to intervene with mixed risk samples.

With adolescent populations, school-based prevention interventions appear to have a great deal of potential in terms of reaching many individuals in a structured community setting. Research currently suggests that these interventions can be further improved in terms of efficacy as well as logistics—particularly by increasing feasibility of implementing such programs (e.g., Sharpe, Schober, Treasure, & Schmidt, 2013). With regard to school-based prevention programs, researchers often study their effects by randomly assigning entire classrooms to receive either the intervention of interest or class as usual (e.g., Richardson, Paxton, & Thomson, 2009; Wilksch, Durbridge, & Wade, 2008). In some cases, the control condition is assessment only/wait-list. Although use of classrooms as the unit of randomization may create some limitations in terms of generalizability, such studies also can shed light on factors that may contribute to future success and/or failure of implementation. We may then evaluate these programs in distinct ways, including efficacy/ effectiveness in reducing risk factors, how feasible they are to implement in various settings (e.g., schools and community spaces), and acceptability by participants.

Research has identified several structural factors that are commonly associated with increased efficacy of ED prevention programs. For instance, a meta-analysis of ED prevention programs conducted by Stice and Shaw (2004) found that selective programs (i.e., those programs targeting individuals with a higher risk) produced larger effects compared to universal programs (i.e., programs employed without any consideration of an individual's level of risk). Stice and Shaw also found that selected intervention programs prevented the future development of eating pathology that was observed in control groups. These findings are promising in that the intervention programs not only decreased initial eating disturbances but also future development of syndromes. In terms of the success of selected interventions, the authors suggest that the distress experienced by the selected high-risk individuals may encourage or motivate such participants to actively engage in the program. It also is possible, however, that increased base rates of risk factors in selective programs makes it easier to find larger effects secondary to regression to the mean and/or a reduction in problems with floor effects. It also should be noted that some have argued that a majority of new cases will emerge from lower- and middle-risk samples because of differences in sample sizes in the general population (see Austin, 2001). Thus, there remain good reasons to continue universal prevention efforts with EDs.

Alcohol-intervention research conducted by Larimer and Cronce (2002) initially demonstrated that psychoeducational interventions (i.e., those programs that focused on information and education) were not as effective as interventions during which participants actively engaged in receiving feedback and developing skills. Stice and Shaw's meta-analysis replicated this finding with EDs, indicating that interactive programs (i.e., programs that required active participation) may be more effective compared to didactic/psychoeducational programs. A possible explanation for this finding is that interactive prevention programs facilitate engaged and active participants and in doing so, increase participant compliance with program materials. This engagement assists in the development of new ideas and skills, and encourages behavioral and attitudinal change.

Additionally, programs that used validated measures to track changes in participants yielded greater effects (Stice & Shaw, 2004). The use of validated measures may be advantageous as they are more sensitive in assessing dependent variables and are better indicators of areas in which participants have room to improve. Finally, multi-session intervention programs were more effective compared to single session programs (Stice & Shaw, 2004). Multi-session programs may allow individuals to properly learn skills and reflect upon material between sessions. Program leaders may also be able to provide feedback to participants who would like to improve upon learned skills from session to session.

A great deal of ED prevention programs have borrowed from these identified factors by designing interactive, multi-session programs that use validated measures to evaluate change. In addition to intervention structure, however, Stice and Shaw's (2004) meta-analysis further suggested that certain targeted risk factors (e.g., body dissatisfaction, thin-ideal internalization) and actual program content (e.g., dissonance-based, cognitive behavioral interventions) may associated with greater effect sizes.

14.4 Risk Factors for EDs

There are a number of identified risk factors for the development of EDs. Prevention focuses on altering modifiable risk factors (i.e., those that can be changed) versus fixed markers that put individuals at risk for developing an ED but cannot be altered (see Jacobi, Hayward, de Zwaan, Kraemer, & Agras, 2004). For example, research indicates that females at are a higher risk for developing an ED (e.g., Newman et al., 1996). Because gender is a marker that cannot be changed, however, prevention programs do no seek to intervene with this factor. Fixed markers are, however, helpful in identifying high-risk populations that may benefit from such programs. For instance, Stice and Shaw's meta-analysis (2004) found that intervention effects were significantly larger in programs that focused solely on females compared to programs that included males.

14.4.1 Fixed Markers

Both gender and ethnicity have been studied as fixed markers for the development of EDs. Research on ethnicity remains mixed, however, and future research is warranted to determine whether or not it is a true marker for ED development.

14.4.1.1 Gender

Females are at a higher relative risk for developing an ED, most likely due to both biological and sociocultural factors. As a result, many prevention programs have been designed with a female population in mind, though efforts are being made to address the prevention of EDs in males. From a biological perspective, differences in gonadal steroid hormone concentrations (e.g., estradiol, testosterone, progesterone) likely affect gender-biased prevalence rates across the ED spectrum. Gender-biased hormonal differences may occur at both the organizational (i.e., prenatal) and activational (i.e., postnatal) level (Klump et al., 2006). For example, lower levels of prenatal testosterone exposure, and higher levels of estradiol in puberty are associated with increased levels of disordered eating, indicating females are at a biologically higher risk for developing an ED, due to disparate endocrine function (Klump et al., 2006). These biological risk factors may then be exacerbated by cultural body messages that, in particular, target females and increase some of the modifiable risk factors discussed below (e.g., body dissatisfaction, thin-ideal internalization, self-objectification). More specifically, females experience significant cultural pressure to conform to the thin-ideal standard of female beauty (i.e., a figure that is very thin, with low body fat, narrow hips, long lean limbs, and large breasts). Because the thin-ideal is unachievable for the vast majority of females and because most girls move further away from the thin-ideal during puberty (i.e., experience increases in body fat), adolescence is a prime time for increasing body dissatisfaction. Adolescent girls also may experience significant increases in sexual objectification compared to younger girls (see Calogero, Tantleff-Dunn, & Thompson, 2011; Smolak & Murnen, 2011 for objectification review; see below for discussion of self-objectification).

14.4.1.2   Ethnicity

Research, involving ethnically diverse samples, though limited, has also identified ethnicity as a potential fixed marker for the development of certain types of EDs. Hispanic populations, for example, are postulated to be at a greater risk for developing disorders characterized by episodes of binge eating (e.g., BN and BED; Reyes-Rodríguez & Bulik, 2010), and Caucasian populations appear to be at greater risk than African-American women for developing AN and BN (Striegel-Moore et al., 2003). The McKnight Investigators (2003) additionally found that Hispanic girls at one site in their study were at a greater risk for developing an ED. It is important to note that more research on ethnicity is needed, as the literature on ethnicity and eating disorders is quite mixed. Further, Smolak and Striegel-Moore (2001) suggest it may be difficult to disentangle the relationship between ethnicity and EDs due to the fact that ethnicity is a summary variable encompassing various experiences (e.g., discrimination, immigration status). In summary, although existing research suggests that ethnicity may be a fixed marker for some EDs, additional research involving diverse samples is warranted to untangle the relationship between ethnicity and EDs.

14.4.2   Variable Risk Factors

14.4.2.1   Body Dissatisfaction

One of the most established risk factors for the development of an ED (see Jacobi & Fittig, 2010 for review), body dissatisfaction impacts up to 70 % of female adolescents (Levine & Smolak, 2004). Body dissatisfaction includes concerns that individuals have about weight and shape and may also relate to specific areas of the body. Body dissatisfaction has been shown to predict a multitude of negative outcomes in addition to full threshold EDs. These include depression and low self-esteem (e.g., Johnson & Wardle, 2005). Additionally, a study conducted by Neumark-Sztainer et al. (2006) found that higher levels of body dissatisfaction were associated with unhealthy versus healthy weight management behaviors in adolescent males and females. As such, programs targeting body dissatisfaction theoretically have the potential to reduce both EDs and other concerns (see Becker, Plasencia, Kilpela, Briggs, & Stewart, 2014 for further discussion), which may be one reason why many programs target this risk factor.

14.4.2.2   Dieting/Dietary Restriction

Severe dieting/dietary restriction also has been identified as a variable risk factor in the development of an ED (e.g., Fairburn, Welch, Doll, Davies, & O'Connor, 1997). Patton, Selzer, Coffey, Carlin, and Wolfe (1999) explored this risk factor in a longitudinal study of nearly 2000 Australian secondary school students. Results indicated that 8 % of adolescent females (age 15) reported dieting at severe levels and 60 % at moderate levels. Severe dieters were 18 times more likely to develop an ED within 6 months and at 12 months severe dieters had a one in five chance of developing a new ED. Additionally, moderate dieters were five times more likely to develop an ED within 6 months, and after 12 months, had a 1 in 40 chance of developing a new ED compared to participants who did not diet. Apart from level of dieting, type of dieting also may predict the onset of an ED. For instance, research suggests that depressed and feeling-fat dieters, versus vanity and over-weight dieters (i.e., those who diet to avoid adverse health consequences), are more likely to report having a lifetime ED (Isomaa, Isomaa, Marttunen, Kaltiala-Heino, & Björkqvist, 2010). Some research also suggests that fasting is a particular form of dieting that may confer increased risk for EDs (Stice, Davis, Miller, & Marti, 2008).

14.4.2.3   Negative Affect

Research also supports the role of negative affect in the development of bulimic behaviors (e.g., Stice, 2001; Stice & Agras, 1998). For instance, the dual pathway model, which is supported by research, proposes that body dissatisfaction increases both negative affect and dietary restraint, which in turn increase risk for EDs (Stice, 2001; Stice, Nemeroff, & Shaw, 1996). It is important to recognize, however, that the relationship between body dissatisfaction and negative affect, and EDs is likely complicated and multidirectional.

14.4.2.4   Self-Esteem

Low self-esteem also may serve as a risk factor for BN (e.g., Jacobi & Fittig, 2010). More specifically, research suggests that self-esteem may interact with other risk factors (e.g., perfectionism, body dissatisfaction) to predict bulimic pathology (Vohs, Bardone, Joiner, & Abramson, 1999; see Stice, 2002 for review). Isomaa et al. (2010) also found that depressed and feeling-fat dieters reported lower levels of self-esteem than other types of dieters and were 15 times more likely to develop an ED by age 18. In addition to being a risk factor, research has shown that high self-esteem may serve as a protective factor against the development of an ED (Cervera et al., 2003).

14.4.2.5   Self-Objectification

Self-objectification refers to the extent to which women internalize society's objec-tifying gaze of their bodies (i.e., views women's bodies as sexual objects) and begin to evaluate themselves in those terms (Fredrickson & Roberts, 1997). According to objectification theory, self-objectification increases body-related shame which in turn increases risk for both EDs and depression (Fredrickson & Roberts, 1997). Cross-sectional research supports the relationship between self-objectification and disordered eating (Greenleaf, 2005; see Tiggemann, 2011 for review). It is important to note, however, that objectification theory has not yet received robust longitudinal support (Becker, Hill, Greif, Han, & Stewart, 2013). As such, it is unclear if self-objectification is a risk factor or correlate of disordered eating.

14.4.2.6 Thin-Ideal Internalization

Defined as the extent to which individuals believe in/internalize the media's thin-ideal standards of beauty (e.g., Thompson & Stice, 2001), thin-ideal internalization may be viewed as a risk factor for other risk factors (e.g., body dissatisfaction and negative affect and dietary restraint; Stice, 2001; Stice, Schupak-Neuberg, Shaw, & Stein, 1994). Research has investigated both the direct and indirect role of thin-ideal internalization on ED pathology. For example, research by Stice et al. (1994) indicates that exposure to media predicts greater gender-role endorsement, which is associated with greater thin-ideal internalization. Thin-ideal internalization also predicts greater body dissatisfaction, which is both a correlate and risk factor for ED pathology. Thus, thin-ideal internalization mediates the effects of exposure to idealized images in the media on the development of ED pathology. Additional research has indicated that thin-ideal internalization prospectively predicts body dissatisfaction, dieting, and negative affect (Stice, 2001). Research also suggests that internalization of appearance-ideals in the media are associated with greater self-objectification (Calogero, Davis, & Thompson, 2005).

14.4.2.7 Perfectionism

Perfectionism also has been shown to predict and even maintain subclinical or full criteria EDs. More specifically, in a review of cross-sectional, longitudinal, and retrospective studies in the ED literature, Jacobi et al. (2004) concluded that perfectionism should be considered a risk factor for EDs. Research is mixed as to whether perfectionism differentially predicts the development of, or maintains, specific EDs. However, it is known to be present before onset of AN and BN, and may lead other known risk factors (e.g., severe dieting; Fairburn, Cooper, Doll, & Welch, 1999).

14.4.3 Environmental Factors

14.4.3.1 Family Mealtime Interactions

Various studies have explored the role that structured family meals and family mealtime interactions play in the development of disordered eating (Godfrey, Rhodes, & Hunt, 2013; Hamilton & Wilson, 2009). For instance, Neumark-Sztainer and colleagues (Neumark-Sztainer, Eisenberg, Fulkerson, Story, & Larson, 2008) concluded that families play a protective role in disordered eating behaviors among girls. More specifically, at 5-year follow-up girls whose families had regular family meals, engaged in less weight control behaviors, including self-induced vomiting, and use of diet pills or laxatives (Neumark-Sztainer et al., 2008). To our knowledge, however, prevention programs have yet to include components incorporating parents, but future work may seek to do so.

14.4.3.2 Peer Influences

A number of sociocultural models of disordered eating identify peers as a formative sociocultural influence that impacts body dissatisfaction among adolescents (Linville, Stice, Gau, & O'Neil, 2011; Shroff & Thompson, 2006). Studies support that notion that peers, directly and indirectly, may promote appearance-related norms, beauty ideals, and the importance of appearance. For instance, in a study with 433 adolescent girls, Jones, Vigfusdottir, and Lee (2004) found that appearance conversations with friends increased body dissatisfaction, with the relationship being mediated by appearance-ideal internalization. In addition, peer appearance criticism both indirectly (i.e., mediated by appearance-ideal internalization) and directly impacted body dissatisfaction. In the same study, with a sample of 347 boys, Jones et al. (2004) found that peer appearance criticism had the strongest association with body dissatisfaction. It is important to note, however, that this research was cross-sectional versus longitudinal. Moreover, although longitudinal research has partially supported the role of peers in later body dissatisfaction, that pattern appears to be complicated with the association varying across age groups (see Paxton, Eisenberg, & Neumark-Sztainer, 2006).

14.5 Common Components of Prevention Interventions for Adolescents

In addressing risk factors and certain environmental influences, there are several components that are common to many prevention programs aimed at adolescents. Media literacy is perhaps the most common, and entails learning about the unrealistic thin-ideal standard of beauty promoted in western culture's media (e.g., Wilksch & Wade, 2009). This component sheds light on photo editing, lighting, and the manner in which many images presented by the media are unattainable constructions of a profiting industry. Education on media literacy is based on social inoculation theory (McGuire, 1964; see Turner & Shepherd, 1999 for review), which aims to help participants build skills to resist social persuasions and pressures. A second component involves learning about interactions with peers and social comparisons. Usually, these sessions include lessons about "fat talk" (Nichter & Nichter, 2009) or any speech that implicitly or explicitly reinforces the thin-ideal.

An example of this negative body talk may be, "Does this dress make me look fat?" or, "You look so great. Have you lost weight?" Participants learn that these commonplace phrases and comparisons perpetuate the thin-ideal standard of beauty and are encouraged to eliminate this speech themselves in addition to preventing fat talk from occurring within their friend groups. Finally, many, though not all, adolescent prevention programs have a material devoted to self-esteem, which is put in place to not only buffer the development of EDs, but provide adolescents with a general tool for healthy and happy development across a time period marked by radical changes.

Although programs may vary in content, mode of delivery, theoretical basis, and duration, many prevention programs carry some or all of the above components. Below we describe a selection of programs that have been developed and tested by researchers. Many are evaluated when delivered in school or university settings. Note that it is beyond the scope of this chapter to review all programs available.

14.6 Programs Targeting Early Adolescence (11–13 Years of Age)

14.6.1 Me, You, and Us

The program *Me, You, and* Us (Sharpe et al., 2013) is a 6-session program that covers various topics including media literacy on standards of beauty, peer interactions such as fat talk, and sessions based on positive psychology principles (e.g., noticing one's strengths, increasing self-esteem). This program has been evaluated when delivered by teachers in school settings. In a recent study with adolescent girls in UK secondary schools grades 8–9, or girls approximately 12–14 years of age, this program was found to increase body esteem and reduce thin-ideal internalization (Sharpe et al., 2013). Both of these effects were maintained 3 months after intervention. However, *You, Me, and Us* was not found to produce any differences in eating pathology, peer factors, or depression (Sharpe et al., 2013), and the finding with regard to eating pathology raises concerns about its ability to actually prevent EDs.

14.6.2 BodyThink

BodyThink is the Australian version of a workshop developed by the Dove Self-Esteem Project (formerly the Dove Self-Esteem Fund). Other contributors included the Butterfly Foundation in Australia, Girls Scouts of the USA and BEAT (the UK ED association). In the UK, the program is distributed under the name *BodyTalk*. *BodyThink* focuses on media literacy, self-esteem, and seeks to reduce factors such as appearance teasing, thin-ideal internalization, and appearance, or body comparisons. Richardson et al. (2009) evaluated this program with 277 students in grade 7 (mean age = 12 years) from four secondary schools in Australia. This study was unusual in that it included males in its sample. In order to evaluate the program, researchers assigned entire classes to the intervention group or the control group. Participants in the intervention group completed four 50-min interactive sessions of *BodyThink*. Outcome variables were assessed baseline, postintervention, and 3-month follow-up.

Results revealed that girls in the intervention group had higher media literacy on a majority of specified content and lower thin-ideal internalization. However, Richardson et al. (2009) found no significant differences on measures of body dissatisfaction, dietary restraint, or bulimic symptoms raising concerns about the programs efficacy. These findings are particularly problematic given the widespread dissemination of this program. For instance by June of 2008, 40,000 adolescents had participated in the program (Richardson et al., 2009).

14.6.3 Media Smart

Wilksch and Wade (2009) evaluated the effectiveness of *Media Smart*, a media literacy program, compared to a control condition in grade 8 students (mean age = 13.62; $N = 540$) when delivered in a universal fashion. The program consists of eight 50-min sessions designed to be interactive through the use of group work. Participants received two lessons per week in this study. Wilksch and Wade sought to reduce weight and shape concern, though dieting, body dissatisfaction, media internalization, perceived pressure, ineffectiveness, depression, and self-esteem also were evaluated. Entire classes were randomly assigned to receive either *Media Smart* or a control condition. Data was collected at pre-intervention, postintervention (i.e., 1 month after the intervention), and 6-month follow-up. This study also included 30-month follow-up, the longest follow-up in this age group for this type of program.

The group receiving *Media Smart* had lower mean scores for shape and weight concerns, dieting, body dissatisfaction, feelings of ineffectiveness, and depression at post-intervention, 6-month follow-up, and 30-month follow-up. When evaluated by gender, girls receiving *Media Smart* reported lower feelings of ineffectiveness at posttest, and lower shape and weight concern than controls at 30-month follow-up. Boys had lower rates of body dissatisfaction, feelings of ineffectiveness, and dieting at posttest. At 6-month follow-up, boys reported lower weight and shape concern. Although girls receiving *Media Smart* reported lower weight and shape concern at a 30-month follow-up, attrition had reached approximately 46% at this time point, and this finding was not present at post or 6-month follow-up. Limitations of this study included the fact that the control group did not receive an alternate intervention, there was no assessment of disordered eating habits, and there was missing data from almost half of study participants at 30-month follow-up. It should be noted that a preliminary trial of *Media Smart* with 15 year-olds (see below for review) indicated that it was comparable to a control condition (i.e., class as usual) and was not as effective as a perfectionism-based intervention. Overall, replication trials are needed to ascertain the effectiveness of *Media Smart* in adolescent populations.

14.6.4   Cognitive-Dissonance-Based Prevention

A recent study by Halliwell and Diedrichs (2014) evaluated a cognitive-dissonance-based intervention delivered to 12- and 13-year-old girls in a school setting. The theory of cognitive dissonance (Festinger, 1957) proposes that psychological discomfort arises when an individual's beliefs and behaviors are misaligned. In order to mitigate this discomfort, individuals typically alter beliefs to comply with behaviors and actions. Dissonance-based programs aimed at ED prevention aim to have participants speak and act against the thin-ideal, which should lower investment in the thin-ideal. This theoretically creates a cascading effect reducing body dissatisfaction, negative affect, dietary restraint, and early stage eating disorder pathology (see Stice, Rohde, & Shaw, 2013 for review of dissonance-based programs). Research does provide support for the theoretical mechanism of action of this type of program (see Stice, Becker, & Yokum, 2013).

Though cognitive-dissonance-based approaches have received substantial empirical support in older populations (e.g., females 14 years of age or older, see Becker, Mackenzie, & Stewart, in press for review), this type of intervention has only recently been examined with younger samples. To test the younger adolescent version of the dissonance-based intervention, Halliwell and Diedrichs assigned two classes to receive the intervention and two classes to attend class as usual. The intervention was administered once per week for 4 weeks by a doctoral student or one of the authors. Each session was 20 min long. Four weeks after the intervention, participants took part in a media exposure task in which they were asked to rate the effectiveness of four advertisements featuring models or control images.

Results indicated that participants receiving the intervention reported lower levels of body dissatisfaction and thin-ideal internalization from pre- to posttest. Additionally, these participants experienced no changes in body satisfaction after being exposed to images of models vs. control images, whereas control participants reported greater body dissatisfaction after viewing advertisements containing models. Longer, more controlled trials, however are needed to ultimately determine the degree to which this program is efficacious for this age group.

In summary, research is at a relatively young stage for this age group when it comes to ED prevention. Although there have been some promising advances, no study to date has demonstrated true prevention effects, and even risk-factor reduction effects need improving. Further, replication of positive findings is needed, ideally with better controlled and longer trials.

14.7 Programs Targeting Mid to Late Adolescents (14–19 Years)

14.7.1 Media Literacy vs. Perfectionism-Based Prevention

Research by Wilksch et al. (2008) evaluated two, 8-lesson programs that focused on either media literacy (note: this was an early version *Media Smart*) or perfectionism versus a control group receiving no intervention. Both interventions were interactive and involved some group work. Participants with a mean age of 15 years were randomly assigned by class to receive either of the interventions or the control. Data was collected at pre, post, and 3-month follow-up. Some classes received 8 sessions over 8 weeks while other classes received 8 sessions over 4 weeks. Dependent variables included concern over mistakes, weight and shape concerns, and personal standards.

Participants receiving the perfectionism-based intervention had lower scores on concern over mistakes than the other two groups at a 3-month follow-up. Additionally, they reported significantly lower mean scores on personal standards compared to the media literacy group. Regarding concern over mistakes, high-risk participants in the perfectionism-based intervention also scored lower than high-risk individuals the other groups at 3-month follow-up. Results indicated that high-risk individuals receiving the perfectionism-based intervention experienced the most improvement.

There were no interaction outcomes for weight and shape concern for any group, suggesting the programs had little impact on this key risk factor. On the positive side, this study demonstrated that high-risk individuals may benefit from a universal program. This is important because universal programs can be more convenient to implement in school settings where it may be less desirable (i.e., more stigmatizing) to separate high-risk participants from their peers. On the negative side, the effects of the media literacy-based intervention largely were comparable to the control group. Limitations of this study included the fact that the control group did not receive a placebo intervention, the short follow-up, no ED behaviors were measured, and there was a difference in the timing of delivery of the intervention. However, this study demonstrates that perfectionism-focused programs may decrease some, but not all, risk factors with mid adolescents (e.g., 15-year-olds).

14.7.2 My Body My Life

In a series of studies, Paxton and colleagues investigated related internet-based programs for adult women and adolescent girls. The first program, *Set Your Body Free* consisted of eight, 90-min sessions provided weekly, which included psychoeducation along with interactive activities in order to improve body image, reduce ED symptomatology, and regulate eating patterns in women reporting higher levels of body dissatisfaction (Gollings & Paxton, 2006). *Set Your Body Free* also includes motivational interviewing and provides information on monitoring eating and body dissatisfaction. Later sessions focus on body image and self-esteem, social comparisons, and the importance of thinness to one's self-concept. The final session is devoted to relapse prevention and strategies to help participants overcome slips.

Set Your Body Free has been tested in both face-to-face formats as well as synchronously via the Internet. The preliminary trial was aimed at young adult women including older adolescents. Results from this trial indicated that women experienced improvements in body dissatisfaction, eating behaviors, self-esteem, depression, and anxiety (Gollings & Paxton, 2006). These results were maintained at a 2-month follow-up. A later trial (Paxton, McLean, Gollings, Faulkner, & Wertheim, 2007) including a control group demonstrated that *Set Your Body Free* improved body dissatisfaction, eating attitudes and behaviors, and depression in body-dissatisfied women, with results maintained at a 6-month follow-up. Although face-to-face delivery was superior to the Internet-delivered program at post-intervention, the two delivery modes produced similar results at 6-month follow-up.

My Body My Life (Heinicke, Paxton, McLean, & Wertheim, 2007) explicitly targets adolescent girls. Like *Set Your Body Free, My Body My Life* combines psycho-education and self-help intervention activities. This program is delivered online over 6 sessions with a 2-month follow-up session, and incorporates information and activities about social pressures, fat talk, teasing, and social comparison all of which are postulated to be very relevant to adolescents (Heinicke et al., 2007). Relative to a delayed intervention control group, girls (mean age 14.4 years) who participated in *My Body My Life* reported significantly greater improvements in body dissatisfaction and disordered eating symptoms at post-intervention. Improvements in disordered eating symptoms were maintained through 6-month follow-up (Heinicke et al., 2007).

14.7.3   Student Bodies

An internet-based cognitive-behavioral intervention, *Student Bodies* seeks to improve body image and to reduce unhealthy weight control behaviors and binge eating (Winzelberg et al., 2000; Zabinski, Wilfley, Calfas, Winzelberg, & Taylor, 2004). This program involves a psycho-educational component regarding EDs as well as body-image-related content and cognitive-behavioral strategies to improve body satisfaction. The program consists of both mandatory and optional homework assignments, which include contributing to an online discussion group designed to foster emotional support among participants. It has been tested using both asynchronous and synchronous moderation, typically with high-risk college-aged women including older adolescents.

In a series of trials (e.g., Celio et al., 2000; Winzelberg et al., 2000; Zabinski et al., 2004; see Sinton & Taylor, 2010 for review) researchers demonstrated that *Student Bodies* improves body image and self-esteem, drive for thinness, eating pathology, and weight and shape concern among female adolescents and adults.

After observing early results, Taylor et al., 2006, tested *Student Bodies* against a wait-list control in an RCT including 480 participants with high weight and shape concerns. This trial indicated that *Student Bodies* was effective in reducing shape and weight concerns among college age women at a high risk for developing an ED out to 12-month follow-up (Taylor et al., 2006). Importantly, this was the first trial to find some evidence of true prevention effects. Although Taylor et al. (2006) did not find a significant difference in ED onset in the intervention versus control group when the full sample was analyzed, *Student Bodies* did decrease the onset of ED cases in participants with a higher BMI and, at one site, participants that engaged in compensatory behaviors prior to receiving the intervention.

14.7.4   The Body Project

The *Body Project* is a small group, cognitive dissonance-based intervention developed by Stice and colleagues. Based on the dual pathway model of ED etiology, the *Body Project* encourages participants to actively challenge the thin-ideal through activities, group discussion, and homework. Theoretically, anti-thin-ideal statements and behaviors result in cognitive dissonance that decreases thin-ideal internalization with cascading effects in body dissatisfaction, negative affect, dietary restraint, and ED pathology. As noted above, research supports the theoretical basis of the Body Project (Stice et al., 2013).

The Body Project is supported by a substantial research base. After preliminary studies supported the risk-factor reduction effects of the Body Project (e.g., Stice, Mazotti, Weibel, & Agras, 2000; Stice, Trost, & Chase, 2003), Stice and colleagues conducted a large-scale investigation of the program's efficacy with over 400 high-risk female students recruited from both high schools and colleges. Results indicated that the Body Project reduced thin-ideal internalization, body dissatisfaction, dieting, negative affect, and bulimic symptoms at post-intervention and 6-month follow-up. Many effects were maintained at 1-year follow-up (Stice, Shaw, Burton, & Wade, 2006). At 3-year follow-up, compared to an assessment only control condition, Body Project participants reported decreased body dissatisfaction, negative affect, and psychosocial impairment (Stice, Marti, Spoor, Presnell, & Shaw, 2008). Perhaps most importantly, at 3-year follow-up the Body Project reduced onset of EDs relative to the control condition by 60 %, demonstrating true prevention effects for the full sample.

To date, the Body Project has amassed more support than any other ED prevention program. For instance, it has repeatedly produced superior effects compared to both active control interventions and assessment-only groups (Becker, Smith, & Ciao, 2006; Stice et al., 2001, 2003, 2006, 2008; Stice, Rohde, Gau, & Shaw, 2009) and is supported by studies conducted by labs independent from the intervention developers (e.g., Becker, Smith, & Ciao, 2005; Green, Scott, Diyankova, & Gasser, 2005; Matusek, Wendt, & Wiseman, 2004; Roehrig, Thompson, Brannick, & Van den Berg, 2006). Empirical research has additionally identified the *Body Project* as a program with favorable effects when implemented in a universal/selective fashion using lower cost providers. For instance, research by Becker and colleagues (Becker et al., 2006, 2010; Becker, Bull, Schaumberg, Cauble, & Franco, 2008) investigated whether or not the *Body Project* could feasibly be run by peer leaders in sororities using a "task-shifting" model (Fairburn & Patel, 2014). This research evaluated if the Body Project would still be effective when provided on a mandatory basis to all members of a community (i.e., universal approach) using low-cost providers (i.e., peers). Even when delivered by peer leaders to participants who were required to participate, results indicated that the *Body Project* yielded significant changes in thin-ideal internalization, body dissatisfaction, dietary restraint, and ED pathology. This line of research provides preliminary support for its dissemination.

14.7.5   Healthy Weight

The *Healthy Weight* intervention was originally developed by Stice and colleagues as placebo intervention to be tested against the *Body Project.* In addition to a psychoeducational component, the most recently modified version of the *Healthy Weight* program incorporates elements of motivational interviewing and behavior modification in order to promote healthy weight management that, in turn, reduces risk of engaging in unhealthy weight management behaviors (e.g., binging and purging, extreme dieting, and exercise). After finding that this program led to reductions in dieting, negative affect, and ED symptoms in females with body image concerns (Stice, Chase, Stormer, & Appel, 2001), Stice and colleagues decided to test it as an actual intervention (Stice et al., 2003, 2006, 2008). In the previously discussed large-scale prevention trial (see *Body Project*), *Healthy Weight* was found to significantly reduce ED risk factors and bulimic symptoms at 1-year follow-up. At 3 years, *Healthy Weight* significantly reduced thin-ideal internalization, body dissatisfaction, negative affect, and bulimic symptoms. Importantly, *Health Weight* produced similar reductions in ED onset compared to assessment only as the Body Project. Thus, *Healthy Weight* also produces true ED prevention effects. Research also suggests that implementation of this small group intervention can be task-shifted to undergraduate peer leaders if the protocol is sufficiently modified to meet their needs as providers (Becker et al., 2010).

14.8   Conclusion

Although significant progress has been made in reducing ED risk factors, to date only three programs have any data to support their ability to actually prevent EDs. Further, many trials are underpowered, lack adequate control groups, and need longer follow-up periods. Future research should aim to address these limitations in the existing literature in addition to investigating strategies for disseminating existing programs with documented efficacy/effectiveness. Additional research also is needed to identify better strategies for younger adolescents. Notably, no trial has prevented any eating disorders in this population. Future work also could further tailor programs to address gender-specific concerns regarding body image with a focus on greater inclusion of males.

References

Agras, W. S. (2001). The consequences and costs of the eating disorders. *Psychiatric Clinics of North America, 24*(2), 371–379.

Agras, W. S., Brandt, H. A., Bulik, C. M., Dolan-Sewell, R., Fairburn, C. G., Halmi, K. A., … Wilfley, D. E. (2004). Report of the National Institutes of Health workshop on overcoming barriers to treatment research in anorexia nervosa. *International Journal of Eating Disorders, 35*(4), 509–521.

Agras, W. S., Walsh, T., Fairburn, C. G., Wilson, G. T., & Kraemer, H. C. (2000). A multicenter comparison of cognitive-behavioral therapy and interpersonal psychotherapy for bulimia nervosa. *Archives of General Psychiatry, 57*(5), 459–466.

American Psychiatric Association. (2013). *Diagnostic and statistical manual of mental disorders* (5th ed.). Arlington, VA: American Psychiatric.

Arcelus, J., Mitchell, A. J., Wales, J., & Nielsen, S. (2011). Mortality rates in patients with anorexia nervosa and other eating disorders: A meta-analysis of 36 studies. *Archives of General Psychiatry, 68*(7), 724–731.

Austin, S. B. (2001). Population-based prevention of eating disorders: An application of the Rose prevention model. *Preventive Medicine, 32*, 268–283.

Becker, C. B., Bull, S., Schaumberg, K., Cauble, A., & Franco, A. (2008). Effectiveness of peer-led eating disorders prevention: A replication trial. *Journal of Consulting and Clinical Psychology, 76*(2), 347–354.

Becker, C. B., Hill, K., Greif, R., Han, H., & Stewart, T. (2013). Reducing self-objectification: Are dissonance-based methods a possible approach? *The Journal of Eating Disorders, 1*(10), doi:10.1186/2050-2974-1-10

Becker, C. B., Mackenzie, K., & Stewart, T. (in press). Cognitive and behavioral approaches to the prevention of eating disorders. In M. Levine & L. Smolak (Eds.), *Wiley-Blackwell handbook of eating disorders*. Hoboken: Wiley.

Becker, C. B., Plasencia, M., Kilpela, L. S., Briggs, M., & Stewart, T. (2014). Changing the course of comorbid eating disorders and depression: What is the role of public health interventions in targeting shared risk factors? *Journal of Eating Disorders, 2*(1), 15.

Becker, C. B., Smith, L. M., & Ciao, A. C. (2005). Reducing eating disorder risk factors in sorority members: A randomized trial. *Behavior Therapy, 36*, 245–253.

Becker, C. B., Smith, L. M., & Ciao, A. C. (2006). Peer-facilitated eating disorder prevention: A randomized effectiveness trial of cognitive dissonance and media advocacy. *Journal of Consulting and Clinical Psychology, 53*(4), 550–565.

Becker, C. B., Wilson, C., Williams, A., Kelly, M., McDaniel, L., & Elmquist, J. (2010). Peer-facilitated cognitive dissonance versus healthy weight eating disorders prevention: A randomized comparison. *Body Image, 7*(4), 280–288.

Beumont, P. J., & Touyz, S. W. (2003). What kind of illness is anorexia nervosa? *European Child & Adolescent Psychiatry, 12*(1), i20–i24.

Calogero, R. M., Davis, W. N., & Thompson, J. K. (2005). The role of self-objectification in the experience of women with eating disorders. *Sex Roles, 52*(1–2), 43–50.

Calogero, R. M., Tantleff-Dunn, S. E., & Thompson, J. K. (2011). Objectification theory: An introduction. In R. M. Calogero, S. E. Tantleff-Dunn, & J. K. Thompson (Eds.), *Self-objectification in women: Causes, consequences, and counteractions* (pp. 3–22). Washington, DC: American Psychological Association.

Celio, A. A., Winzelberg, A. J., Wilfley, D. E., Eppstein-Herald, D., Springer, E. A., Dev, P., & Taylor, C. B. (2000). Reducing risk factors for eating disorders: Comparison of an internet-and a classroom-delivered psychoeducational program. *Journal of Consulting and Clinical Psychology, 68*(4), 650–657.

Cervera, S., Lahortiga, F., Martínez-González, M. A., Gual, P., Irala-Estévez, J. D., & Alonso, Y. (2003). Neuroticism and low self-esteem as risk factors for incident eating disorders in a prospective cohort study. *International Journal of Eating Disorders, 33*(3), 271–280.

Fairburn, C. G., Cooper, Z., Doll, H. A., & Welch, S. L. (1999). Risk factors for anorexia nervosa: Three integrated case-control comparisons. *Archives of General Psychiatry, 56*(5), 468–476.

Fairburn, C. G., & Patel, V. (2014). The global dissemination of psychological treatments: A road map for research and practice. *American Journal of Psychiatry, 171*(5), 495–498.

Fairburn, C. G., Welch, S. L., Doll, H. A., Davies, B. A., & O'Connor, M. E. (1997). Risk factors for bulimia nervosa: A community-based case-control study. *Archives of General Psychiatry, 54*(6), 509–517.

Festinger, L. (1957). *A theory of cognitive dissonance.* Stanford, CA: Stanford University Press.

Fredrickson, B. L., & Roberts, T. A. (1997). Objectification theory. *Psychology of Women Quarterly, 21*(2), 173–206.

Godfrey, K., Rhodes, P., & Hunt, C. (2013). The relationship between family mealtime interactions and eating disorder in childhood and adolescence: A systematic review. *Australian and New Zealand Journal of Family Therapy, 34*, 54–74.

Gollings, E. K., & Paxton, S. J. (2006). Comparison of internet and face-to-face delivery of a group body image and disordered eating intervention for women: A pilot study. *Eating Disorders, 14*(1), 1–15.

Green, M., Scott, N., Diyankova, I., & Gasser, C. (2005). Eating disorder prevention: An experimental comparison of high level dissonance, low level dissonance, and no-treatment control. *Eating Disorders, 13*(2), 157–169.

Greenleaf, C. (2005). Self-objectification among physically active women. *Sex Roles, 52*(1–2), 51–62.

Halliwell, E., & Diedrichs, P. H. (2014). Testing a dissonance body image intervention among young girls. *Health Psychology, 33*(2), 201–204.

Hamilton, S. K., & Wilson, J. H. (2009). Family mealtimes: Worth the effort? *Infant, Child and Adolescent Nutrition, 1*, 346–350.

Heinicke, B. E., Paxton, S. J., McLean, S. A., & Wertheim, E. H. (2007). Internet-delivered targeted group intervention for body dissatisfaction and disordered eating in adolescent girls: A randomized controlled trial. *Journal of Abnormal Child Psychology, 35*(3), 379–391.

Herpertz-Dahlmann, B., Bühren, K., & Remschmidt, H. (2013). Growing up is hard: Mental disorders in adolescence. *Deutsches Ärzteblatt International, 110*(25), 432.

Herzog, D. B., Greenwood, D. N., Dorer, D. J., Flores, A. T., Ekeblad, E. R., Richards, A., … Keller, M. B. (2000). Mortality in eating disorders: A descriptive study. *International Journal of Eating Disorders, 28*(1), 20–26.

Hudson, J. I., Hiripi, E., Pope, H. G., Jr., & Kessler, R. C. (2007). The prevalence and correlates of eating disorders in the national comorbidity survey replication. *Biological Psychiatry, 61*(3), 348–358.

Isomaa, R., Isomaa, A., Marttunen, M., Kaltiala-Heino, R., & Björkqvist, K. (2010). Psychological distress and risk for eating disorders in subgroups of dieters. *European Eating Disorders Review, 18*(4), 296–303.

Jacobi, C., & Fittig, E. (2010). Psychosocial risk factors for eating disorders. In W. S. Agras (Ed.), *The Oxford handbook of eating disorders* (pp. 123–136). New York, NY: Oxford University Press.

Jacobi, C., Hayward, C., de Zwaan, M., Kraemer, H. C., & Agras, W. S. (2004). Coming to terms with risk factors for eating disorders: Application of risk terminology and suggestions for a general taxonomy. *Psychological Bulletin, 130*(1), 19–65.

Jáuregui-Garrido, B., & Jáuregui-Lobera, I. (2012). Sudden death in eating disorders. *Vascular Health and Risk Management, 8*, 91.

Johnson, F., & Wardle, J. (2005). Dietary restraint, body dissatisfaction, and psychological distress: A prospective analysis. *Journal of Abnormal Psychology, 114*(1), 119–125.

Jones, J. M., Bennett, S., Olmsted, M. P., Lawson, M. L., & Rodin, G. (2001). Disordered eating attitudes and behaviours in teenaged girls: A school-based study. *Canadian Medical Association Journal, 165*(5), 547–552.

Jones, D. C., Vigfusdottir, T. H., & Lee, Y. (2004). Body image and the appearance culture among adolescent girls and boys an examination of friend conversations, peer criticism, appearance magazines, and the internalization of appearance ideals. *Journal of Adolescent Research, 19*(3), 323–339.

Klump, K. L., Burt, S. A., McGue, M., & Iacono, W. G. (2007). Changes in genetic and environmental influences on disordered eating across adolescence: A longitudinal twin study. *Archives of General Psychiatry, 64*(12), 1409–1415.

Klump, K. L., Gobrogge, K. L., Perkins, P. S., Thorne, D., Sisk, C. L., & Breedlove, S. (2006). Preliminary evidence that gonadal hormones organize and activate disordered eating. *Psychological Medicine, 36*(04), 539–546.

Klump, K. L., McGue, M., & Iacono, W. G. (2003). Differential heritability of eating attitudes and behaviors in prepubertal versus pubertal twins. *International Journal of Eating Disorders, 33*(3), 287–292.

Larimer, M. E., & Cronce, J. M. (2002). Identification, prevention and treatment: A review of individual-focused strategies to reduce problematic alcohol consumption by college students. *Journal of Studies on Alcohol and Drugs Supplement, 63*, 148–164.

Levine, M. P., & Smolak, L. (2004). Body image development in adolescence. In T. F. Cash & T. Pruzinsky (Eds.), *Body image: A handbook of theory, research, and clinical practice* (pp. 74–82). New York, NY: Guilford Press.

Linville, D., Stice, E., Gau, J., & O'Neil, M. (2011). Predictive effects of mother and peer influences on increases in adolescent eating disorder risk factors and symptoms: A 3-year longitudinal study. *International Journal of Eating Disorders, 44*(8), 745–751.

Matusek, J. A., Wendt, S. J., & Wiseman, C. V. (2004). Dissonance thin-ideal and didactic healthy behavior eating disorder prevention programs: Results from a controlled trial. *International Journal of Eating Disorders, 36*, 376–388.

McGuire, W. (1964). Inducing resistance to persuasion. In L. Berkowitz (Ed.), *Advances in experimental social psychology* (pp. 191–229). New York, NY: Academic Press.

McKnight Investigators. (2003). Risk factors for the onset of eating disorders in adolescent girls: Results of the McKnight longitudinal risk factor study. *American Journal of Psychiatry, 160*(2), 248–254.

Mrazek, P. J., & Haggerty, R. J. (Eds.). (1994). *Reducing risks for mental disorders: Frontiers for preventive intervention research.* Washington, DC: National Academies Press.

Neumark-Sztainer, D., Eisenberg, M. E., Fulkerson, J. A., Story, M., & Larson, N. I. (2008). Family meals and disordered eating in adolescents: Longitudinal findings from project EAT. *Archives of Pediatrics & Adolescent Medicine, 162*(1), 17–22. doi:10.1001/archpediatrics.2007.9.

Neumark-Sztainer, D., Paxton, S. J., Hannan, P. J., Haines, J., & Story, M. (2006). Does body satisfaction matter? Five-year longitudinal associations between body satisfaction and health behaviors in adolescent females and males. *Journal of Adolescent Health, 39*(2), 244–251.

Newman, D. L., Moffitt, T. E., Caspi, A., Magdol, L., Silva, P. A., & Stanton, W. R. (1996). Psychiatric disorder in a birth cohort of young adults: Prevalence, comorbidity, clinical significance, and new case incidence from ages 11 to 21. *Journal of Consulting and Clinical Psychology, 64*, 552–562.

Nichter, M., & Nichter, M. (2009). *Fat talk: What girls and their parents say about dieting.* Cambridge, MA: Harvard University Press.

Patton, G. C., Selzer, R., Coffey, C., Carlin, J. B., & Wolfe, R. (1999). Onset of adolescent eating disorders: Population based cohort study over 3 years. *British Medical Journal, 318*(7186), 765–768.

Paxton, S. J., Eisenberg, M. E., & Neumark-Sztainer, D. (2006). Prospective predictors of body dissatisfaction in adolescent girls and boys: A five-year longitudinal study. *Developmental Psychology, 42*(5), 888.

Paxton, S. J., McLean, S. A., Gollings, E. K., Faulkner, C., & Wertheim, E. H. (2007). Comparison of face-to-face and Internet interventions for body image and eating problems in adult women: An RCT. *International Journal of Eating Disorders, 40*, 692–704.

Reyes-Rodríguez, M. L., & Bulik, C. M. (2010). Hacia una adaptación cultural del tratamiento de trastornos alimentarios para Latinos residentes en Estados Unidos. *Revista Mexicana de Trastornos Alimentarios, 1*(1), 27–35.

Richardson, S. M., Paxton, S. J., & Thomson, J. S. (2009). Is *BodyThink* an efficacious body image and self-esteem program? A controlled evaluation with adolescents. *Body Image, 6*(2), 75–82.

Roehrig, M., Thompson, J. K., Brannick, M., & Van den Berg, P. (2006). Dissonance-based eating disorder prevention program: A preliminary dismantling investigation. *International Journal of Eating Disorders, 39*, 1–10.

Sharpe, H., Schober, I., Treasure, J., & Schmidt, U. (2013). Feasibility, acceptability and efficacy of a school-based prevention programme for eating disorders: Cluster randomised controlled trial. *The British Journal of Psychiatry, 203*(6), 428–435.

Shroff, H., & Thompson, J. K. (2006). Peer influences, body-image dissatisfaction, eating dysfunction and self-esteem in adolescent girls. *Journal of Health Psychology, 11*(4), 533–551.

Sinton, M., & Taylor, C. B. (2010). Prevention: Current status and underlying theory. In W. E. Agras (Ed.), *Oxford handbook of eating disorders* (pp. 307–333). New York, NY: Oxford University Press.

Sisk, C. L., & Zehr, J. L. (2005). Pubertal hormones organize the adolescent brain and behavior. *Frontiers in Neuroendocrinology, 26*(3), 163–174.

Smolak, L., & Murnen, S. K. (2011). The sexualization of girls and women as a primary antecedent of self-objectification. In R. M. Calogero, S. E. Tantleff-Dunn, & J. K. Thompson (Eds.), *Self-objectification in women: Causes, consequences, and counteractions* (pp. 53–75). Washington, DC: American Psychological Association.

Smolak, L., & Striegel-Moore, R. H. (2001). Challenging the myth of the golden girl: Ethnicity and eating disorders. In R. H. Striegel-Moore & L. Smolak (Eds.), *Eating disorders: Innovative directions in research and practice* (pp. 111–132). Washington, DC: American Psychological Association.

Steiner, H., Kwan, W., Shaffer, T. G., Walker, S., Miller, S., Sagar, A., & Lock, J. (2003). Risk and protective factors for juvenile eating disorders. *European Child & Adolescent Psychiatry, 12*(1), 38–46.

Stice, E. (2001). A prospective test of the dual-pathway model of bulimic pathology: Mediating effects of dieting and negative affect. *Journal of Abnormal Psychology, 110*(1), 124.

Stice, E. (2002). Risk and maintenance factors for eating pathology: A meta-analytic review. *Psychological Bulletin, 128*(5), 825.

Stice, E., & Agras, W. S. (1998). Predicting onset and cessation of bulimic behaviors during adolescence: A longitudinal grouping analysis. *Behavior Therapy, 29*(2), 257–276.

Stice, E., Becker, C. B., & Yokum, S. (2013). Eating disorder prevention: Current evidence-base and future directions. *International Journal of Eating Disorders, 46*(5), 478–485.

Stice, E., Chase, A., Stormer, S., & Appel, A. (2001). A randomized trial of a dissonance-based eating disorder prevention program. *International Journal of Eating Disorders, 29*(3), 247–262.

Stice, E., Davis, K., Miller, N. P., & Marti, C. N. (2008). Fasting increases risk for onset of binge eating and bulimic pathology: A 5-year prospective study. *Journal of Abnormal Psychology, 117*(4), 941.

Stice, E., Marti, C. N., Shaw, H., & Jaconis, M. (2009). An 8-year longitudinal study of the natural history of threshold, subthreshold, and partial eating disorders from a community sample of adolescents. *Journal of Abnormal Psychology, 118*(3), 587.

Stice, E., Marti, C. N., Spoor, S., Presnell, K., & Shaw, H. (2008). Dissonance and healthy weight eating disorder prevention programs: Long-term effects from a randomized efficacy trial. *Journal of Consulting and Clinical Psychology, 76*(2), 329.

Stice, E., Mazotti, L., Weibel, D., & Agras, W. S. (2000). Dissonance prevention program decreases thin ideal internalization, body dissatisfaction, dieting, negative affect, and bulimic symptoms: A preliminary experiment. *International Journal of Eating Disorders, 27*(2), 206–217.

Stice, E., Nemeroff, C., & Shaw, H. E. (1996). Test of the dual pathway model of bulimia nervosa: Evidence for dietary restraint and affect regulation mechanisms. *Journal of Social and Clinical Psychology, 15*(3), 340–363.

Stice, E., Presnell, K., & Bearman, S. K. (2001). Relation of early menarche to depression, eating disorders, substance abuse, and comorbid psychopathology among adolescent girls. *Developmental Psychology, 37*(5), 608.

Stice, E., Rohde, P., Gau, J., & Shaw, H. (2009). An effectiveness trial of a dissonance-based eating disorder prevention program for high-risk adolescent girls. *Journal of Consulting and Clinical Psychology, 77*(5), 825.

Stice, E., Rohde, P., & Shaw, H. (2013). *The body project: A dissonance-based eating disorder prevention intervention.* New York, NY: Oxford University Press.

Stice, E., Schupak-Neuberg, E., Shaw, H. E., & Stein, R. I. (1994). Relation of media exposure to eating disorder symptomatology: An examination of mediating mechanisms. *Journal of Abnormal Psychology, 103*(4), 836.

Stice, E., & Shaw, H. (2004). Eating disorder prevention programs: A meta-analytic review. *Psychological Bulletin, 130*(2), 206.

Stice, E., Shaw, H., Burton, E., & Wade, E. (2006). Dissonance and healthy weight eating disorder prevention programs: A randomized efficacy trial. *Journal of Consulting and Clinical Psychology, 74*(2), 263.

Stice, E., Trost, A., & Chase, A. (2003). Healthy weight control and dissonance based eating disorder prevention programs: Results from a controlled trial. *International Journal of Eating Disorders, 33*(1), 10–21.

Striegel-Moore, R. H., Dohm, F. A., Kraemer, H. C., Taylor, C. B., Daniels, S., Crawford, P. B., & Schreiber, G. B. (2003). Eating disorders in white and black women. *American Journal of Psychiatry, 160*(7), 1326–1331.

Sullivan, P. F. (1995). Mortality in anorexia nervosa. *American Journal of Psychiatry, 152*(7), 1073–1074.

Taylor, C. B., Bryson, S., Luce, K. H., Cunning, D., Doyle, A. C., Abascal, L. B., … & Wilfley, D. E. (2006). Prevention of eating disorders in at-risk college-age women. *Archives of General Psychiatry, 63*(8), 881–888.

Thompson, J. K., & Stice, E. (2001). Thin-ideal internalization: Mounting evidence for a new risk factor for body-image disturbance and eating pathology. *Current Directions in Psychological Science, 10*(5), 181–183.

Tiggemann, M. (2011). Mental health risks of self-objectification: A review of the empirical evidence for disordered eating, depressed mood, and sexual dysfunction. In R. M. Calogero, S. Tantleff-Dunn, & J. K. Thompson (Eds.), *Self-objectification in women: Causes, consequences, and counteractions* (pp. 139–159). Washington, DC: American Psychological Association.

Turner, G., & Shepherd, J. (1999). A method in search of a theory: Peer education and health promotion. *Health Education Research, 14*(2), 235–247.

Vohs, K. D., Bardone, A. M., Joiner, T. E., Jr., & Abramson, L. Y. (1999). Perfectionism, perceived weight status, and self-esteem interact to predict bulimic symptoms: A model of bulimic symptom development. *Journal of Abnormal Psychology, 108*(4), 695.

Wentz, E., Gillberg, I. C., Anckarsäter, H., Gillberg, C., & Råstam, M. (2009). Adolescent-onset anorexia nervosa: 18-year outcome. *The British Journal of Psychiatry, 194*(2), 168–174.

Wilksch, S. M., Durbridge, M. R., & Wade, T. D. (2008). A preliminary controlled comparison of programs designed to reduce risk of eating disorders targeting perfectionism and media literacy. *Journal of the American Academy of Child & Adolescent Psychiatry, 47*(8), 939–947.

Wilksch, S. M., & Wade, T. D. (2009). Reduction of shape and weight concern in young adolescents: A 30-month controlled evaluation of a media literacy program. *Journal of the American Academy of Child & Adolescent Psychiatry, 48*(6), 652–661.

Winzelberg, J., Eppstein, D., Eldredge, K. L., Wilfley, D., Dasmahapatra, R., Dev, P., & Taylor, C. B. (2000). Effectiveness of an internet-based program for reducing risk factors for eating disorders. *Journal of Consulting and Clinical Psychology, 68*, 346–350.

World Health Organization. (2002). The World health report: 2002: Reducing the risks, promoting healthy life, Geneva.

Zabinski, M. F., Wilfley, D. E., Calfas, K. J., Winzelberg, A. J., & Taylor, C. B. (2004). An interactive psychoeducational intervention for women at risk of developing an eating disorder. *Journal of Consulting and Clinical Psychology, 72*(5), 914–919.

Chapter 15
Partnering with Adolescents, Parents, Researchers, and Family Medicine Clinics to Address Adolescent Weight and Weight-Related Behaviors

Jerica M. Berge, Katharine Didericksen, Michaela Bucchianeri, Shailendra Prasad, and Dianne Neumark-Sztainer

15.1 Prevalence of Adolescent Obesity and Disordered Eating Behaviors

While the prevalence of adolescent obesity may have started to plateau (Bethell, Simpson, Stumbo, Carle, & Gombojav, 2010; NIH, 2007; Ogden, Carroll, Curtin, Lamb, & Flegal, 2010; Ogden, Lamb, Carroll, & Flegal, 2010; Wilson, 2009), adolescent obesity has more than tripled over the last three decades and remains one of the most serious health problems facing youth (Ogden et al., 2006; Ogden, Carroll, et al., 2010; Ogden, Lamb, et al., 2010). Additionally, adolescent weight status strongly tracks into adulthood and has been linked to increased risk for cardiovascular disease, type II diabetes, cancer, and poor mental health as an adult (Daniels, 2006; Gordon-Larsen, The, & Adair, 2009; Merten, 2010; Pi-Sunyer, 2002; Popkin, 2007; Stovitz et al., 2010; Whitaker, Wright, Pepe, Seidel, & Dietz, 1997). Similarly, disordered eating behaviors (e.g., binge eating and using unhealthy weight control practices such as fasting, self-induced vomiting, or use of diet pills) are prevalent in adolescence. In a national sample of adolescents, 45 % of girls and 20 % of boys reported having dieted, and 13 % of girls and 7 % of boys had engaged

J.M. Berge, Ph.D., M.P.H. (✉) • S. Prasad, M.D., M.P.H.
Department of Family Medicine and Community Health, University of Minnesota Medical School, Minneapolis, MN, USA
e-mail: jberge@umn.edu; pras0054@umn.edu

K. Didericksen, Ph.D., LMFT
Child Development and Family Relations, East Cardina University, Grennville, NC, USA
e-mail: didericksenk14@ecu.edu

M. Bucchianeri, Ph.D. • D. Neumark-Sztainer, Ph.D., M.P.H., R.D.
Division of Epidemiology and Community Health, School of Public Health, University of Minnesota, Minneapolis, MN, USA
e-mail: mmbucchia@gmail.com; neuma011@umn.edu

© Springer Science+Business Media New York 2016
M.R. Korin (ed.), *Health Promotion for Children and Adolescents*,
DOI 10.1007/978-1-4899-7711-3_15

in some sort of disordered eating behavior (Neumark-Sztainer & Hannan, 2000). Dieting and disordered eating behaviors pose serious risks to adolescents' physical and psychosocial development as they are predictive of health concerns such as depression (Crow, Eisenberg, Story, & Neumark-Sztainer, 2008; Katzman, 2005; Stice, Hayward, Cameron, Killen, & Taylor, 2000) and clinical eating disorders (Keel, Fulkerson, & Leon, 1997; Neumark-Sztainer et al., 2006; Neumark-Sztainer, Wall, Larson, Eisenberg, & Loth, 2011; Patton, Selzer, Coffey, Carlin, & Wolfe, 1999). Thus, it is critical to target disordered eating and weight-related behaviors in adolescents to reduce the risks they pose for serious health conditions.

Prevalences of obesity (Bethell et al., 2010; NIH, 2007; Ogden, Carroll, et al., 2010; Ogden, Lamb, et al., 2010; Wilson, 2009), unhealthy dieting practices (Austin et al., 2011; Neumark-Sztainer et al., 2011; Neumark-Sztainer, Wall, Eisenberg, Story, & Hannan, 2006) and disordered eating behaviors (Austin et al., 2011; Neumark-Sztainer, Wall, Eisenberg, et al., 2006, Neumark-Sztainer, Wall, Guo, et al., 2006 ; Neumark-Sztainer et al., 2011) are disturbingly high in adolescents across race/ethnicity and socioeconomic status (SES). For example, national data indicate that the prevalence of obesity is 42 % among those of Hispanic ethnicity and 41 % among Non-Hispanic black youth compared to 30 % among Non-Hispanic White youth; these high prevalences and disparities are of public health concern (Ogden, Carroll, Kit, & Flegal, 2012). A large, community-based sample found that weight-related concerns and behaviors, such as body dissatisfaction, chronic dieting, binge eating, and extreme weight control behaviors, were prevalent across adolescents from different ethnic/racial backgrounds, with some notable differences across groups. In comparison to White girls, African American girls tended to report fewer weight-related concerns and disordered eating behaviors, while Hispanic, Asian American, and Native American girls tended to report similar and more weight-related concerns and behaviors. Among boys, weight-related concerns and behaviors were equally or more prevalent among all non-Whites than among Whites.

15.2 Intervention Research to Date on Adolescent Obesity and Disordered Eating

The majority of obesity interventions targeted to youth have been carried out in schools, or specialty healthcare clinics (Caballero et al., 2003; Story et al., 2003) with a focus on youth individual-level behaviors or school-level nutrition policies and practices. Although schools and specialty healthcare clinics are a logical context for intervening, results have shown low to moderate success with reducing body mass index (BMI) percentile and obesity using these types of interventions (Davison & Birch, 2001; Ebbeling, Pawlak, & Ludwig, 2002; Livingstone, McCaffrey, & Rennie, 2006; Rao, 2008). In response to the limited success with interventions for adolescent weight and weight-related behaviors, expert panels, researchers, and the National Institutes of Health (NIH) have called for family-level and community-based interventions in order to address the multi-level systems in which youth reside and by which they are primarily influenced when addressing weight and weight-related behaviors ("Expert Committee Recommendations on the Assessment, Prevention, & Treatment of Child and Adolescent Overweight and Obesity," 2007; Lindsay, Sussner, Kim, & Gortmaker, 2006; Rhee, De Lago, Arscott-Mills, Mehta, & Davis, 2005).

Additionally, research has shown that intervention programs targeting established risk factors for disordered eating generally exhibit moderate success with reducing adolescent disordered eating behaviors (Ciao, Loth, & Neumark-Sztainer, 2014; Neumark-Sztainer et al., 2006; Stice, Becker, & Yokum, 2013). Findings from one meta-analysis suggest that effects may be strongest when intervention programs target high-risk individuals, feature interactive content, focus on risk factors shown to predict future onset of eating disorders (e.g., body dissatisfaction), and follow a multisession structure (Stice, Shaw, & Marti, 2007). Thus, there is a need for intervention research that incorporates lessons learned from earlier intervention studies on adolescent weight and weight-related behaviors and that utilizes new approaches that can increase the likelihood of success and sustainability of interventions aimed at changing weight and weight-related behaviors in adolescents.

15.3   Can Obesity and Disordered Eating Be Intervened on Simultaneously?

Research has suggested that weight-related behaviors connected to overweight (e.g., binge eating) and disordered eating (e.g., fasting, purging) may not necessarily be distinct and instead overlap on a continuum of weight-related problems (Neumark-Sztainer, 2005a; Neumark-Sztainer et al., 2007). Furthermore, research has suggested that it may be possible and useful to develop interventions to simultaneously prevent a spectrum of weight-related problems such as obesity and disordered eating (Neumark-Sztainer, 2005a; Neumark-Sztainer et al., 2007). For example, theoretically and practically it makes sense to teach the concept of body image to adolescents who struggle with overweight/obesity or adolescents who are challenged with disordered eating behaviors in order to increase body satisfaction and promote healthful eating behaviors. Thus, creating interventions that can simultaneously target weight-related problems for both overweight and disordered eating in adolescents may be more successful.

Given the high prevalence and disparities of different types of weight-related problems in adolescents, including both obesity and disordered eating across youth from different racial/ethnic and SES backgrounds (Ogden et al. 2006, 2012; Ogden, Carroll, et al., 2010), and the low to moderate success with prevention and treatment interventions to date, it is crucial to continue to explore new strategies for addressing these problems among populations at greatest risk. Strategies important to consider include: (1) intervention strategies that address a broad spectrum of weight-related problems and take into account the overall well-being of the adolescent; (2) the involvement of family members; (3) community involvement via community-based participatory research (CBPR) methods in the design of relevant interventions; and (4) the implementation of interventions within community clinics where access is easy and healthcare providers are more likely to be attuned to participant needs. An example (i.e., UMatter) of an adolescent weight and weight-related prevention intervention is presented later in the chapter to illustrate how to incorporate all of the above mentioned strategies.

15.4   Utilizing Community-Based Participatory Research (CBPR) Methods to Address Adolescent Weight and Weight-Related Behaviors

15.4.1   Overview of CBPR

Community-based participatory research (CBPR) methods are one way to create novel and more sustainable prevention interventions because they engage community members, family members, community organizations/leaders, and researchers in co-creating interventions that address problems of importance to the community as a whole in order to have high potential for sustainability (Berge, Mendenhall, & Doherty, 2009; Minkler & Wallerstein, 2003; Peterson & Gubrium, 2011). Hierarchical differences that can arise between academic researchers and participants are flattened through this partnership and everyone works together to co-create knowledge and effect change throughout all aspects of the research process (Berge et al., 2009; Israel et al., 2003; Minkler & Wallerstein, 2003). Each person contributes unique strengths and knowledge to improve the health and well-being of community members (Berge et al., 2009; Israel et al., 2003).

Several core assumptions permeate CBPR projects, including:

- Recognition of the community as the principal unit of identity
- Democratic and equitable partnership between all project members (e.g., parents, families, community stakeholders, healthcare providers, academic researchers) as collaborators through every stage of the project or study (e.g., developing research questions, data collection, carrying out the intervention, data analysis, presentation, and publication of results)
- Building on the strengths and resources within the community
- Promoting co-learning and capacity-building between and among partners
- Deep investment in change that carries with it an element of challenging the status quo and improving the lives of members in a community or clinical practice
- Iterative process(es) wherein problems are identified, solutions are developed within the context(s) of the community's existing resources, interventions are implemented, outcomes are evaluated according to what participants view as important, and interventions are revised and improved in accord with new information as indicated

- Project members' humility and flexibility to accommodate necessary changes across any part of a project or study
- Disseminating findings and new knowledge to all partners and constituents in the investigative process
- Recognition that CBPR partnerships can be slow and messy, especially during initial phases of development; and
- Long-term engagement and commitment to the work (Berge et al., 2009; Israel et al., 2003; Mendenhall et al., 2010)

Given the core assumptions of CBPR, this approach may be especially useful in addressing adolescent weight and weight-related behaviors because parents and adolescents bring expertise in relation to day-to-day barriers/challenges and successes with addressing weight and weight-related behaviors and community organizations and academic researchers bring expertise with regard to evidence-based findings related to adolescent weight and weight-related behaviors (Berge et al., 2009). Bringing these different types of expertise together can work synergistically in finding new ways to address adolescent weight and weight-related behaviors within a family- and community-based context.

15.4.2   Prior Studies Utilizing CBPR Methods

CBPR methods are new to the field of obesity and disordered eating prevention (Berge et al., 2009; Israel, Eng, Schulz, & Parker, 2005). Few studies have utilized a true CBPR framework from study inception to data collection, intervention delivery, and data analysis (Berge et al., 2016; Davison, Jurkowski, Li, Kranz, & Lawson, 2013). However, there are a couple of exceptions that focus on child and adolescent obesity. A study carried out by Davison and colleagues (Davison et al., 2013) utilized CBPR to partner with parents of children attending Head Start programs. Parents and researchers developed a childhood obesity prevention intervention to be carried out in Head Start. They began by carrying out a community assessment to determine parent needs with regard to addressing childhood obesity. Based on the community assessment, parents and researchers created an intervention that included the following elements: (1) revisions to letters sent home to families reporting child body mass index (BMI); (2) a communication campaign to raise parents' awareness of their child's weight status; (3) the integration of nutrition counseling into Head Start family engagement activities; and (4) a 6-week parent-led program to strengthen parents' communication skills, conflict resolution, resource-related empowerment for healthy lifestyles, social networks, and media literacy (Davison et al., 2013). Results of the study showed increased child fruit and vegetable intake and hours of physical activity and reduced body mass index. The authors concluded that the CBPR approach was effective in their sample and may be a promising approach for childhood obesity prevention interventions going forward.

Another study using CBPR methods in relation to childhood obesity was conducted with a slightly older group of children (ages 8–16). This study was called "Play it Forward" (Berge et al., 2016). Parents, researchers and community leaders (e.g., school social worker, YMCA director, health store owner) partnered together to co-create a neighborhood-level healthy living program that would help the next generation of children become more active. This group also started with a needs assessment of community strengths and challenges with regard to child and family health. The CBPR group created both planned and spontaneous activities at the local park that families would come to in order to engage in family-level physical activity to promote physical activity in their children (Berge et al., 2016). Feasibility results indicate high feasibility and satisfaction of parents, children, and neighbors in the "Play it Forward" intervention.

Although CBPR methods are relatively new to the field of childhood obesity and almost nonexistent to the field of disordered eating, the approach is not new to other fields, such as chronic disease management. For example, several studies have been conducted using CBPR methods to address type II diabetes, type I diabetes, asthma, and cardiovascular disease (Berge et al., 2009; Israel et al., 2003, 2005). The CBPR approach has been well received by participants in these studies and results have indicated significant changes in health behaviors, such as better hemoglobin A1C levels (diabetes), better asthma control, and more healthful eating (Doherty, Mendenhall, & Berge, 2010; Mendenhall et al., 2010). Thus, while there is evidence to suggest a CBPR approach may be effective in childhood obesity prevention studies and in other general health conditions, more research is needed to confirm its effectiveness in reducing childhood obesity and disordered eating behaviors and improving child and family health.

15.4.3 Medical Homes

Family Medicine clinics that are Patient Centered Medical Homes (PCMH), also known as "Medical Homes," may be an ideal place to address adolescent weight-related issues because they provide direct access to parents and adolescents; are in a convenient location typically situated within the community where families live; and usually create a feeling of trust or safety for families because adolescents and parents have preexisting relationships with providers and staff. Additionally, because they are physically located within communities, these sites provide a perfect setting for carrying out CBPR methods.

PCHMs are a comprehensive, interprofessional, and community-based model of primary care delivery, in which patients receive care coordination and a team-based approach to care ("Minnesota Department of Health," 2014; Rittenhouse, Casalino, Gillies, Shortell, & Lau, 2008). Medical homes have received renewed attention since the passage of the Patient Protection and Affordable Care Act of 2010 (PPACA). According to Section 3502 of the PPACA, PCMHs should "develop and implement interdisciplinary, interprofessional care plans that integrate clinical and community preventive and health promotion services for patients" (i.e., Patient Centered Medical Homes). Provisions in the legislation supporting the integration of PCMHs into the US healthcare system include financing for Medicare and Medicaid PCMH pilot programs, along with community-based collaborative care networks for low-income populations.

15.5 The UMatter Program: Using CBPR to Address Adolescent Healthy Eating, Physical Activity and Weight

The "UMatter" (i.e., You Matter!) program, aimed at reducing obesity and other weight-related problems, was created using concepts from CBPR methods (Berge et al., 2009; Minkler & Wallerstein, 2003; Peterson & Gubrium, 2011) and research evidence supporting the simultaneous targeting of overweight and disordered eating behaviors within the same intervention (Neumark-Sztainer, 2005a; Neumark-Sztainer et al., 2007). The intervention was also implemented within a PCMH setting. Relying on these key components increased the likelihood that targeting adolescent weight and weight-related behaviors would be relevant to adolescents and their parents and would increase the chances of sustainability over time because the intervention was implemented within a Medical Home setting. Additionally, the intervention was carried out within a low income and racially diverse population in order to target adolescent populations at high risk for overweight/obesity and disordered eating behaviors. First, focus groups were conducted with adolescents, peers, parents, primary care physicians, and primary care staff to tap expertise from all potential levels of influence in an adolescent's life (e.g., individual, family/parent, community). Next, the UMatter intervention was refined, based on focus group feedback, and the first round of UMatter was carried out. Process evaluations were conducted at the conclusion of the UMatter pilot study via individual interviews with mothers and daughters to further tailor the intervention to the mother/daughter population being targeted in UMatter. Finally, the second round of UMatter piloting was carried out.

15.5.1 UMatter: An Overview

The guiding philosophy of the UMatter program is to provide an environment that supports adolescent girls in establishing self-confidence so that they will want to take care of their bodies through physical activity and healthy eating on a long-term basis (see Fig. 15.1). This philosophy emerged from empirical research on eating and weight-related problems with adolescents, which has suggested the importance of a positive body image in order to facilitate healthful eating and physical activity behaviors as a way of simultaneously targeting weight-related behaviors that are

UMatter Conceptual Model

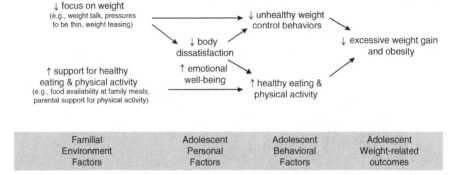

Fig. 15.1 UMatter conceptual model

present in adolescents who are overweight/obese and/or who engage in disordered eating behaviors (Neumark-Sztainer, 2005a, 2005b; Neumark-Sztainer, Paxton, Hannan, Haines, & Story, 2006). The specific content and format of delivery of UMatter was further informed by input gathered from participants themselves (i.e., adolescent girls, mothers, primary care physicians, and staff) and additional evidence-based research findings in the adolescent obesity field (Berge, 2009; Berge et al., 2013; Berge & Everts, 2011; Neumark-Sztainer 2004, 2009a, 2009b; Neumark-Sztainer et al. 2007, 2012). UMatter is grounded in Social Cognitive Theory (Bandura, 1977, 1986) and targets factors at the socio-ecological (e.g., family support), personal (e.g., body image), and behavioral (e.g., goal setting) levels to facilitate positive health behavior change.

Specifically, UMatter aims to: (1) facilitate positive change at the personal and family levels with regard to healthy eating and physical activity, (2) help girls feel good about themselves, and (3) help girls avoid unhealthy weight control behaviors. The UMatter intervention has seven behavioral objectives for girls and their parents, based on evidence in the field of adolescent obesity (Berge, 2009; Berge & Everts, 2011; Neumark-Sztainer, 2009a; Neumark-Sztainer et al., 2010; Neumark-Sztainer, Flattum, Story, Feldman, & Petrich, 2008): (1) decrease parent weight talk, teasing, and encouragement to diet, (2) increase frequency of family meals, (3) increase availability of healthy foods in the home, (4) increase parent support for physical activity, (5) decrease girls' body dissatisfaction, (6) decrease girls' unhealthy weight control behaviors, and (7) increase girls' healthy eating and physical activity.

Comprised of various integrated components, the UMatter intervention was designed to provide girls with a consistent set of messages and supportive resources across multiple domains (e.g., individual goal setting, peer engagement, family support) that would help them to achieve these behavioral goals. The intervention comprised (1) adolescent- and parent-specific group sessions at a primary care clinic, (2) in-home visits to tailor messages delivered in group sessions, and (3) a social media component (i.e., Google+).

15.5.2 Focus Groups

Focus groups were conducted separately for adolescents, parents, physicians, and primary care staff (e.g., medical assistants, nurses, front desk staff, administrative staff) at the same Family Medicine clinic where the UMatter intervention was going to be carried out. Within the focus groups six main areas of focus emerged: (1) healthy eating, (2) physical activity, (3) self-image/body image, (4) weight talk/teasing, (5) intervention delivery with same-sex groups (i.e., girls did not want boys to attend groups with them), and (6) importance of intervention targeting both parents and daughters (i.e., daughters wanted their mothers to come with them). Parents identified challenges they were experiencing regarding their own and their daughter's eating patterns, weight status, body image, and concerns about eating and weight issues in African American girls in general. Adolescent girls talked about challenges with weight talk/teasing, body image, self-image, and general dislike for physical activity. Additionally, adolescent girls mentioned the importance of making intervention sessions active and fun. Physicians and Family Medicine clinic staff identified challenges they had experienced when working with African American girls and their mothers in the clinic such as eating patterns, physical activity patterns, and parent/daughter relationship issues. Across all groups, participants identified the importance of bringing girls and mothers together when carrying out an intervention.

Additionally during the focus groups, facilitators presented visuals of specific proposed components of the UMatter intervention (e.g., educational sessions at the Family Medicine clinic, in-home visits, social media via Google+), taken from evidence-based findings in the field of obesity prevention and disordered eating (Neumark-Sztainer, 2009a), in order for participants to give feedback regarding the relevance of the topics, feasibility of covering the topics, and delivery modality of the topics. In general, focus group participants were supportive of the proposed UMatter program, with the majority indicating that there was a need for this type of group within their community.

15.5.3 Group Visit Component

The group visit component of the UMatter program took place in a community Family Medicine clinic within which program participants were already connected. Each group visit consisted of separate classes for girls and, on select weeks, their mothers; a brief goal-setting session; physical activity; and, on weeks when mothers were present, a family meal. Each class was based on feedback received from adolescents, mothers, Family Medicine physicians, and staff (see above) and focused on a specific topic of relevance to the girls or their mothers, such as body image, healthy eating, not dieting, family meals, physical activity, and communication about weight. In addition to communicating intervention content, a primary goal of the classes was to create a positive and safe environment in which participants felt comfortable raising questions and discussing their own challenges and insecurities regarding body image and healthy choices. Infused with activities designed to provide concrete and relatable illustrations of the intervention messages, these classes also gave participants the opportunity to practice skills that can help them make positive changes in their own lives, outside of the program.

At the end of each class session, participants were invited to set a new goal for the following week, based on the content covered in class. For example, following the class on "Physical Activity," a participant might choose to increase by a certain amount the number of minutes she is physically active each day, or try one new activity before the next class. Program staff facilitated participants' goal-setting process, offering supportive guidance and clarification as needed using the SMART (Specific, Measureable, Achievable, Relevant, Time-bound) goal framework (Doran, 1981). At the start of each new class, program staff conducted a brief check-in on participants' progress toward their goal from the previous class.

In order to reinforce the intervention messages regarding physical activity, girls (and, when present, their mothers) were given the opportunity to experience a variety of types of movement during group visits at the clinic. For some participants, certain types of activities may have been familiar; for others, this represented their first exposure to a given type or movement. Physical activities engaged in during the program included yoga, dance, and relay races, and ranged from approximately 15 min (at most group visits) to 45 min (at the group visit in which the "Physical Activity" class was presented).

15.5.4 In-home Visit Component

At several points throughout the intervention, program staff joined participants for an in-home visit. These visits provided staff with the opportunity to tailor intervention messages, using Motivational Interviewing Techniques (Emmons & Rollnick, 2001; Gance-Cleveland & Oetzel, 2010; Miller & Rollnick, 2002; Resnicow et al., 2002; Resnicow, Davis, & Rollnick, 2006), specifically to the needs of each participant, as well as engage girls and their parents in a discussion of goals, barriers, and facilitators of healthy behavior change at the family level. In addition, these visits allowed families to host program staff informally for a brief time, and to communicate important information about their home environment that might not otherwise be captured in group visits at the clinic.

15.5.5 Social Media Component

To bridge group visit class content together, as well as help participants apply intervention messages to their everyday lives, the UMatter program included a social media component on Google+. Moderated by program staff, this Google+ group provided an online space where participants could communicate with each other in between group visits, and build community through their posts and conversations about program topics. To provide some structure for these interactions, program staff challenged participants to complete a series of "Try It @ Home" activities, designed to both (1) increase the level of engagement between girls and their mothers and (2) facilitate application of the class content to participants' daily lives. Sample "Try It @ Home" activities included engaging in media literacy (e.g., "Watch a TV or movie together and discuss the types of body-related messages or comments you notice"), building self-efficacy for healthy eating (e.g., "Find a new healthy recipe and cook it together"), and drafting and signing a "Weight-Talk-Free Zone" pledge to post in the home. In addition, participants were encouraged to communicate with each other, and with program staff, via PhotoVoice (Wang & Burris, 1994). For example, participants posted photos of aspects of their neighborhood that either facilitated or impeded their ability to practice healthy behaviors.

15.6   Implications for Future Adolescent Obesity Interventions and Integrating UMatter Model into a Patient-Centered Medical Home

The UMatter intervention may be useful for informing obesity and disordered eating prevention research in general and in particular for Family Medicine/Primary Care settings. First, utilizing a CBPR approach allowed for tailoring of the intervention for adolescents and parents from low income and African American households in order to increase the overall effectiveness of the intervention. Specifically, partnering with adolescents and their parents in creating and adapting the intervention ongoing helped identify specific challenges/barriers adolescents and parents from low income and African American households face, in order to make the intervention relevant and readily applicable for them. Additionally, the CBPR approach increased the likelihood of sustainability of the intervention within the Family Medicine clinic. Specifically, we partnered with Family Medicine physicians and clinic staff in designing the intervention to meet the needs of the clinic and the population they serve.

A second implication of the results of the UMatter intervention is that integrating the UMatter model into a Patient-Centered Medical Home setting (i.e., Family Medicine clinic, Pediatric clinic) may be feasible given how the intervention was designed. Because we partnered with Family Medicine physicians and clinic staff who were aware of the key components needed to qualify to be a certified Patient-Centered Medical Home Home ("Minnesota Department of Health," 2014) all elements of the UMatter intervention are able to be carried out within a Patient-Centered Medical Home. For example, PCMHs are encouraged to have behavioral medicine providers as part of the care team. The UMatter intervention was led by behavioral medicine providers and students. Additionally, PCMHs have "Care Coordinators" who function as "coaches" and "coordinators" of health care for patients. One role a Care Coordinator can engage in is arranging for appropriate in-home visits, which were used in UMatter. The groups sessions facilitated at the Family Medicine clinics may be able to be reimbursable as group preventive healthcare visits.

Table 15.1 Recommendations to help youth avoid excessive weight gain and disordered eating behaviors

1. Inform young people that dieting, and particularly unhealthy weight control behaviors, may be counterproductive. Instead encourage positive eating and physical activity behaviors that can be maintained on a regular basis
2. Promote body satisfaction in youth. Help young people care for their bodies so that they will want to nurture them through healthy eating, physical activity, and positive self-talk
3. Encourage families to have regular, and enjoyable, family meals and to provide a home environment in which the healthy choices are the easy choices
4. Encourage families to avoid weight talk. Instead encourage families to do more to provide a home environment in which it is easier to make healthful food choices and to be physically active
5. Assume overweight children have experienced weight teasing and other forms of weight mistreatment. Discuss with children and their families and explore ways to decrease at home

Source: Preventing obesity and eating disorders in adolescents: What can healthcare providers do? Neumark-Sztainer D. Journal of Adolescent Health. 2009;44:206–213

Third, adolescent obesity researchers and healthcare providers may be able to use results from the UMatter intervention when working with adolescents and parents to address weight and weight-related behaviors. For example, the five recommendations that guided the UMatter intervention (Table 15.1) may be used to guide discussions with adolescents and their parents when targeting weight and weight-related issues.

Additionally, adolescent girls and their mothers felt that it was helpful and positive to address these issues as a team; thus, including mothers, daughters, and healthcare providers may be a useful approach to addressing weight and weight-related issues in adolescents.

15.7 Future Directions for Obesity and Disordered Eating Research and Interventions

Although research simultaneously targeting adolescent obesity and disordered eating behaviors using a CBPR approach has been limited to date, it has a high potential for success (Berge et al., 2016; Davison et al., 2013; Israel et al., 2003, 2005). Future research should continue to develop programs or interventions using a CBPR framework in order to increase the effectiveness of the intervention and the overall sustainability of the program. Additionally, developing programs and interventions that simultaneously target overweight/obesity and disordered eating behaviors is important as many of the weight-related behaviors that are present in both types of conditions overlap (Neumark-Sztainer et al., 2007) Overall, programs and interventions that include the following strategies are most likely to have the highest success with intervening in weight and weight-related behaviors conditions in youth:

- Intervention strategies that address a broad spectrum of weight-related problems and take into account the overall well-being of the adolescent
- Involvement of parents and family members

- Community involvement via community-based participatory research (CBPR) methods in the design of relevant interventions
- Implementation of interventions within community clinics where access is easy and healthcare providers are more likely to be attuned to participant needs

15.8 Conclusions

Obesity and disordered eating behaviors are prevalent among adolescents. There are also disparities in obesity and disordered eating behaviors among low income and minority adolescent populations. It is important to use intervention strategies that address a broad spectrum of weight-related problems and take into account the overall well-being of the adolescent, involve family members, use community-based participatory research (CBPR) approaches to increase success and sustainability of the intervention, and to implement interventions within community clinics where access is easy and healthcare providers are more likely to be attuned to participant needs. Using approaches with all of these elements may be promising in designing future obesity and disordered eating behavior prevention interventions for adolescents and their families.

References

Austin, S., Spadano-Gasbarro, J., Greaney, M., Richmond, T., Feldman, H., Osganian, S., ... Peterson, K. (2011). Disordered weight control behaviors in early adolescent boys and girls of color: An under-recognized factor in the epidemic of childhood overweight. *Journal of Adolescent Health, 48*(1), 109–112.

Bandura, A. (1977). *Social learning theory*. Englewood Cliffs, NJ: Prentice Hall.

Bandura, A. (1986). *Social foundations of thought and action: A social cognitive theory*. Englewood Cliffs, NJ: Prentice-Hall.

Berge, J. M. (2009). A review of familial correlates of child and adolescent obesity: What has the 21st century taught us so far? *International Journal of Adolescent Medicine and Health, 21*(4), 457–483.

Berge, J. M., & Everts, J. (2011). Family-based interventions targeting childhood obesity: A meta-analysis. *Childhood Obesity, 7*(2), 110–121.

Berge, J., Jin, S., Hanson, C., Doty, J., Jagaraj, K., Braaten, K., ... Doherty, W. J. (2016). Play it forward: A community-based participatory research approach to childhood obesity prevention. *Families, Systems and Health, 34*(1), 15–30.

Berge, J. M., Maclehose, R., Loth, K. A., Eisenberg, M., Bucchianeri, M. M., & Neumark-Sztainer, D. (2013). Parent conversations about healthful eating and weight: Associations with adolescent disordered eating behaviors. *JAMA Pediatrics, 167*(8), 746–753. doi:10.1001/jamapediatrics.2013.78.

Berge, J. M., Mendenhall, T. J., & Doherty, W. J. (2009). Using community-based participatory research (CBPR) to target health disparities in families. *Family Relations, 58*(4), 475–488. doi:10.1111/j.1741-3729.2009.00567.x.

Bethell, C., Simpson, L., Stumbo, S., Carle, A. C., & Gombojav, N. (2010). National, state and local disparities in childhood obesity. *Health Affairs, 29*(3), 347–356.

Caballero, B., Clay, T., Davis, S. M., Ethelbah, B., Rock, B. H., Lohman, T., … Stevens, J. (2003). Pathways: A school-based, randomized controlled trial for the prevention of obesity in American Indian schoolchildren. *American Journal of Clinical Nutrition, 78*(5), 1030–1038.

Ciao, A., Loth, K., & Neumark-Sztainer, D. (2014). Preventing eating disorder pathology: Common and unique features of successful eating disorders prevention programs. *Current Psychiatry Reports, 16*(7), 453. doi:10.1007/s11920-014-0453-02.

Crow, S. J., Eisenberg, M. E., Story, M., & Neumark-Sztainer, D. (2008). Are body dissatisfaction, eating disturbances, and body mass index predictors of suicidal behavior in adolescents? A longitudinal study. *Journal of Consulting and Clinical Psychology, 76,* 887–892.

Daniels, S. R. (2006). The consequences of childhood overweight and obesity. *Future of Children, 16*(1), 47–67.

Davison, K. K., & Birch, L. L. (2001). Childhood overweight: A contextual model and recommendations for future research. *Obesity Reviews, 2,* 159–171.

Davison, K. K., Jurkowski, J. M., Li, K., Kranz, S., & Lawson, H. A. (2013). A childhood obesity intervention developed by families for families: Results from a pilot study. *International Journal of Behavioral Nutrition and Physical Activity, 10,* 3. doi:10.1186/1479-5868-10-3.

Doherty, W. J., Mendenhall, T. J., & Berge, J. M. (2010). The families and democracy and citizen health care project. *Journal of Marital and Family Therapy, 36*(4), 389–402. doi:10.1111/j.1752-0606.2009.00142.x.

Doran, G. (1981). There's a S.M.A.R.T. way to write management's goals and objectives. *Management Review, 70*(11), 36–36.

Ebbeling, C. B., Pawlak, D. B., & Ludwig, D. S. (2002). Childhood obesity: Public-health crisis, common sense cure. *Lancet, 360,* 473–482.

Emmons, K. M., & Rollnick, S. (2001). Motivational interviewing in health care settings. Opportunities and limitations. *American Journal of Preventive Medicine, 20*(1), 68–74.

Expert Committee Recommendations on the Assessment, Prevention, and Treatment of Child and Adolescent Overweight and Obesity. (2007). Retrieved August 27, 2007, from http://www.ama-assn.org/ama1/pub/upload/mm/433/ped_obesity_recs.pdf

Gance-Cleveland, B., & Oetzel, K. B. (2010). Motivational interviewing for families with an overweight child. *Childhood Obesity, 6*(4), 198–200.

Gordon-Larsen, P., The, N. S., & Adair, L. S. (2009). Longitudinal trends in obesity in the United States from adolescence to the third decade of life. *Obesity, 18*(9), 1801–1804.

Israel, B. A., Eng, E., Schulz, A. J., & Parker, E. A. (2005). *Methods in community-based participatory research for health.* San Francisco: Wiley.

Israel, B., Schultz, A. J., Parker, E. A., Becker, A. B., Allen, A. J., & Guzman, J. R. (2003). Critical issues in developing and following community based participatory research principals. In M. Minkler & N. Wallerstein (Eds.), *Community-based participatory research for health* (pp. 53–76). San Francisco: Jossey-Bass.

Katzman, D. K. (2005). Medical complications in adolescents with anorexia nervosa: A review of the literature. *International Journal of Eating Disorders, 37*(Suppl), S52–S59.

Keel, P. K., Fulkerson, J. A., & Leon, G. R. (1997). Disordered eating precursors in pre- and early adolescent girls and boys. *Journal of Youth and Adolescence, 26,* 203–206.

Lindsay, A. C., Sussner, K. M., Kim, J., & Gortmaker, S. (2006). The role of parents in preventing childhood obesity. *Future of Children, 16*(1), 169–186.

Livingstone, M. B., McCaffrey, T. A., & Rennie, K. L. (2006). Childhood obesity prevention studies: Lessons learned and to be learned. *Public Health Nutrition, 9*(8A), 1121–1129.

Mendenhall, T. J., Berge, J. M., Harper, P., GreenCrow, B., LittleWalker, N., WhiteEagle, S., & BrownOwl, S. (2010). The Family Education Diabetes Series (FEDS): Community-based participatory research with a midwestern American Indian community. *Nursing Inquiry, 17*(4), 359–372. doi:10.1111/j.1440-1800.2010.00508.x.

Merten, M. J. (2010). Weight status continuity and change from adolescence to young adulthood: Examining disease and health risk conditions. *Obesity (Silver Spring), 18*(7), 1423–1428. doi:10.1038/oby.2009.365. oby2009365 [pii].

Miller, W. R., & Rollnick, S. (2002). *Motivational interviewing: Preparing people for change* (2nd ed.). New York: Guilford Press.

Minkler, M., & Wallerstein, N. (2003). *Community-based participatory research for health*. San Francisco: Jossey-Bass.

Minnesota Department of Health. (2014). *Health care homes*. Retrieved from www.health.state.mn.us

Neumark-Sztainer, D. (2004). *New moves: Obesity prevention among adolescent girls: Grant proposal*. Bethesda, MD: National Institutes of Health.

Neumark-Sztainer, D. (2005a). Can we simultaneously work toward the prevention of obesity and eating disorders in children and adolescents. *International Journal of Eating Disorders, 38*, 220–227. doi:10.1002/eat.20181.

Neumark-Sztainer, D. (2005b). Preventing the broad spectrum of weight-related problems: Working with parents to help teens achieve a healthy weight and a positive body image. *Journal of Nutrition Education and Behavior, 37*(Suppl 2), S133–S140.

Neumark-Sztainer, D. (2009a). Preventing obesity and eating disorders in adolescents: What can health care providers do? *Journal of Adolescent Health, 44*(3), 206–213.

Neumark-Sztainer, D. (2009b). *New moves online*. Retrieved January 26, 2010, from http://www.newmovesonline.com

Neumark-Sztainer, D., Flattum, C. F., Story, M., Feldman, S., & Petrich, C. A. (2008). Dietary approaches to healthy weight management for adolescents: The new moves model. *Adolescent Medicine: State of the Art Reviews, 19*(3), 421–430.

Neumark-Sztainer, D., Friend, S. E., Flattum, C. F., Hannan, P. J., Story, M., Bauer, K. W., ... Petrich, C. A. (2010). New moves-preventing weight-related problems in adolescent girls: A group-randomized study. *American Journal of Preventive Medicine, 39*(5), 421–432.

Neumark-Sztainer, D., & Hannan, P. J. (2000). Weight-related behaviors among adolescent girls and boys: Results from a national survey. *Archives of Pediatrics and Adolescent Medicine, 154*(6), 569–577.

Neumark-Sztainer, D., Levine, M. P., Paxton, S. J., Smolak, L., Piran, N., & Wertheim, E. H. (2006). Prevention of body dissatisfaction and disordered eating: What next? *Eating Disorders, 14*(4), 265–285.

Neumark-Sztainer, D., Maclehose, R., Loth, K., Fulkerson, J. A., Eisenberg, M. E., & Berge, J. (2012). What's for dinner? Types of food served at family dinner differ across parent and family characteristics. *Public Health Nutrition, 17*, 145–155. doi:10.1017/s1368980012004594.

Neumark-Sztainer, D., Paxton, S. J., Hannan, P. J., Haines, J., & Story, M. (2006). Does body satisfaction matter? Five-year longitudinal associations between body satisfaction and health behaviors in adolescent females and males. *Journal of Adolescent Health, 39*, 244–251.

Neumark-Sztainer, D., Wall, M., Eisenberg, M. E., Story, M., & Hannan, P. J. (2006). Overweight status and weight control behaviors in adolescents: Longitudinal and secular trends from 1999–2004. *Preventive Medicine, 43*(1), 52–59.

Neumark-Sztainer, D., Wall, M., Guo, J., Story, M., Haines, J., & Eisenberg, M. (2006). Obesity, disordered eating, and eating disorders in a longitudinal study of adolescents: How do dieters fare five years later? *Journal of the American Dietetic Association, 106*, 559–568.

Neumark-Sztainer, D., Wall, M., Haines, J., Story, M., Sherwood, N., & van den Berg, P. (2007). Shared risk and protective factors for overweight and disordered eating in adolescents. *American Journal of Preventive Medicine, 33*, 359–369.

Neumark-Sztainer, D., Wall, M., Larson, N. I., Eisenberg, M. E., & Loth, K. (2011). Dieting and disordered eating behaviors from adolescence to young adulthood: Findings from a 10-year longitudinal study. *Journal of the American Dietetic Association, 111*(7), 1004–1011. doi:10.1016/j.jada.2011.04.012. S0002-8223(11)00425-1 [pii].

NIH. (2007). *Reducing health disparities among children: Strategies and programs for health plans*. Washington, DC: NIHCM.

Ogden, C., Carroll, M., Curtin, L., Lamb, M., & Flegal, K. (2010). Prevalence of high body mass index in US children and adolescents, 2007–2008. *Journal of the American Medical Association, 303*(3), 8.

Ogden, C. L., Carroll, M. D., Curtin, L. R., McDowell, M. A., Tabak, C. J., & Flegal, K. M. (2006). Prevalence of overweight and obesity in the United States, 1999–2004. *JAMA, 295*(13), 1549–1555.

Ogden, C., Carroll, M. D., Kit, B. K., & Flegal, K. M. (2012). Prevalence of obesity and trends in body mass index among US children and adolescents, 1999–2010. *Journal of the American Medical Association, 307*(5), 483–490. doi:10.1001/jama.2012.40.

Ogden, C., Lamb, M., Carroll, M., & Flegal, K. (2010). Obesity and Socioeconomic status in children and adolescents: United Stated, 2005–2008. *NCHS Data Brief, 51*, 1–8.

Patient Centered Medical Homes. Retrieved from http://www.hhs.gov/healthcare/rights/law/index.html

Patton, G. C., Selzer, R., Coffey, C., Carlin, J. B., & Wolfe, R. (1999). Onset of adolescent eating disorders: Population based cohort study over 3 years. *BMJ, 318*(7186), 765–768.

Peterson, J. C., & Gubrium, A. (2011). Old wine in new bottles? The positioning of participation in 17 NIH-funded CBPR projects. *Health Communication, 26*(8), 724–734. doi:10.1080/1041 0236.2011.566828.

Pi-Sunyer, F. X. (2002). The obesity epidemic: Pathophysiology and consequences of obesity. *Obesity Research, 10*(Suppl 2), 97S–104S.

Popkin, B. M. (2007). Understanding global nutrition dynamics as a step towards controlling cancer incidence. *Nature Reviews Cancer, 7*, 61–67.

Rao, G. (2008). Childhood obesity: Highlights of AMA expert committee recommendations. *American Family Physician, 78*(1), 56–63.

Resnicow, K., Davis, R., & Rollnick, S. (2006). Motivational interviewing for pediatric obesity: Conceptual issues and evidence review. *Journal of the American Dietetic Association, 106*(12), 2024–2033.

Resnicow, K., DiIorio, C., Soet, J. E., Ernst, D., Borrelli, B., & Hecht, J. (2002). Motivational interviewing in health promotion: It sounds like something is changing. *Health Psychology, 21*(5), 444–451.

Rhee, K. E., De Lago, C. W., Arscott-Mills, T., Mehta, S. D., & Davis, R. K. (2005). Factors associated with parental readiness to make changes for overweight children. *Pediatrics, 116*(1), e94–e101.

Rittenhouse, D. R., Casalino, L. P., Gillies, R. R., Shortell, S. M., & Lau, B. (2008). Measuring the medical home infrastructure in large medical groups. *Health Affairs, 27*(5), 1246–1258.

Stice, E., Becker, C., & Yokum, S. (2013). Eating disorder prevention: Current evidence-base and further directions. *International Journal of Eating Disorders, 46*(5), 478–485.

Stice, E., Hayward, C., Cameron, R. P., Killen, J. D., & Taylor, C. B. (2000). Body-image and eating disturbances predict onset of depression among female adolescents: A longitudinal study. *Journal of Abnormal Psychology, 109*(3), 438–444.

Stice, E., Shaw, H., & Marti, C. N. (2007). A meta-analytic review of eating disorder prevention programs: Encouraging findings. *Annual Review of Clinical Psychology, 3*, 207–231. doi:10.1146/annurev.clinpsy.3.022806.091447.

Story, M., Sherwood, N. E., Himes, J. H., Davis, M., Jacobs, D. R., Jr., Cartwright, Y., … Rochon, J. (2003). An after-school obesity prevention program for African-American girls: The Minnesota GEMS pilot study. *Ethnicity & Disease, 13*(Suppl 1), S54–S64.

Stovitz, S., Hannan, P., Lytle, L., Demerath, E., Pereira, M., & Himes, J. (2010). Child height and the risk of young-adult obesity. *American Journal of Preventive Medicine, 38*(1), 74–77.

Wang, C., & Burris, M. (1994). Empowerment through Photo Novella: Portraits of participants. *Health Education and Behavior, 21*(2), 171–186.

Whitaker, R. C., Wright, J. A., Pepe, M. S., Seidel, K. D., & Dietz, W. H. (1997). Predicting obesity in young adulthood from childhood and parental obesity. *New England Journal of Medicine, 25*(337), 869–873.

Wilson, D. K. (2009). New perspectives on health disparities and obesity interventions in youth. *Journal of Pediatric Psychology, 34*(3), 231–244.

Part VI
Children and Adolescents in the Health Care System

Chapter 16
Wellness Promotion in Children with Chronic Physical Illness

Katharine Thomson and Simona Bujoreanu

16.1 Introduction

The percentage of US children living with a chronic physical condition has increased dramatically over the past three decades (The National Center for Chronic Disease Preventions and Health Promotion, 2009; Van Cleave, Gortmaker, & Perrin, 2010), not only due to medical advances supporting survival rates, but also due to the increase in risk factors for chronic physical conditions, such as obesity (Halfon & Newacheck, 2014). It is estimated that 10 % of children in the United States are affected by a chronic physical condition that has a moderate to severe impact on their health-related quality of life and functioning (Newacheck & Taylor, 1992).

There are numerous ways to categorize chronic physical conditions. Given that physical illness affects psychological functioning and well-being, Rolland's typology of illness seems most inclusive (Rolland, 1984), as it categorizes illnesses based on onset, course, outcome, and level of functional impairment from a psychosocial perspective. For example, some chronic physical conditions present episodically and are not necessarily life-shortening (e.g., asthma, inflammatory bowel disease, epilepsy), while other conditions can be debilitating, chronic, progressive, and potentially life-shortening (e.g., cystic fibrosis, cancer, diabetes, cerebral palsy, congenital heart disease, sickle cell anemia). It is important to consider these disease characteristics, including the nature of the child's treatment, when anticipating the emotional and psychosocial needs of both youth and families living with chronic medical conditions (Herzer et al., 2010).

Health behaviors are multifaceted and contextual, and the relationships between personal, interpersonal, cultural, and environmental factors in the context of coping with chronic illness are both dynamic and bidirectional (Wilson & Lawman, 2009).

K. Thomson, Ph.D. (✉) • S. Bujoreanu, Ph.D.
Harvard Medical School, Boston Children's Hospital, Boston, MA, USA
e-mail: katharine.thomson@children.harvard.edu

© Springer Science+Business Media New York 2016
M.R. Korin (ed.), *Health Promotion for Children and Adolescents*,
DOI 10.1007/978-1-4899-7711-3_16

A biopsychosocial approach to working with physically ill children allows for comprehensive understanding of each child's symptoms and ability to adapt and cope based on their age and developmental levels. This approach—which considers biological, psychological, and social aspects of illness development and management—gives a multidimensional picture of the child as part of various systems (i.e., family, cultural, institutional, community), goes beyond diagnostic labels and medical explanations, and puts forward hypotheses about underlying causes and perpetuating factors of the presenting problems as well as strength and resiliency factors to consider. The use of the biopsychosocial framework allows opportunities for providers to identify not only points of intervention, but also areas of strength and resilience in each individual and in their life context (Shaw & DeMaso, 2010). Mental health clinicians, such as pediatric psychologists and child psychiatrists, are trained in health psychology and behavioral medicine and are equipped to conduct these evaluations and consult with patients, families, and medical providers (Phelps, 2006; Willen, 2007).

There is considerable research regarding risk factors for children with chronic illnesses, though the majority of research is disease-specific and does not compare across clinical groupings (Sawyer, Drew, Yeo, & Britto, 2007). Comprehensive and empirically based reviews of the psychosocial impact of various physical illnesses on pediatric patients and their families, as well as available treatments to minimize such impacts, are available (Roberts & Steele, 2009; Shaw & DeMaso, 2010). This chapter will focus on various protective and wellness-promoting factors across disease groups by summarizing available knowledge about key aspects related to adjustment and coping with a chronic physical illness. This chapter will use an ecological framework to identify biopsychosocial elements at individual, family, cultural, and community levels that increase physical and mental health among pediatric patients. Using Bronfenbrenner's ecological systems theory (Bronfenbrenner, 2005), this chapter will highlight the ways in which a child's ability to manage and cope with chronic illness is influenced by multiple factors at each level. Additionally, this chapter will discuss knowledge and resources that youth, families and caregivers, educators, policy makers, as well as medical and other allied health providers can use to promote health and wellness.

16.2   Individual Wellness-Promoting Factors

16.2.1   Psychoeducation

Knowledge about one's illness is an important aspect of healthy coping for physically ill children and their families. Psychoeducation interventions provide structured information about an illness, its treatment, and have been used successfully across many illness types and age groups to target youths' understanding of their disease and treatments, leading to positive behavioral changes via teaching illness management skills. Psychoeducation has been shown to increase youth self-efficacy and self-advocacy skills, improve psychological adaptation to illness, and decrease physical symptoms and treatment side effects (Barlow & Ellard, 2004; Beale, Bradlyn, & Kato, 2003; Kirk et al., 2013; Plante, 2001), with positive effects on both short- and long-term health outcomes (Grey, Boland, Davidson, Li, & Tamborlane, 2000). Many research studies have shown better outcomes for psychoeducational efforts in a group-based setting, as opposed to individual settings (Kirk et al., 2013), likely due to the opportunity to also provide normalization, support, and networking for youth with chronic physical illness and their families. Interventions that involve patients and families together, along with community-based follow-up, add to the effectiveness and impact of acquired knowledge and skills (Kirk et al., 2013).

Delivering psychoeducation in a culturally responsive manner is vital (Center for Mental Health Services, 2009). Culture impacts the way patients and families view an illness and the proposed treatments and influences how families chose to cope with stressors (Suzuki, White, & Velez, 2010). As providers, educators, and policy makers, being aware of one's own cultural values helps to buffer against biases; when developing a psychoeducational plan, it is important to consider cultural elements such as youth's and family's religious beliefs, level of acculturation, gender relations, family member roles, and notions of privacy and independence/ interdependence in the youth's social network. Information should be provided in a language that is accessible to the patient and family member. If necessary, trained interpreters are most appropriate and it is of outmost importance that children should not serve as interpreters for their parents (Flores, 2005).

Computer- and internet-based psychoeducational programs are growing in popularity given their availability for patients who might not have access to in-person psychoeducational resources (Ritterband et al., 2003); benefits include accessibility, low cost, ease of updating, and ability to be highly individualized and interactive (Bradlyn, Beale, & Kato, 2003). Online interventions have demonstrated positive outcomes related to improved illness-related knowledge, symptoms, self-care autonomy, health outcomes, and quality of life (Lewis, 1999; Mulvaney et al., 2011; Whittemore et al., 2013). For example, a psychoeducational initiative in the form of a video game created for pediatric cancer patients demonstrated improved adherence and cancer-related self-efficacy and knowledge (Kato, Cole, Bradlyn, & Pollock, 2008).

16.2.2   Treatment Adherence

Children with chronic physical conditions have complex and time-consuming medical regimens that may include medications, medical interventions, frequent medical appointments, and diet and activity restrictions. Poor adherence to these treatments has been linked with higher health care costs and utilization, increased symptoms, and higher mortality rates (McGrady & Hommel, 2013; Pai & Ostendorf, 2011; Simons, McCormick, Mee, & Blount, 2009). Adherence is well researched among particular age groups and illness populations, particularly among those in which poor adherence is especially dangerous (e.g., cardiac disease, organ transplant, diabetes) (Chapman, 2004; Ittenbach, Cassedy, Marino, Spicer, & Drotar, 2009; Simons, Gilleland, et al., 2009; Simons, McCormick, et al., 2009).

From a biopsychosocial perspective, it is well known that adherence has a developmental trajectory where various factors are relevant at different ages (e.g., parent coping and distress are most predictive of adherence during childhood; social support and peer factors are very influential on adherence throughout adolescence; lack of preparation for the transition from pediatric to adult care teams also reduces adherence). Therefore, interventions are often tailored to target unique developmental stages (Pai & Ostendorf, 2011; Quittner, Barker, Marciel, & Grimley, 2009). For example, an important barrier to adherence is forgetfulness (Lemanek & Ranalli, 2009), and there are many technologies available to assist adolescents as they learn to take on more responsibility in their medical care, such as applications on smartphones, text message reminders, and interactive adherence "games" online (Castano, Stockwell, & Malbon, 2013). Overall, psychoeducation combined with behavioral skills training has proven to be the most successful approach for increasing adherence (Dean, 2010; Grey et al., 2000; Kahana, Drotar, & Frazier, 2008; Williams, 2010) and using patient- and family-centered approaches is ideal (Simons, McCormick, et al., 2009). Adolescents, for example, respond particularly well to cognitive behavioral therapy, self-monitoring, stress management training, behavioral techniques, social support, and motivational interviewing (Quittner et al., 2009; Wysocki et al., 2007; Wysocki, Buckloh, & Greco, 2009). Family factors that have been found to promote adherence in children include the use of behavioral family systems therapy with educational support, flexibility in problem-solving, active coping strategies, adequate family and peer social support, and specific and concrete recommendations (e.g., "Drink two liters of water per day" versus "Stay hydrated") (Lemanek & Ranalli, 2009, Wysocki et al., 2007, 2009).

16.2.3 Coping with Medical Procedures

While promoting adjustment to the illness and minimizing its impact on daily living are important goals for youth with chronic physical illness, helping children cope effectively with medical procedures also influences long-term health behaviors. Studies have shown that increased medical fears and perceived procedural pain during childhood predict poorer coping overall (Blount et al., 2009) and significant procedural anxiety in adulthood (Kuppenheimer & Brown, 2002), above and beyond the burden of the illness itself. Coping strategies require a patient- and family-centered approach, and when planning interventions, the biopsychosocial perspective integrates factors such as a child's age, sex, developmental level and temperament, past experiences with medical care, parental distress levels, cultural factors, and available family and community resources (Blount et al., 2009).

Giving sufficient warning time prior to a procedure is important—adolescents do best when involved in treatment planning from the beginning, whereas school-age children do well with 5–7 days warning, and preschool children only need 1–2 days. While the provision of printed materials and narrative preparations are most commonly used (Blount et al., 2009), they are not the most effective preparation strategies. Video preparation, medical play with equipment that will be used during the procedure (using equipment in fun and nontypical ways such as painting with syringes or "playing doctor" where the child can administer the injection to a doll), parent coaching on how to support their child during procedure, and parent psycho-education are effective in both reducing patient and parent anxiety and increasing compliance during the procedure (Cohen, Bernard, Greco, & McClellan, 2002; Kain et al., 2007).

During the procedure, active or solution-focused coping strategies (Brannon & Feist, 2009) such as active distraction, relaxation skills, and hypnosis have been shown to be helpful in reducing pain-related behaviors and self-reported pain levels during medical procedures (Nilsson, Enskär, Hallqvist, & Kokinsky, 2013). Passive or emotion-focused coping strategies such as avoidance, lead to increased distress and higher levels of depressive symptoms (Snow-Turek, Norris, & Tan, 1996). Encouragingly, studies have shown that many physically ill children cope with everyday stressors more effectively when compared to their healthy peers, suggesting that the coping skills they develop related to illness management may transfer beyond the medical arena (Hampel, Rudolph, Stachow, Lass-Lentzsch, & Petermann, 2005). The same coping skills that are effective in helping children during medical procedures are also very helpful in addressing mood changes and anxiety associated with chronic physical illness.

Parents and medical staff can have a direct and immediate impact on a child's response to acute and chronic pain and medical procedures. Research shows that caregiver behavior during procedures accounts for over half of the variance in the level of distress in the child (Frank, Blount, Smith, Manimala, & Martin, 1995). While the most common vocalizations from adults tend to be reassurance-based (e.g., "Everything is okay, you're going to be alright"), a child's distress is significantly greater when parents reassure, criticize, or apologize compared to when they distract the child (Manimala, Blount, & Cohen, 2000; Walker et al., 2006). The most effective family-centered coping techniques include coping-promoting coaching (e.g., parent reminding the child to take deep breaths or taking deep breaths with the youth), non-procedural based distraction (visual, auditory, tactile, or cognitive engagement such as story building and memory tasks), and humor (Cohen et al., 2002; Kain et al., 2007; Manimala et al., 2000). Distraction is particularly effective for younger children or when minimal preparation time is available (Doellman, 2003). Ongoing coaching is important, as research indicates that gains made by younger children in pain management techniques are not maintained during a painful procedure if the trained coach is withdrawn during the medical context (Cohen et al., 2002). Individually tailored coping kits created by youth and parents in collaboration with psychosocial and medical providers, which include items for distraction, procedural coping, supportive messages from staff and family, as well as booklets describing the procedure and common responses, are helpful for children with significant distress during medical procedures (Drake, Johnson, Stoneck, Martinez, & Massey, 2012).

The risk of medical trauma during procedures can be minimized with the appropriate use of local or systemic anesthesia or psychotropic medications (Duff & Bliss, 2005). Finally, various complementary and alternative medical interventions have been effective in reducing distress and perceived pain levels during procedures, both alone and when coupled with psychopharmacological interventions (Landier & Tse, 2010). Biofeedback has demonstrated significant effects in the treatment of chronic pain, anxiety, and hypertension (Palermo, Eccleston, Lewandowski, Williams, & Morley, 2010; Yucha & Montgomery, 2008).

16.2.4   Coping with Hospitalizations

Some children may need to stay in the hospital frequently and/or for extended periods of time due to medical management therefore missing developmentally appropriate life experiences and school for weeks or months at a time (Reuben & Pastor, 2013). There are several hospital-specific stressors, in addition to the illness-associated stress, that children with chronic illness describe, including trouble sleeping because of physical discomfort and/or frequent medical cares (vital signs, medication administration), high stimulation and noise levels, changes in daily routine, and adjustment to hospital food or diet limitations (Spirito, Stark, & Tyc, 1994). Creating a daily schedule with the youth can help to minimize unexpected medical events, regulate the sleep/wake cycle, and offset challenging medical procedures and treatments with pleasurable activities and calm intervals. The schedule should mimic aspects of the youth's home life, such as bedtime routines, "quiet time," meal times, and cultural and religious elements, which will help to maximize predictability and familiarity during hospitalization. It is beneficial for children if medical staff respect established quiet times (e.g., door signs can be used to signal when a child is napping or when a family is praying) as much as is feasible. Providing children with developmentally appropriate decisional control in managing the illness can help to promote a sense of agency and actively involve the child in developing skills around adherence and medical care. Additionally, the patient's hospital room should be maintained as safe place, free from medical procedural anxiety and pain; when possible, it is helpful for medical treatments to occur in a separate treatment room rather than at bedside.

Psychosocial support has been found to be one of the most helpful factors for youth during hospitalizations (Dodds, 2010) and can be available via family support (e.g., presence of at least one caregiver at bedside and regular contact with other family members, including siblings); communication, strong rapport, and trust with medical providers; peer contact (e.g., in person or via phone/online/ cards); and regular access to other services in the hospital (e.g., child life, social work, psychiatry, psychology, volunteers, interfaith chaplaincy, interpreters, and cultural liaisons) (Suzuki & Kato, 2003). It is helpful to create opportunities for youth to maintain their identity from outside the hospital, beyond that of being a medical patient, by bringing favorite items from home, hanging personalized signs on the walls of the hospital room, displaying pictures of pets or family or cultural or religious items as desired, and providing tutoring for schoolwork if appropriate. Cultural considerations are paramount; factors such as availability of parents and extended family support, parents' understanding of roles and expectations (both of themselves and of staff during hospitalizations), access to resources, access to/ understanding of medical information (e.g., language, education level, background), and the role of faith and religion in healing may vary greatly by patient and family.

16.2.5 Psychiatric Treatments

The stress of chronic physical illness manifests in many ways, such as psychological reactions involving somatic symptoms (e.g., pain, dizziness, fatigue), behavioral changes (e.g., acting out, non-adherence, lifestyle alterations), emotional states (e.g., fear, sadness, anxiety), and/or developmental challenges (e.g., incorporating medical information in one's identity at different developmental stages), and can add to the complexity of managing a medical condition. Similarly, both the direct effects (i.e., physiological effects of the illness and treatment) and the indirect effects (e.g., hospitalizations, lifestyle changes) of the health condition need to be considered when working with pediatric patients in order to understand the impact on a patient's functioning (Sawyer et al., 2007). Pediatric psychosomatic medicine (including behavioral medicine, pediatric psychology, and consultation-liaison psychiatry) has developed as a specialty to support children and their families in coping with the emotional and behavioral impacts of chronic illness using both psychological and pharmacological treatments (Sawyer et al., 2007) and is available in all settings, from community mental health centers, to primary care, specialty clinics, and hospitals.

There appears to be a subset of children with chronic illness who are particularly at risk for psychiatric difficulties, such as those who have a history of trauma (medical or otherwise), past behavioral or emotional problems, and/or a lack of social support (National Traumatic Child Stress Network, 2004). These youth may require extra attention and assistance over and above the areas outlined above. For example, cognitive behavioral therapy is an evidence-based treatment to assist children struggling with depression, anxiety, or non-adherence in the context of chronic health conditions (Powers, Manne, Blount, et al., 1999), and can be administered during inpatient hospitalizations by mental health clinicians available on consultation services, or via outpatient therapists in the community.

16.3 Family Wellness-Promoting Factors

16.3.1 Assessing Family Functioning

Families of children with chronic physical conditions must balance day-to-day activities and typical developmental tasks with symptom management and treatment needs of their chronically ill child (Kazak, Rourke, & Navsaria, 2009). Families may need to learn to adapt differently based on specific characteristics of a child's condition; a chronic, progressive, life-shortening medical condition may leave families with minimal, if any, periods of respite, while nonlife shortening and episodic illnesses may require families to adapt quickly between periods of relative stability and stress. Given that family functioning has been shown to play a vital role in the psychological adjustment of pediatric patients (Wallander, Thompson, & Alriksson-Schmidt, 2003) and poor family functioning is associated with increased symptoms and disease severity (Alderfer & Stanley, 2012; Barakat et al., 2007), it is key that healthcare providers identify families in need and provide the necessary supports. Therefore, assessing for family functioning via the biopsychosocial model—including strengths and protective factors as well as cultural considerations—is an essential component of a healthcare team's ability to meet a family "where they are" (Nabors & Lehmkuhl, 2004; Rolland, 1987).

It is widely accepted that families of physically ill children experience high levels of stress, which has the potential to impact family functioning (Barakat & Alderfer, 2011; Herzer et al., 2010; Kazak, 2001). However, contrary to past belief, research has shown that the majority of families of children with chronic health conditions adapt relatively well and do not have significantly different levels of family functioning when compared to families of healthy children (Kazak et al., 2009; McClellan & Cohen, 2007). In a study comparing family functioning across disease types and control groups concluded that approximately one third of *all* families, regardless of disease status, present with elements of "unhealthy" family functioning (Herzer et al., 2010). However, having older children, fewer children in the home, and a lower household income were risk factors for poor family functioning across both groups. An additional factor that has been found to increase stress and undermine family functioning among those with physically ill children is the presence of comorbid depression or learning disability in the child (Bujoreanu, Ibeziako, & Demaso, 2011), underlining the need for comprehensive developmentally informed biopsychosocial evaluations for each child. Targeted supports and intervention—such as family therapy to improve family communication and problem-solving skills, spousal support, social support, and parent respite—can have a significant positive impact on parents' ability to support their child.

16.3.2 Supporting Siblings

Not surprisingly, siblings of physically ill children are at risk for behavioral and mental health issues; however, social support and high family cohesion can help to mitigate these risks (Barrera, Chung, & Fleming, 2004; Williams et al., 1999). Family-based interventions that provide psychoeducation for siblings are effective in decreasing siblings' emotional symptoms, perceived stress, and use of avoidance coping strategies (e.g., denial, withdrawal, isolation), as well as improving family time and routines (Giallo & Gavidia-Payne, 2008). Siblings who participate in psychosocial support groups demonstrate increased knowledge about illness, social support, self-esteem, and mood, as well as decreased behavior problems (Williams et al., 2003). Interventions that focus on helping siblings to identify positive outcomes and areas of personal growth in the face of their sibling's illness (i.e., "benefit finding") may also be helpful (Kamibeppu et al., 2010; Packman, 1999).

16.3.3 Parent Education

Parent education is an effective way to disseminate health-promoting information. Since parents are typically responsible for gauging their child's physical health and managing treatment on a daily basis, it is important to build a sense of agency for parents so that they feel equipped to support their child. Parental empowerment has been correlated not only with lower stress levels in parents, but self-efficacy has also been related to youth's increased treatment adherence (Barlow & Ellard, 2004; Melnyk et al., 2004). Psychoeducation regarding psychological functioning is equally important in helping parents to understand the potential for mood/anxiety changes, monitor for psychiatric comorbidities, and learn about developmental phases and possible reactions their child may experience as a result of any life changes imposed by the illness. Since parental presence and behavior account for a large portion of the variance in child distress around medical care, it is important to offer parents specific behavioral strategies to coach and manage their children in the context of medical struggles (e.g., adherence, during medical procedures or hospitalizations, etc.) (Barlow & Ellard, 2004). Of course, this information is most effectively provided with cultural and linguistic considerations in mind; parents are the experts on their unique child and can be encouraged to co-create plans of care for maximum effectiveness.

Disease-specific support groups, online chat forums, and having a strong rapport with medical providers are effective methods for providing parent education (Kieckhefer et al., 2014; Mason & Vazquez, 2007; Van Servellen, Fongwa, & Mockus D'Errico, 2006). As with youth educational programs, a combination of techniques in addition to education, such as video modeling, parent coaching, or parent-direction home-based exposure programs, have been the most successful. (Kain et al., 2007).

16.4 Institutional Wellness-Promoting Factors

16.4.1 Biopsychosocial Evaluation

Families and providers can utilize developmental biopsychosocial assessments in order to identify a child's individual risk and protective factors and capture the complexity of a child's unique vulnerabilities due to their health challenges (Shaw & DeMaso, 2010; Winters, Hanson, & Stoyanova, 2007). Several chronic conditions and their treatment sequelae are associated with cognitive vulnerabilities (e.g., epilepsy, cancer, cardiac disease); therefore, cognitive and academic testing must be considered for these children as unidentified problems may hinder adjustment in school and social environments (Bujoreanu et al., 2011). A thorough neuropsychological assessment may be indicated in order to identify additional subtle cognitive changes associated with certain illnesses or treatments (Bellinger et al., 2011; Hocking & Alderfer, 2012; Kupst, 1999). Developmentally informed biopsychosocial evaluations can lead to tailored patient- and/or family-centered interventions that are culturally responsive and work to promote strengths and address any risk factors.

Since children with chronic illness are at particular risk for emotional distress when compared with healthy peers (Wallander et al., 2003), early identification of mental health struggles is key. As a growing trend, many medical centers and primary care clinics now are beginning to integrate mental health clinicians into their practices (e.g., Massachusetts Child Psychiatry Access Project: http://www.mcpap.com/) (Kelly & Coons, 2012). Increasing awareness among medical providers about the epidemiology of pediatric mental health disorders, developmentally matched signs and symptoms of depression or anxiety, and effective treatment approaches empowers these providers to identify and manage their patients' emotional needs or refer families to mental health services. Given time constraints and lack of appropriate mental health resources in some medical settings, computer-based screeners have shown promise in reducing some of the burden associated with psychosocial assessments (Chisolm, Gardner, Julian, & Kelleher, 2008).

16.4.2 Integrated Care and Family-Centered Care

In integrated care, patients are viewed as more than the sum of their illnesses and care is based on communication and collaboration between providers with the goal of wellness-promotion across all levels of medical institutions—from primary care (e.g., medical homes) and community clinics to hospitals. Family- and patient-centered care is now the recommended standard (Drotar et al., 2001) and represents a significant departure from the past philosophy where care was more healthcare provider-focused (King, Teplicky, King, & Rosenbaum, 2004; Kuo, Houtrow, et al., 2012; Kuo, Sisterhen, et al., 2012). For individuals with chronic physical conditions, continuity of patient care via ongoing relationships with consistent medical teams has been linked with improved functioning, quality of life, and satisfaction with medical services (Van Servellen et al., 2006).

Building on the importance of a solid alliance with medical providers, family-centered care has led to initiatives both on outpatient and inpatient medical settings. This approach is associated with less delayed health care, fewer unmet service needs, reduced out-of-pocket costs, stable health care needs, reduced odds of emergency room visits, and increased odds of doctor visits for triage and appropriate use of services (Kuo, Bird, & Tilford, 2011). For example, the "Collaborative Family Healthcare Association" (CFHS; http://www.cfha.net/) views parents, patients, and medical providers as equal participants in the healthcare process. Utilizing the expertise of families of physically ill children has shown benefits for pediatric patients requiring medical admissions. The practice of family-centered rounds, described as "interdisciplinary work rounds at the bedside in which patient and family share the control of the management plan," (Sisterhen, Blaszak, Woods, & Smith, 2007) has increased dramatically in popularity in pediatric facilities in the past decade (Kuo, Houtrow, et al., 2012; Kuo, Sisterhen, et al., 2012) and is associated with families receiving more consistent medical information and feeling more respected by the medical team (Kuo, Houtrow, et al., 2012; Kuo, Sisterhen, et al., 2012). Other initiatives that involve partnering with patients and families exist in pediatric palliative medical education programs (Browning & Solomon, 2005) and in the design and planning of pediatric centers (Coad & Coad, 2008). Furthermore, many pediatric hospitals in the country now have patient and parent focus groups involved in the development and revision of hospital protocols of care (Popper, Anderson, Black, Ericson, & Peck, 1987).

16.4.3   Transition to Adult Care

Given that many youth with chronic diseases are now living longer (e.g., cystic fibrosis), the transition to adult care is recognized as a crucial step in assuring successful adjustment to new medical providers and centers, potential changes in medical regimens, and different lifestyles and demands (Crowley, 2011; Quittner et al., 2009; Steinbeck, Brodie, & Towns, 2008). The adult medical system often includes a variety of specialists across multiple hospital sites and places the expectation for coordination of care on the patient; thus, the transition from one comprehensive pediatric team providing integrated care to the adult system can be challenging and potentially traumatic for young adults. Without sufficient preparation and support, this transition can undermine adherence to medical treatment, health status, and overall quality of life due to increased stress (Lemanek & Ranalli,

2009; Pai & Ostendorf, 2011; Quittner et al., 2009; Rodrigue & Zelikovsky, 2009). Studies within the last decade have identified several major stages of transition to adult care, such as gradual shift of primary care and treatment decisions from the parent to the youth, long-term preparation mirroring the developmentally informed involvement of youth in their medical decision-making and care (starting as early as 12 years of age), gradual transition of care from the child-focused institution to medical providers in an adult center with the help of a continuity provider, and assigning adult care physicians who have a preestablished and ongoing collaborative relationship with the pediatric providers (Wallis, 2007). In addition, other elements that promote a positive transition include the presence and involvement of uniquely specialized transition coordinators, peer group support and life skills training (including psychoeducation on topics such as health insurance and functioning of health care systems), culturally sensitive approaches, and long-term mentoring and support (Lemanek & Ranalli, 2009; Pai & Ostendorf, 2011; Quittner et al., 2009; Rodrigue & Zelikovsky, 2009).

16.5 Community Wellness-Promoting Factors

16.5.1 Schools

Schools are the main community institutions responsible for the socialization and education of children, and youth with chronic illness may spend weeks, months, or even years out of community-based schools (Thies, 1999). Schools play a vital role in creating effective individual-centered educational plans for youth in order to assure access to learning while accounting for the unique cognitive, emotional, behavioral, and physical needs due to medical conditions and associated treatment consequences (Drotar, 2001; Dupaul, Power, & Shapiro, 2009). In support of this claim, studies have shown that children with chronic physical conditions who are able to remain connected academically and socially with their school, teachers, and classmates during medical treatments and hospitalizations demonstrate improved academic functioning and report significant social support (Nabors & Lehmkuhl, 2004; Reuben & Pastor, 2013). Advances in technology help such children remain engaged with their peers and their schooling during hospitalizations and home-based treatments through video conferencing (Di Fiore, Jorissen, Van Reeth, et al., 2008) and even robot avatars for distance learning (e.g., www.vgocom.com).

When children are ready to return to community-based schools in person, there are a number of evidence-based school reintegration programs that are accessible to staff and families to promote a smooth transition and adjustment (Dupaul et al., 2009). Mental health clinicians and special education staff working in schools can provide academic, cognitive, and emotional assessments and interventions via 504 plans or Individual Educational Plans (www.drcnh.org/IDEA504.pdf), support, counseling and guidance, cognitive retraining (i.e., skills related to attention, problem-solving, decision-making, and higher level cognitive abilities), and social skills training (Nabors & Lehmkuhl, 2004) for children with chronic medical conditions and their families (Perry & Flanagan, 1986), and can implement effective programs focused on teacher and peer education.

16.5.2 Communities

From a biopsychosocial perspective, "exosystemic" (Bronfenbrenner, 2005) approaches are needed in order to make lasting change in the area of wellness-promotion, especially related to reducing barriers to healthcare. There is limited research regarding community-based interventions for children with chronic conditions, as the lack of resources makes large-scale community-based studies challenging (Wilson & Lawman, 2009); however, it has been shown that community-level interventions, such as via local media, churches, supermarkets, and even restaurants, can influence health behaviors and promote awareness for the general population (Wilson & Lawman, 2009). It is important that interventions are adapted to specific cultural considerations by consulting with community and/or religious members and using cultural liaisons where possible. It is known from research on protective factors and posttraumatic growth in the context of potentially medically traumatizing events experienced by children and their families that social support (both at family and community levels) has a positive impact on psychosocial adjustment (Picoraro, Womer, Kazak, & Feudtner, 2014). Summer camps for children with chronic health conditions are an example of supports available in the community that have shown to help medically involved youth foster independence, feel more hopeful, and become more confident in their ability to accomplish goals (Woods, Mayes, Bartley, Fedele, & Ryan, 2013; Wu, Prout, Roberts, Parikshak, & Amylon, 2011).

16.5.3 Health Advocacy

Successful interventions for youth and families target both health-compromising behaviors as well as health-promoting behaviors (Wilson & Lawman, 2009). "Health literacy" has been introduced as an important aspect of health promotion and is defined as a person having the "capacity to obtain, process, and understand basic health information and services to make appropriate health decisions" (www.cdc.gov/healthliteracy/). Given that individuals with chronic illnesses are required to navigate complex medical systems frequently, health literacy is especially salient among this population. Unfortunately, wellness promotion and services are less defined and less studied for children, adolescents, and young adults with chronic medical conditions (Massey, Prelip, Calimlim, Quiter, & Glik, 2012), perhaps because the focus of care is understandably placed on the management of the chronic disease and it may be assumed that children are not able to take charge of their complex medical care.

However, not including children as active participants in their health care in developmentally appropriate ways can have negative consequences during transition to adult care where medical providers expect self-initiative and independence.

Youth with chronic medical conditions tend to have lower self-esteem when compared to their healthy peers and are as likely or more likely to undertake risky behaviors than their healthy peers (Pinquart, 2013; Suris & Parera, 2005). As a result of the unique challenges that youth with chronic illness face, it is important to empower these youth to self-advocate in order to help them develop into healthy and conscious adults who are informed consumers in the medical world and active players in policy development. Youth of color may benefit from additional support in this area as research has demonstrated that ethnicity and health disparities (Centers for Disease Control, 2010) may play a role in self-advocacy in a medical setting (Wiltshire, Cronin, Sarto, & Brown, 2006). Psychoeducational interventions might include dimensions such as understanding one's rights and responsibilities, engaging in preventive care, becoming an active presence in one's care by seeking out information and skill mastery, and building a trusting patient–provider relationship (Massey et al., 2012). That said, the degree of expected or typical independence from a youth or young adult may vary by culture (and by gender within cultures); medical teams should work with patients and families to create developmentally and culturally appropriate goals for each patient.

Health advocacy has helped change policies and effect large-scale changes in health care systems, and youth with chronic medical conditions may be in a strong position to advocate for change given their regular contact with the medical system. Examples of important movements in health advocacy for children with chronic illness and their families include legislation regarding transplant allocation in pediatric populations, the Family and Medical Leave Act, health care reform, and obesity prevention programs (Kazak et al., 2009). The increased awareness among providers of medical trauma is another example of a prevention-based initiative that can be tracked over the years: initial clinical observations of medically traumatized children branched into targeted psychoeducational programs for providers and medical trauma is now common knowledge among pediatric providers with national-level committees and resources available (e.g., www.NCTSN.org/medtoolkit).

16.6 Summary and Conclusions

Perhaps the most important "take-home" message regarding health-promotion for children with chronic physical conditions is the concept that effective and healthy coping for patients and their families requires systemic support across individual, family, institutional, and community levels. Patients, parents, providers, educators, communities, and policy makers can work together to support physically ill children by promoting illness-prevention and health-promotion while recognizing individual strengths and cultural values and minimizing impacts on typical development. Children's experience of the medical and educational systems can have lasting effects on outcomes related to their health, health-related quality of life, and well-being as adults.

References

Alderfer, M. A., & Stanley, C. M. (2012). Health and illness in the context of the family. In A. Baum, T. A. Revenson, & J. Singer (Eds.), *Handbook of health psychology* (2nd ed., pp. 493–516). New York: Psychology Press.

Barakat, L. P., & Alderfer, M. A. (2011). Introduction to special issue: Advancing the science of family assessment in pediatric psychology. *Journal of Pediatric Psychology, 36,* 489–493. doi:10.1093/jpepsy/jsq110.

Barakat, L. P., Patterson, C. A., Weinberger, B. S., Simon, K., Gonzalez, E. R., & Dampier, C. (2007). A prospective study of the role of coping and family functioning in health outcomes for adolescents with sickle cell disease. *Journal of Pediatric Hematology, 29,* 752–760.

Barlow, J. H., & Ellard, D. R. (2004). Psycho-educational interventions for children with chronic disease, parents and siblings: An overview of the research evidence base. *Child: Care, Health and Development, 30,* 637–645. doi:10.1111/j.1365-2214.2004.00474.x.

Barrera, M., Chung, J., & Fleming, C. (2004). A group intervention for siblings of pediatric cancer patients. *Journal of Psychosocial Oncology, 22,* 21–39.

Beale, I. L., Bradlyn, A. S., & Kato, P. M. (2003). Psychoeducational interventions with pediatric cancer patients: Part II. Effects of information and skills training on health-related outcomes. *Journal of Child and Family Studies, 12*(4), 385–397. doi:10.1023/A:1026007922274.

Belar, C. (2003). Models and concepts. In S. Llewelyn & P. Kennedy (Eds.), *Handbook of clinical health psychology.* San Francisco: Wiley.

Bellinger, D. C., Wypij, D., Rivkin, M. J., DeMaso, D. R., Robertson, R. L., Jr., Dunbar-Masterson, C., … Newburger, J. W. (2011). Adolescents with d-transposition of the great arteries corrected with the arterial switch procedure: Neuropsychological assessment and structural brain imaging. *Circulation, 124,* 1361–1369. doi:10.1161/CIRCULATIONAHA.111.026963.

Blount, R. L., Zempsky, W. T., Jaaniste, T., Evans, S., Cohen, L. L., Devine, K. A., & Zeltzer, L. K. (2009). Management of pediatric pain and distress due to medical procedures. In M. C. Roberts & R. G. Steele (Eds.), *Handbook of pediatric psychology* (4th ed., pp. 171–188). New York: Guilford Press.

Bradlyn, A. S., Beale, I. L., & Kato, P. M. (2003). Psychoeducational interventions with pediatric cancer patients: Part I. Patient information and knowledge. *Journal of Child and Family Studies, 12,* 257–277.

Brannon, L., & Feist, J. (2009). Defining, measuring, and managing stress. In: *Health psychology: An introduction to behavior and health* (7th ed., p. 592). Belmont, CA: Cengage Learning.

Bronfenbrenner, U. (2005). Ecological systems theory. In *Making human beings human: Bioecological perspectives on human development* (pp. 106–173). Thousand Oaks: Sage.

Browning, D. M., & Solomon, M. Z. (2005). The initiative for pediatric palliative care: An interdisciplinary educational approach for healthcare professionals. *Journal of Pediatric Nursing, 20,* 326–334. doi:10.1016/j.pedn.2005.03.004.

Bujoreanu, I. S., Ibeziako, P., & Demaso, D. (2011). Psychiatric concerns in pediatric epilepsy. *Child and Adolescent Psychiatric Clinics of North America, 58*(4), 973–988, xii. doi:10.1016/j.chc.2010.01.001.

Castano, P. M., Stockwell, M. S., & Malbon, K. M. (2013). Using digital technologies to improve treatment adherence. *Clinical Obstetrics and Gynecology, 56*(3), 434–445.

Center for Mental Health Services. (2009). *Family psychoeducation: Getting started with evidence-based practices.* Rockville, MD: Author.

Centers for Disease Control. (2010). *Establishing a holistic framework to reduce inequities in HIV, viral hepatitis, STDs, and tuberculosis in the United States.* An NCHHSTP white paper on social determinants of health.

Chapman, J. R. (2004). Compliance: The patient, the doctor, and the medication? *Transplantation, 77,* 782–786.

Chisolm, D., Gardner, W., Julian, T., & Kelleher, K. (2008). Adolescent satisfaction with computer-assisted behavioural risk screening in primary care. *Child and Adolescent Mental Health, 13,* 163–168.

Coad, J., & Coad, N. (2008). Children and young people's preference of thematic design and colour for their hospital environment. *Journal of Child Health Care, 12*, 33–48. doi:10.1177/1367493507085617.

Cohen, L. L., Bernard, R. S., Greco, L. A., & McClellan, C. B. (2002). A child-focused intervention for coping with procedural pain: Are parent and nurse coaches necessary? *Journal of Pediatric Psychology, 27*, 749–757. doi:10.1093/jpepsy/27.8.749.

Crowley, R. (2011). Improving the transition between paediatric and adult healthcare: A systematic review. *Archives of Disease in Childhood, 96*(6), 548–553.

Dean, A. J. (2010). A systematic review of interventions to enhance medication adherence in children and adolescents with chronic illness. *Archives of Disease in Childhood, 95*, 717–723.

Di Fiore, F., Jorissen, P., Van Reeth, F., Lombaert, E., Valcke, M., Vansichem, G., Veevaete, P., and Hauttekeete, L. (2008). ASCIT sick children again at my school by fostering communication through interactive technologies for long-term sick children. *Advanced Technology for Learning, 5*, 68–78. doi:10.2316/Journal.208.2008.1.208-1105.

Dodds, H. (2010). Meeting the needs of young people in the hospital. *Paediatric Nursing, 22*(9), 14–18.

Doellman, D. (2003). Pharmacological versus nonpharmacological techniques in reducing venipuncture psychological trauma in pediatric patients. *Journal of Infusion Nursing, 26*, 103–109.

Drake, J., Johnson, N., Stoneck, A. V., Martinez, D. M., & Massey, M. (2012). Evaluation of a coping kit for children with challenging behaviors in a pediatric hospital. *Pediatric Nursing, 38*, 215–221.

Drotar, D. (2001). Promoting comprehensive care for children with chronic health conditions and their families: Introduction to the special issue. *Children's Services: Social Policy, Research, and Practice, 4*, 157–163.

Drotar, D., Walders, N., Burgess, E., et al. (2001). Recommendations to enhance comprehensive care for children with chronic health conditions and their families. *Children's Services: Social Policy, Research, and Practice, 4*, 251–265.

Duff, A., & Bliss, A. (2005). Reducing distress during venepuncture. *Recent Advances in Paediatrics, 22*, 149–165.

Dupaul, G., Power, T., & Shapiro, E. (2009). Schools and integration/reintegration into schools. In *Handbook of pediatric psychology* (4th ed., pp. 689–702). New York: Guilford Press.

Flores, G. (2005). The impact of medical interpreter services on the quality of health care: A systematic review. *Medical Care Research and Review, 62*, 255–299. doi:10.1177/1077558705275416.

Frank, N., Blount, R., Smith, A., Manimala, M., & Martin, J. (1995). Parent and staff behavior, previous child medical experience, and maternal anxiety as they relate to child procedural distress and coping (English). *Journal of Pediatric Psychology, 20*, 277–289.

Giallo, R., & Gavidia-Payne, S. (2008). Evaluation of a family-based intervention for siblings of children with a disability or chronic illness. *Advanced Mental Health, 7*, 84–96. doi:10.5172/jamh.7.2.84.

Grey, M., Boland, E. A., Davidson, M., Li, J., & Tamborlane, W. V. (2000). Coping skills training for youth with diabetes mellitus has long-lasting effects on metabolic control and quality of life. *Journal of Pediatrics, 137*, 107–113. doi:10.1067/mpd.2000.106568.

Halfon, N., & Newacheck, P. W. (2014). Evolving notions of childhood chronic illness. *Journal of the American Medical Association, 303*, 1–2. doi:10.1136/jech.2008.082842.16.

Hampel, P., Rudolph, H., Stachow, R., Lass-Lentzsch, A., & Petermann, F. (2005). Coping among children and adolescents with chronic illness. *Anxiety, Stress, and Coping, 18*, 145–155. doi:10.1080/10615800500134639.

Herzer, M., Godiwala, N., Hommel, K. A., Driscoll, K., Mitchell, M., Crosby, L. E., … Modi, A. C. (2010). Family functioning in the context of pediatric chronic conditions. *Journal of Developmental and Behavioral Pediatrics, 31*, 26–34. doi:10.1097/DBP.0b013e3181c7226.

Hocking, M. C., & Alderfer, M. A. (2012). Neuropsychological sequelae of childhood cancer. In Kreitler, S., Ben-Arush, M. W., & Martin, A. (Eds.), *Pediatric psycho-oncology: Psychosocial aspects and clinical interventions* (pp. 177–186). Oxford: Wiley-Blackwell.

Ittenbach, R. F., Cassedy, A. E., Marino, B. S., Spicer, R. L., & Drotar, D. (2009). Adherence to treatment among children with cardiac disease. *Cardiology in the Young, 19*, 545–551. doi:10.1017/S1047951109991260.

Kahana, S., Drotar, D., & Frazier, T. (2008). Meta-analysis of psychological interventions to promote adherence to treatment in pediatric chronic health conditions. *Journal of Pediatric Psychology, 33*, 590–611.

Kain, Z., Caldwell-Andrews, A., Mayes, L., Weinberg, M. E., Wang, S. M., MacLaren, J. E., & Blount, R. L. (2007). Family-centered preparation for surgery improves perioperative outcomes in children: A randomized controlled trial. *Anesthesiology, 106*, 65–74.

Kamibeppu, K., Sato, I., Honda, M., Ozono, S., Sakamoto, N., Iwai, T., & Ishida, Y. (2010). Mental health among young adult survivors of childhood cancer and their siblings including posttraumatic growth. *Journal of Cancer Survivorship: Research and Practice, 4*, 303–312. doi:10.1007/s11764-010-0124-z.

Kato, P. M., Cole, S. W., Bradlyn, A. S., & Pollock, B. H. (2008). A video game improves behavioral outcomes in adolescents and young adults with cancer: A randomized trial. *Pediatrics, 122*, 305–317. doi:10.1542/peds.2007-3134.

Kazak, A. E. (2001). Comprehensive care for children with cancer and their families: A social ecological framework guiding research, practice, and policy. *Children's Services: Social Policy, Research, and Practice, 4*, 217–233. doi:10.1207/S15326918CS0404_05.

Kazak, A. E., Rourke, M. T., & Navsaria, N. (2009). Families and other systems in pediatric psychology. In M. C. Roberts & R. G. Steele (Eds.), *Handbook of pediatric psychology* (4th ed., pp. 656–671). New York: Guilford Press.

Kelly, J. F., & Coons, H. L. (2012). Integrated health care and professional psychology: Is the setting right for you? *Professional Psychology Research and Practice, 43*, 586–595.

Kieckhefer, G. M., Trahms, C. M., Churchill, S. S., Kratz, L., Uding, N., & Villareale, N. A. (2014). A randomized clinical trial of the building on family strengths program: An education program for parents of children with chronic health conditions. *Maternal and Child Health Journal, 18*(3), 563–574. doi:10.1007/s10995-013-1273-2.

King, S., Teplicky, R., King, G., & Rosenbaum, P. (2004). Family-centered service for children with cerebral palsy and their families: A review of the literature. *Seminars in Pediatric Neurology, 11*, 78–86. doi:10.1016/j.spen.2004.01.009.

Kirk, S., Beatty, S., Callery, P., Gellatly, J., Milnes, L., & Pryjmachuk, S. (2013). The effectiveness of self-care support interventions for children and young people with long-term conditions: A systematic review. *Child: Care, Health and Development, 39*, 305–324. doi:10.1111/j.1365-2214.2012.01395.x.

Kuo, D., Bird, T., & Tilford, J. (2011). Associations of family-centered care with health care outcomes for children with special health care needs. *Maternal and Child Health Journal, 15*(6), 794–805.

Kuo, D., Houtrow, A. J., Arango, P., Kuhlthau, K. A., Simmons, J. M., & Neff, J. M. (2012). Family-centered care: Current applications and future directions in pediatric health care. *Maternal and Child Health Journal, 16*, 297–305. doi:10.1007/s10995-011-0751-7.

Kuo, D. Z., Sisterhen, L. L., Sigrest, T. E., Biazo, J. M., Aitken, M. E., & Smith, C. E. (2012). Family experiences and pediatric health services use associated with family-centered rounds. *Pediatrics, 130*, 299–305.

Kuppenheimer, W. G., & Brown, R. T. (2002). Painful procedures in pediatric cancer: A comparison of interventions. *Clinical Psychology Review, 22*, 753–786.

Kupst, M. J. (1999). Assessment of psychoeducational and emotional functioning. In R. Brown (Ed.), *Cognitive aspects of chronic illness in children* (pp. 25–44). New York: Guilford Press.

Landier, W., & Tse, A. M. (2010). Use of complementary and alternative medical interventions for the management of procedure-related pain, anxiety, and distress in pediatric oncology: An integrative review. *Journal of Pediatric Nursing, 25*, 566–579. doi:10.1016/j.pedn.2010.01.009.

Lemanek, K. L., & Ranalli, M. (2009). Sickle cell disease. In M. C. Roberts & R. G. Steele (Eds.), *Handbook of pediatric psychology* (4th ed., pp. 303–318). New York: Guilford Press.

Lewis, D. (1999). Computer-based approaches to patient education: A review of the literature. *Journal of the American Medical Informatics Association, 6,* 272–282. doi:10.1136/jamia.1999.0060272.

Manimala, M. R., Blount, R. L., & Cohen, L. L. (2000). The effects of parental reassurance versus distraction on child distress and coping during immunizations. *Children's Health Care, 29*(3), 161–177.

Mason, S., & Vazquez, D. (2007). Making positive changes: A psychoeducation group for parents with HIV/AIDS. *Social Work with Groups, 30*(2), 27–40. doi:10.1300/J009v30n02-04.

Massey, P. M., Prelip, M., Calimlim, B. M., Quiter, E. S., & Glik, D. C. (2012). Contextualizing an expanded definition of health literacy among adolescents in the health care setting. *Health Education Research, 27,* 961–974.

McClellan, C. B., & Cohen, L. L. (2007). Family functioning in children with chronic illness compared with healthy controls: A critical review. *Journal of Pediatrics, 150,* 221–223, 223. e1–2. doi: 10.1016/j.jpeds.2006.11.063.

McGrady, M. E., & Hommel, K. A. (2013). Medication adherence and health care utilization in pediatric chronic illness: A systematic review. *Pediatrics, 132,* 730–740. doi:10.1542/peds.2013-1451.

Melnyk, B. M., Alpert-Gillis, L., Feinstein, N. F., Crean, H. F., Johnson, J., Fairbanks, E., … Corbo-Richert, B. (2004). Creating opportunities for parent empowerment: Program effects on the mental health/coping outcomes of critically ill young children and their mothers. *Pediatrics, 113,* e597–607.

Mulvaney, S. A., Rothman, R. L., Osborn, C. Y., Lybarger, C., Dietrich, M. S., & Wallston, K. A. (2011). Self-management problem solving for adolescents with type 1 diabetes: Intervention processes associated with an Internet program. *Patient Education and Counseling, 85,* 140–142. doi:10.1016/j.pec.2010.09.018.

Nabors, L. A., & Lehmkuhl, H. D. (2004). Children with chronic medical conditions: Recommendations for school mental health clinicians. *Journal of Developmental and Physical Disabilities, 16,* 1–15. doi:10.1023/B:JODD.0000010036.72472.55.

National Traumatic Child Stress Network. (2004). *Pediatric medical traumatic stress: A comprehensive guide.* Los Angeles, CA: Author.

Newacheck, P. W., & Taylor, W. R. (1992). Childhood chronic illness: Prevalence, severity, and impact. *American Journal of Public Health, 82,* 364–371.

Nilsson, S., Enskär, K., Hallqvist, C., & Kokinsky, E. (2013). Active and passive distraction in children undergoing wound dressings. *Journal of Pediatric Nursing, 28,* 158–166. doi:10.1016/j.pedn.2012.06.003.

Packman, W. (1999). Psychosocial impact of pediatric BMT on siblings. *Bone Marrow Transplantation, 24*(7), 701–706.

Pai, A., & Ostendorf, H. M. (2011). Treatment adherence in adolescents and young adults affected by chronic illness during the health care transition from pediatric to adult health care: A literature review. *Children's Health Care, 40,* 16–33. doi:10.1080/02739615.2011.537934.

Palermo, T. M., Eccleston, C., Lewandowski, A. S., Williams, A. C., & Morley, S. (2010). Randomized controlled trials of psychological therapies for management of chronic pain in children and adolescents: An updated meta-analytic review. *Pain, 148,* 387–397.

Perry, J. D., & Flanagan, W. K. (1986). Pediatric psychology: Applications to the school needs of children with health disorders. *Techniques, 2,* 333–340.

Phelps, L. (Ed.). (2006). *Chronic health-related disorders in children: Collaborative medical and psychoeducational interventions.* Washington: American Psychological Association.

Picoraro, J. A., Womer, J. W., Kazak, A. E., & Feudtner, C. (2014). Posttraumatic growth in parents and pediatric patients. *Journal of Palliative Medicine, 17,* 209–218. doi:10.1089/jpm.2013.0280.

Pinquart, M. (2013). Self-esteem of children and adolescents with chronic illness: A meta-analysis. *Child: Care, Health and Development, 39,* 153–161. doi:10.1111/j.1365-2214.2012.01397.x.

Plante, W. A. (2001). Review of group interventions for pediatric chronic conditions. *Journal of Pediatric Psychology, 26,* 435–453. doi:10.1093/jpepsy/26.7.435.

Popper, B., Anderson, B., Black, A., Ericson, E., & Peck, D. (1987). A case study of the impact of a parent advisory committee on hospital design and policy. *Children's Environments Quarterly, 4,* 12–17.

Powers, S. W., Manne, S., Blount, R. L., et al. (1999). Empirically supported treatments in pediatric psychology: Procedure-related pain. Commentaries: Special series on empirically supported. *Journal of Pediatric Psychology, 24,* 131–154.

Quittner, A., Barker, D., Marciel, K., & Grimley, M. (2009). Cystic fibrosis: A model for drug discovery and patient care. In M. C. Roberts & R. G. Steele (Eds.), *Handbook of pediatric psychology* (4th ed., pp. 271–286). New York: Guilford Press.

Reuben, C. A., & Pastor, P. N. (2013). The effect of special health care needs and health status on school functioning. *Disability Health Journal, 6*(4), 325–332.

Ritterband, L. M., Gonder-Frederick, L. A., Cox, D. J., Clifton, A. D., West, R. W., & Borowitz, S. M. (2003). Internet interventions: In review, in use, and into the future. *Professional Psychology: Research and Practice., 34*(5), 527–553.

Roberts, M. C., & Steele, R. G. (2009). *Handbook of pediatric psychology* (4th ed.). New York: Guilford Press.

Rodrigue, J. R., & Zelikovsky, N. (2009). Pediatric organ transplantation. In M. C. Roberts & R. G. Steele (Eds.), *Handbook of pediatric psychology* (4th ed., pp. 392–402). New York: Guilford Press.

Rolland, J. S. (1984). Toward a psychosocial typology of chronic and life-threatening illness. *Family Systems Medicine, 2,* 245–262.

Rolland, J. S. (1987). Chronic illness and the life cycle: A conceptual framework. *Family Process, 26,* 203–221. doi:10.1111/j.1545-5300.1987.00203.x.

Sawyer, S. M., Drew, S., Yeo, M. S., & Britto, M. T. (2007). Adolescents with a chronic condition: Challenges living, challenges treating. *Lancet, 369,* 1481–1489. doi:10.1016/S0140-6736(07)60370-5.

Shaw, R. J., & DeMaso, D. R. (2010). *Textbook of pediatric psychosomatic medicine.* Arlington: American Psychiatric Publishing.

Simons, L., Gilleland, J., Blount, R., Amaral, S., Berg, A., & Mee, L. L. (2009). Multidimensional adherence classification system: Initial development with adolescent transplant recipients. *Pediatric Transplantation, 13,* 590–598. doi:10.1111/j.1399-3046.2008.01038.x.

Simons, L., McCormick, M., Mee, L., & Blount, R. (2009). Parent and patient perspectives on barriers to medication adherence in adolescent transplant recipients. *Pediatric Transplantation, 13,* 338–347. doi:10.1111/j.1399-3046.2008.00940.x.

Sisterhen, L. L., Blaszak, R. T., Woods, M. B., & Smith, C. E. (2007). Defining family-centered rounds. *Teaching and Learning in Medicine, 19,* 319–322. doi:10.1080/10401330701366812.

Snow-Turek, A. L., Norris, M. P., & Tan, G. (1996). Active and passive coping strategies in chronic pain patients. *Pain, 64,* 455–462.

Spirito, A., Stark, L., & Tyc, V. (1994). Stressors and coping strategies described during hospitalizations by chronically ill children. *Journal of Clinical Child Psychology, 23,* 314–322.

Steinbeck, K. S., Brodie, L., & Towns, S. J. (2008). Transition in chronic illness: Who is going where? *Journal of Paediatrics and Child Health, 44,* 478–482. doi:10.1111/j.1440-1754.2008.01321.x.

Suris, J.-C., & Parera, N. (2005). Sex, drugs and chronic illness: Health behaviours among chronically ill youth. *European Journal of Public Health, 15,* 484–488. doi:10.1093/eurpub/cki001.

Suzuki, L. K., & Kato, P. M. (2003). Psychosocial support for patients in pediatric oncology: The influences of parents, schools, peers, and technology. *Journal of Pediatric Oncology Nursing, 20,* 159–174. doi:10.1177/1043454203254039.

Suzuki, T., White, B., & Velez, I. (2010). Psychoeducation and cultural competence in the primary care setting. In R. A. DiTomasso, B. A. Golden, & H. Morris (Eds.), *Handbook of cognitive behavioral approaches in primary care.* New York: Springer.

The National Center for Chronic Disease Preventions and Health Promotion. (2009). *Chronic diseases: The power to prevent, the call to control.* Atlanta: Author.

Thies, K. (1999). Identifying the educational implications of chronic illness in school children. *Journal of School Health, 69,* 392–397.

Van Cleave, J., Gortmaker, S. L., & Perrin, J. M. (2010). Dynamics of obesity and chronic health conditions among children and youth. *Journal of the American Medical Association, 303*, 623–630. doi:10.1001/jama.2010.104.

Van Servellen, G., Fongwa, M., & Mockus D'Errico, E. (2006). Continuity of care and quality care outcomes for people experiencing chronic conditions: A literature review. *Nursing and Health Sciences, 8*, 185–195.

Walker, L. S., Williams, S. E., Smith, C. A., Garber, J., Van Slyke, D. A., & Lipani, T. A. (2006). Parent attention versus distraction: Impact on symptom complaints by children with and without chronic functional abdominal pain. *Pain, 122*, 43–52. doi:10.1016/j.pain.2005.12.020.

Wallander, J. L., Thompson, R. J. J., & Alriksson-Schmidt, A. (2003). Psychosocial adjustment of children with chronic physical conditions. In M. C. Roberts (Ed.), *Handbook of pediatric psychology* (3rd ed., pp. 141–158). New York: Guilford Press.

Wallis, C. (2007). Transition of care in children with chronic disease. *BMJ, 334*, 1231–1232. doi:10.1136/bmj.39232.425197.BE.

Whittemore, R., Jaser, S. S., Faulkner, M. S., Murphy, K., Delamater, A., Grey, M., & T.R. Group. (2013). Type 1 diabetes eHealth psychoeducation: Youth recruitment, participation, and satisfaction. *Journal of Medical Internet Research, 15*, e15. doi:10.2196/jmir.2170.

Willen, E. (2007). Collaborative practice consultation and collaboration in the care of children and families: The role of the pediatric psychologist. *Journal for Specialists in Pediatric Nursing, 12*(4), 290–293.

Williams, A. (2010). Including a behavioural component into educational interventions may enhance medication adherence in children and adolescents with chronic illness. *Evidence-Based Nursing, 14*, 13–14. doi:10.1136/ebn1123.

Williams, P., Williams, A., Graff, J., Hanson, S., Stanton, A., Hafeman, C., … Sanders, S. (2003). A community-based intervention for siblings and parents of children with chronic illness or disability: The ISEE study. *Journal of Pediatrics, 143*, 386–393.

Williams, P., Williams, A., Hanson, S., Graff, C., Ridder, L., Curry, H., … Karlin-Setter, R. (1999). Maternal mood, family functioning, and perceptions of social support, self-esteem, and mood among siblings of chronically ill children. *Children's Health Care, 28*, 297–310.

Wilson, D. K., & Lawman, H. G. (2009). Health promotion in children and adolescents: An integration of the biopsychosocial model and ecological approaches to behavior change. In M. C. Roberts & R. G. Steele (Eds.), *Handbook of pediatric psychology* (4th ed., pp. 603–617). New York: Guilford Press.

Wiltshire, J., Cronin, K., Sarto, G., & Brown, R. (2006). Self-advocacy during the medical encounter: Use of health information and racial/ethnic differences. *Medical Care, 44*, 100–109.

Winters, N. C., Hanson, G., & Stoyanova, V. (2007). The case formulation in child and adolescent psychiatry. *Child and Adolescent Psychiatric Clinics of North America, 16*, 111–132. doi:10.1016/j.chc.2006.07.010.

Woods, K., Mayes, S., Bartley, E., Fedele, D., & Ryan, J. (2013). An evaluation of psychosocial outcomes for children and adolescents attending a summer camp for youth with chronic illness. *Children's Health Care, 42*, 85–98. doi:10.1080/02739615.2013.753822.

Wu, Y. P., Prout, K., Roberts, M. C., Parikshak, S., & Amylon, M. D. (2011). Assessing experiences of children who attended a camp for children with cancer and their siblings: A preliminary study. *Child & Youth Care Forum, 40*, 121–133.

Wysocki, T., Buckloh, L. M., & Greco, P. (2009). The psychological context of diabetes mellitus in youths. In M. C. Roberts & R. G. Steele (Eds.), *Handbook of pediatric psychology* (4th ed., pp. 287–302). New York: Guilford Press.

Wysocki, T., Harris, M. A., Buckloh, L. M., Mertlich, D., Lochrie, A. S., Mauras, N., & White, N. H. (2007). Randomized trial of behavioral family systems therapy for diabetes: Maintenance of effects on diabetes outcomes in adolescents. *Diabetes Care, 30*, 555–560. doi:10.2337/dc06-1613.

Yucha, C., & Montgomery, D. (2008). *Evidence based practice in biofeedback and neurofeedback.* Wheat Ridge, CO: Association of Applied Psychophysiology.

Chapter 17
Confidentiality in Adolescent Health Care

Carol A. Ford, Abigail English, Nadia Dowshen, and Charles G. Rogers

17.1 Overview

Many adolescents benefit from confidential health services. Concerns about privacy evolve as a normal aspect of adolescent development, and can influence adolescents' willingness to seek health care and share information with their health care providers (English, 1990; Ford, English, & Sigman, 2004). Adolescents may be particularly concerned about privacy related to their sexual behaviors, substance use, and mental health. Adolescent sexual behaviors are linked to unintended pregnancy, high rates of sexually transmitted infections (STIs), and risk of HIV. Substance use is linked to increased risk for injury, death, substance abuse, and addiction.

Depression is common among adolescents and associated with risk of suicide, poor school performance, and participation in a range of health-compromising behaviors. These negative health outcomes encompass the major causes of morbidity and mortality in the adolescent and young adult age group. Effective clinic-based interventions exist to reduce participation in these risk-associated behaviors and treat depression (Council, 2009; Force, 2013). Connecting adolescents who can benefit from these interventions to services depends upon adolescents accessing health care settings and openly communicating with clinicians about sensitive health issues.

Confidentiality protections encourage adolescents to seek care and openly discuss issues related to sexuality, substance use, and mental health concerns—sometimes

C.A. Ford, M.D. (✉) • N. Dowshen, M.D.
The Children's Hospital of Philadelphia, Philadelphia, PA, USA
e-mail: fordc@email.chop.edu

A. English, J.D.
Center for Adolescent Health and the Law, Chapel Hill, NC, USA

C.G. Rogers, M.D.
Naval Medical Center Portsmouth, Portsmouth, VA, USA

© Springer Science+Business Media New York 2016
M.R. Korin (ed.), *Health Promotion for Children and Adolescents*,
DOI 10.1007/978-1-4899-7711-3_17

without parental consent or notification—allowing clinicians to fulfill their role in improving adolescent health. In this chapter we review the ethical principles and laws which support the availability of confidential adolescent health services. We also discuss implementing confidential adolescent health services in clinical settings, and issues important for several specific populations such as adolescents who are: in foster care; in juvenile justice systems; homeless; living with HIV; or being cared for within the context of the military health services.

17.2 Ethical Principles

Ethical principles which support the availability of confidential adolescent health services provide the framework for clinicians making decisions about when they can and cannot provide confidential services for adolescents in health care settings (English, 1990; Ford et al., 2004). Protecting the confidentiality of adolescents' health information is a professional duty that derives from the moral tradition of physicians and the goals of medicine. The goals of medicine include curing disease, prolonging life, relieving suffering, and preventing illness. The basic ethical principles that can help guide health care professionals in their pursuit of these goals include respect for autonomy, beneficence, nonmaleficence, and justice (Beauchamp & Childress, 1994). Each of these principles also has specific relevance to confidentiality protection in adolescent health care as follows:

- Respect for *autonomy* means that patient's own wishes, ideas, and choices are to be supported during the process of helping them. Protection of confidentiality in a health care setting is derived from this principle. It represents an agreement between the patient and the health care professional that information about the patient during encounters will not be shared with others without the patient's permission.
- *Nonmaleficence* means that health care professionals avoid doing harm to the patient. Failing to respect an adolescent's privacy or to honor an agreement of confidentiality might cause harm through disclosure of information to a parent or guardian, even though including parents in an adolescents' care might generally be helpful to the adolescent.
- *Beneficence* is the principle that requires action to further a patient's welfare: doing good for the patient. Protecting confidentiality often enables a health care professional to benefit a patient. Offering confidential care to adolescent patients encourages them to disclose their symptoms and life circumstances fully and completely, thereby increasing the likelihood that they will receive appropriate care and enhancing the clinician's capacity to help them.
- *Justice* requires health care professionals to give adolescents a fair and reasonable opportunity to receive appropriate health care on the same basis as other groups in society. To the extent that the lack of confidentiality protection impedes adolescents' access to health care they need, protection of confidentiality may be necessary to further the principle of justice.

Individual adolescents vary in their levels of psychosocial maturity and economic independence, as well as in their behaviors and family situations. The protection of confidentiality in adolescent health care should be grounded in the ethical principle of respect for autonomy, but must recognize that in specific circumstances it may be permissible or even necessary to breach confidentiality to further other important moral principles, such as beneficence or nonmaleficence.

Both the disclosure of confidential information and the failure to disclose may constitute a clear ethical breach in specific circumstances (English, 1990; Ford et al., 2004). A professional who fails to disclose confidential information, despite a likely benefit to the patient, merely because it would be inconvenient or difficult puts his or her own needs above those of the patient. For example, failure to disclose concerns that a patient is suicidal would be unethical for any reason. Similarly, a professional who breaks confidentiality merely because it seems "good for the patient," without a strong and persuasive specific reason, engages in inappropriate paternalism (i.e., interference with a person's freedom of action based on a wish to benefit them). Neither of these is morally defensible.

A breach of confidentiality—even one that is motivated by paternalism—may damage an adolescent's trust in the health care professional. Therefore, it should be avoided unless a greater good can be achieved by breaching confidentiality. There are circumstances in which breaching confidentiality by disclosing information to an adolescent's parents, caretakers, or others may lead to a greater benefit (for the patient or society). These circumstances might include cases of suicidal or homicidal ideation or acts, serious chemical dependence, and life-threatening eating disorders. "Justified paternalism" in the care of adolescents could be appropriate under these circumstances, provided there is reasonable evidence that an adolescent's capacity for exercising autonomous choice is impaired and protecting the adolescent's life is the central goal (Silber, 1989). In this view, protecting life outweighs the principle of autonomy. Even when a health care professional encounters a circumstance in which "justified paternalism" and disclosure better serves the adolescent, there is still a moral duty to respect the adolescent. This can be accomplished by explaining to the adolescent beforehand the basis of any decision to breach confidentiality and involving the adolescent in the process of identifying how and to whom the information will be disclosed.

17.3 Law

Numerous laws protect the confidentiality of health care information (English & Morreale, 2001). Many of these laws apply to adolescents who are minors as well as to adults. Nevertheless, there are some important differences based on the legal status of adolescents. Adolescents who are under the age of majority (usually age 18) are minors and cannot necessarily expect the same level of confidentiality protection under the law as adults. Adolescents who are age 18 or older are adults and should expect the same confidentiality protection as other adults.

17.3.1 Consent and Confidentiality

The concepts of consent and confidentiality are inextricably intertwined (English, 1990; Ford et al., 2004). First, when a minor's own consent for health care is not legally sufficient, the process of obtaining consent from someone else compromises confidentiality. Second, even when minors are legally authorized to consent, the law may also permit (or require) that a parent or another person or entity be informed. Third, some medical privacy laws explicitly rely on the minor consent laws in delineating who controls the confidentiality of health care information for minors.

The law generally requires the consent of a parent when health care is provided to a minor child, but includes numerous exceptions (Holder, 1985). The exceptions include medical emergencies, care for the "mature minor," and laws authorizing minors to consent to their own care (English, Bass, Boyle, & Eshragh, 2010; Sigman & O'Conner, 1991). Consent may also be required from a legal guardian or conservator for a person who is an adult but severely mentally incapacitated.

A legal basis for minors to consent to their own care also provides a strong foundation for protecting the confidentiality of the care. Every state has statutes that authorize minors to consent to medical care under a variety of circumstances (English et al., 2010). In some statutes, the authorization is based on the minor's status, such as when the minor is emancipated, married, serving in the armed forces, pregnant, a parent, or a high school graduate; is living apart from parents; has attained a certain age; or has qualified as a mature minor. A mature minor is generally one who has the capacity to give an informed consent and has given a voluntary informed consent to low-risk medical care that is within the mainstream of recommended medical treatment. In other statutes, the authorization to consent to health care is based on the type of care needed, such as contraceptive services; pregnancy related care; diagnosis and treatment of STIs, HIV, or reportable diseases; treatment for drug or alcohol problems; care related to a sexual assault; or mental health services. While not every state has statutes covering minors in each of the above status categories or all types of "sensitive" services, every state does have some of these provisions. These minor consent laws reflect judgments that certain minors have attained a level of maturity or autonomy which makes it appropriate for them to make their own medical decisions or that adolescents generally are unlikely to seek certain "sensitive" but essential services unless they are able to do so independently of their parents.

17.3.2 Confidentiality and the HIPAA Privacy Rule

The HIPAA Privacy Rule, issued under the Health Insurance Portability and Accountability Act of 1996, has important implications for the confidentiality of adolescent health care. The Rule contains specific requirements that affect medical records and information pertaining to the care of minors (English & Ford, 2004; Weiss, 2003).

The HIPAA Privacy Rule provides that, in general, when minors legally consent to health care or can receive it without parental consent, or when a parent has assented to an agreement of confidentiality between the minor and the health care provider, the parent does not necessarily have the right to access the minor's health information. Who may do so depends upon "state or other applicable law."

Thus, a health care provider must look to state or other law to determine whether it specifically addresses the confidentiality of a minor's health information. State or other laws that explicitly require, permit, or prohibit disclosure of information to a parent are controlling. If state or other law is silent on the question of parents' access, a health care professional exercising professional judgment has discretion to determine whether or not to grant access. The relevant sources of state or other law that a health care provider must consider include the state minor consent laws, state medical privacy laws, the federal confidentiality rules for the federal Title X family planning program, the federal confidentiality rules for drug or alcohol programs, and court cases interpreting both these laws and the constitutional right of privacy.

17.3.3 Confidentiality Limits

Even when the law protects the confidentiality of adolescents' health information, legal limits apply, in addition to the clinical and ethical limits that exist. The legal limits include, for example, legal obligations to warn intended victims of homicide and to take protective action in cases of suicidal ideation or attempts, any requirements to notify parents in specific circumstances, and laws granting parents explicit access to minors' medical records (English, 1990). In addition, the obligation to report child abuse acts as an overall limit on the scope of confidential care, although there are ongoing questions of interpretation regarding the application of child abuse reporting laws to some adolescent health situations, such as consensual sexual behavior of adolescents (Teare & English, 2002). Also, public health laws that require reporting of communicable diseases, including some STIs, place limits on confidentiality, although the public health reporting and contact tracing system has been structured to minimize breaches of confidentiality and to protect privacy as much as possible.

17.3.4 Confidentiality and Payment

Adolescents often have difficulty obtaining confidential health care unless there is a clear way to pay for the care. Most often, an adolescent's care is paid for by parents or by health insurance. Alternatively, adolescents may be able to receive certain services without charge or at an affordable cost in a variety of settings such as community or migrant health centers, health departments, school-based and school-linked health clinics, and family planning clinics, among others.

A few of these sites operate under laws that provide confidentiality protection for minors as well as adults. For example, since 1970 the federal Title X Family Planning Program has included strong confidentiality protections for adolescents (English, 2000). In Title X clinics there are sliding fee scales based on income and adolescents are permitted to qualify based on their own (rather than their parents') income. Eligible adolescents are also entitled to receive confidential family planning services through Medicaid.

Reliance on health insurance coverage for confidential care can be problematic for an adolescent who wants care to be confidential. Particularly in the private health insurance arena, there are numerous ways in which confidentiality can be breached when an adolescent is covered on a family policy, such as through the sending of explanations of benefits (EOBs) to the policyholder who is generally the parent. The effect of the HIPAA Privacy Rule on adolescents' ability to obtain confidential care through a family insurance policy could be helpful (English & Ford, 2004). For example, the Rule permits individuals, including minors who have consented to their own care, to request specific privacy protections from a health care provider or health plan. A few states have laws that limit disclosure of confidential communications—such as by not requiring the sending of an EOB when there is no remaining financial obligation on the part of the policyholder—but further legal clarification and protection is needed to enable adolescents to seek confidential care and use their health insurance to pay for it.

17.4   Confidential Adolescent Health Services in Clinical Practice

The importance of confidential adolescent health care, within the context of ethical principles and laws described above, has been explicitly acknowledged by all major health care professional organizations including the American Medical Association, the American Academy of Pediatrics, and the Society for Adolescent Health and Medicine for nearly two decades (Ford et al., 2004; Gans, 1993). Private conversations between adolescent patients and health care professionals are developmentally appropriate as children transition through adolescence into young adulthood, because adolescents need to learn skills to become increasingly responsible for their own health and health care. Private conversations with a health care professional also allow discussion of topics or behaviors that adolescents may not disclose or discuss in the presence of a parent. Research has consistently shown that adolescents' concerns about privacy can delay or prevent some adolescents from seeking healthcare, and interfere with open patient–physician communication about issues that need to be discussed because they have a major impact on adolescent health—such as sexual behaviors, substance use, and mental health (Boekeloo, Schamus, Cheng, & Simmens, 1996; Cheng, Savageau, Sattler, & DeWitt, 1993; Ford, 2010; Ford, Bearman, & Moody, 1999; Ford, Best, & Miller, 2001; Ford, Millstein, Halpern-Felsher, & Irwin, 1997; Ginsburg et al.,

1995; Jackson & Hafemeister, 2001; Jones, Purcell, Singh, & Finer, 2005; Klein, Wilson, McNulty, Kapphahn, & Collins, 1999; Marks, Malizio, Hoch, Brody, & Fisher, 1983; Meehan, Hansen, & Klein, 1997; Nowell & Spruill, 1993; Reddy, Fleming, & Swain, 2002; Sugerman et al., 2000; Thrall et al., 2000; Zabin, Stark, & Emerson, 1991).

Health care professionals are always required to balance competing legal and ethical considerations in providing the best health care for their patients. Providing high quality health care to adolescents for sensitive health concerns within the context of the HIPAA Privacy Rule and against the backdrop of other state and federal laws, including requirements related to health insurance claims, is challenging. Furthermore, most organizations of health care professionals who are involved in the care of adolescents have codes of ethics and organizational policies that address issues of confidentiality in adolescents' care (Ford et al., 2004; Gans, 1993). These codes and policies often address the importance of protecting confidentiality as well as the importance of helping adolescents and parents understand both the protections and limits of confidentiality.

From a practical standpoint, a clinician providing adolescent health care must understand and implement both the widespread system and clinical operation changes required by the HIPAA Privacy Rule for all clinical settings, regardless of the age of patients served, and the particular aspects of the rule that are significant for adolescents (English & Ford, 2004; Weiss, 2003). Important implications of the HIPAA Privacy Rule that are most pertinent for clinicians who provide health care to adolescents who are unemancipated minors are summarized as follows:

- Health care professionals must be knowledgeable about state minor consent laws, including any provisions they contain that permit, prohibit, or require disclosure of information to parents.
- Health care professionals must be knowledgeable about state laws regarding privacy of health information and medical records, including any provisions they contain that permit, prohibit, or require disclosure of information to parents, particularly when minors may legally give their own consent for care.
- When state minor consent laws, state health privacy and medical records laws, and other laws are silent or unclear on the question of parents' access to information about care for which minors may legally consent, the HIPAA Privacy Rule makes clear that the covered entity has discretion (that must be exercised by a health care professional) to grant or deny access.
- Many health care professionals have found, based on their clinical experience, that parents are often willing to agree that their adolescent should be able to receive at least some care on a confidential basis. The HIPAA Privacy Rule grants legal significance to such an agreement, providing that when a parent assents to an agreement of confidentiality between a physician and a minor, the minor assumes the rights of the individual with respect to information and records about the care.
- The HIPAA Privacy Rule makes it essential to clarify the location and status of information about health care that students receive in school-based health centers. If the information becomes part of a student's education record, it would

likely be covered by the Family Educational Rights and Privacy Act (FERPA), not the HIPAA Privacy Rule, and FERPA gives parents access to education records (Law, 2010).

- Health care professionals must understand the requirements of the federal Title X Family Planning Program and Medicaid, which protect confidential access to family planning services for adolescents who receive them in Title X funded sites or from Medicaid providers.

Clinicians still face challenges concerning how to maintain their records when the parent has rights with respect to some of the information (about routine, nonsensitive services) and the adolescent has rights with respect to other information (about STIs or substance abuse, for example). Such questions may arise less frequently in settings where an adolescent is seen only for "confidential" care, such as in a family planning clinic, but become increasingly complex in offices where adolescents are seen for a variety of issues, such as a private physician's office or in large institutions with electronic medical records over which individual physicians may have little control.

Further, when third party reimbursement is at stake, the operational challenges of maintaining the appropriate level of confidentiality protection are enormous, even if a minor legally has the rights as an individual under the HIPAA Privacy Rule. Most adolescents are covered by private insurance, but some of them are unwilling or unable to use their insurance coverage for contraceptive services, STI diagnosis and treatment, or other sensitive issues, because they worry that through the billing and insurance claims process their parents will find out. Although the HIPAA Privacy Rule does provide a legal basis for a minor to request that health care providers and health plans restrict disclosure of their protected health information or that they communicate with the minor in a confidential manner, the effective implementation of these provisions requires the willing and active cooperation of both health care providers and third-party payers.

Clinicians continue to face the challenge of conveying the protections and limitations of confidentiality to adolescent patients and their parents. They also still face the challenge of encouraging communication between adolescent patients and their parents in a way that is respectful of both the support parents can provide and the adolescent's need for privacy. Within this context, practical strategies to support the goal of providing confidential adolescent health care when appropriate in primary care settings are described below.

17.4.1 Setting the Stage for Confidential Adolescent Health Care

One strategy for creating an environment where confidential adolescent care can be delivered is to set the stage well in advance of when it is most needed. Despite the acknowledged importance of providing opportunities for private adolescent patient–clinician discussions, existing research shows that this does not occur as frequently as one might hope or expect (Edman, Adams, Park, & Irwin, 2010). It is useful to make spending part of each visit privately with adolescent patients a standard part of clinical practice beginning in late childhood or early adolescence.

The American Academy of Pediatrics, Bright Futures, and the American Medical Association recommend explaining the rationale for private time to parents and patients around age 11 (Hagan, Shaw, & Duncan, 2008; Levenberg & Elster, 1995). The rationale for spending part of each visit alone with *all* adolescents includes that it is developmentally appropriate since young people need to gradually learn to take responsibility for their own health and develop independent patient–clinician relationships over the second decade of life. It is also a time when adolescents can ask the clinician questions about puberty and adolescent health issues that they may not feel comfortable asking other adults. When a clinician has not established a previous relationship with an adolescent patient and family or during episodic care or acute care, it may be useful to explain at the beginning of the visit that standard of care for adolescent patients is that clinicians first talk with the patient and family together, then spend time alone talking to the patient privately and conducting whatever examination needs to be done, and then gathering altogether at the end to discuss clinical impressions and plans. Consistent implementation of these strategies to assure time alone with adolescent patients at each visit can go a long way towards setting the stage for private discussions when needed. Parents often trust clinicians when they convey that time alone with adolescents is standard care, and that the clinicians' motivation is to help parents assure that their adolescent child's health needs are met.

17.4.2 Assurances of Confidentiality

Adolescents who hear assurances about confidentiality are more likely to openly discuss sensitive issues with clinicians and return for future care (Ford et al., 1997). Professional recommendations are to discuss both the protections and limitations of confidentiality (Ford et al., 2004; Gans, 1993). Adolescents are more likely to understand what clinicians are trying to convey when clinicians are very specific about what can and cannot be managed confidentially. Previous research suggests that it is particularly important to emphasize the protections of confidentiality, because adolescents are less aware of the protections of confidentiality than of the limitations (Ford, Thomsen, & Compton, 2001). When limitations to confidentiality are explained, clinicians should consider explaining the limits of confidentiality within the context of caring rather than the law. One example of an assurance of confidentiality that includes specific language addressing both protections and limitations, emphasizes protections, frames limitations within the context of caring for the patient, and acknowledges that clinicians may encourage communication with parents is as follows:

You should know that there are many things I can keep confidential, like if you were having sex, getting birth control, getting tested or treated for STIs, using drugs, or having emotional problems. Some things I can't keep private, like if you are thinking about killing yourself or someone else or if you are being abused. Those are really serious things so if they are going on I hope you would tell me so we can make sure you get some help, and you and I would discuss the best way to get others involved. The main point I am trying to make is that we can handle most things privately. I may encourage you to talk to your parents, but that would be up to you. Any questions?

In addition to discussing confidentiality, adolescents report that it is important for clinicians to behave in a trustworthy manner, and that it may be useful to supplement discussions with information in written clinic materials.

17.4.3   *Encouraging Parental Involvement Without Losing Adolescents' Trust*

Experienced clinicians can often find a way to provide care that respects teens' desire for privacy, is consistent with legal/ethical guidelines, and appropriately involves parents or other responsible adults. Clinicians can give parents clear messages that they should talk to teens about health related issues, and can educate parents and teens about the spectrum of issues they should be discussing. Linking adolescent behaviors to potential health issues helps parents understand the importance of encouraging health promoting behaviors and minimizing risk-associated behaviors. At the end of a clinic visit, clinicians can develop strategies to tailor general counseling to parents and encourage parent–teen communication about behaviors that are currently salient to their adolescent, without betraying specific information the adolescent has disclosed during the visit. For example, if the adolescent patient has disclosed privately that they have been attending parties where alcohol is consumed, the clinician can incorporate general counseling about safety and alcohol use into discussions of anticipatory guidance when the parent and teen are together at the end of the appointment. After explaining that there are several general issues that clinicians discuss with all parents of adolescents their child's age, the clinician can choose to discuss the importance of all families developing an emergency rescue plan that allows a teen to call a parent or other responsible adult and use code words to relay the message that they need to be picked up (e.g., rather than getting into a car with a drunk driver).

There will be circumstances when a clinician's professional opinion is that an adolescent patient needs to have a responsible adult involved in their healthcare, or when clinicians are required by law to break confidentiality. In these situations, it is important to explain to the patient why the clinician thinks it is important to involve a responsible adult. It may be more useful for explanations to be framed within the context of caring and concern about the adolescent patient, rather than legal requirements. Many teens will understand that having a responsible adult (typically a parent) know what is going on will be helpful. Clinicians can discuss with adolescent patients which responsible adult in their life would be the best to involve, the pros and cons of involving a parent, help adolescents reflect on how parents have handled difficult situations in the past, and offer to facilitate discussions with the responsible adult (e.g., Would you like me to tell your mother privately or would you prefer for all of us to be together? If we are together, do you want me to tell your mother, or do you prefer to tell her and I can be here for support?)

17.4.4 Billing

It is important to realize that clinical care generates billing and insurance claims information that will likely be sent to parents (English, Gold, Nash, & Levine, 2012). This can result in unintentional disclosure of confidential adolescent health information. For example, if a bill or EOB sent home itemizes testing, the parent may see that the adolescent received a pregnancy test or STI test within the context of a confidential visit. It is important for clinicians to understand the billing system within the clinic or institution in which they work so that they can be aware of and minimize this risk.

Private insurance companies often generate documents related to claims, such as an EOB, or other notices; in this situation it may be feasible to negotiate with an adolescent patient a strategy for letting parents know what may show up on the bill (e.g., STI testing is a routine part of evaluation for dysmenorrhea in all females). It is also important to work with insurers on strategies to avoid listing sensitive health information in bills and EOBs (English et al., 2012). Medicaid may or may not generate a bill or EOB sent to homes, so it is important to learn typical local procedures. Title X Family Planning clinics, Planned Parenthood clinics, health departments, and some specialized clinics generally do not generate bills and are the locations where adolescents should be referred if they cannot receive needed confidential services in other settings. However, some family planning clinics and other safety net providers are beginning to file insurance claims for patients who are covered by insurance, so confidentiality issues may arise even in those settings.

17.4.5 Release of Medical Information

Adolescents usually should be able to control release of medical records for healthcare to which they have consented (English & Ford, 2004). Policies and procedures to implement this have typically involved segregating adolescent-controlled confidential information in the medical records so that record custodians understand that the minor (rather than the parent) needs to consent before release. Alternatively, clinicians have reviewed and summarized pertinent data to be released, based on whether or not the minor has consented to release. Release of medical information to insurance companies and third-party payers raises separate issues as previously discussed.

17.4.6   Electronic Medical Records

New risks for unintentional disclosure of confidential adolescent health information have emerged with implementation of electronic medical records (EMRs). Strategies used to control access to information in paper charts housed in one location are no longer effective. As health systems using EMRs continually expand and become more integrated, privacy of health information for adolescents and adults becomes more challenging. These challenges influence the ability to protect generally sensitive health information as well as legally protected sensitive health information.

Sensitive health information may be automatically integrated across general EMRs. For example, EMR problem lists may contain sensitive diagnoses (e.g., STIs, HIV, mental illness, genetic disorders), EMRs may provide access to all lab test results (e.g., pregnancy, STI, drug, and genetic testing), and EMR medication lists may contain those prescribed for sensitive health issues (e.g., STIs, HIV, contraception). The content of visits in multiple clinic settings (primary care, emergency rooms, STI/HIV clinics, family planning clinics, mental health clinics) may include sensitive information and be visible across the institution; similar concerns arise with visibility of the content of telephone calls and certain types of clinic appointments. Automatically generated After Visit Summaries (AVS) and discharge summaries may contain sensitive information, and clinicians may not be able to edit them before they are distributed to parents. Patient portals also present unique issues for parents and minor adolescent patients.

As a result of these changes, a much wider range of clinicians within clinics and institutions will likely have access to sensitive adolescent health information integrated into adolescent patient EMRs. These clinicians may be unfamiliar with the legal protections that minors have for confidential adolescent health care, or lack the fundamental knowledge and/or skills to appropriately manage sensitive adolescent health information. Health information exchange between institutions will only intensify these challenges. Furthermore, there will be more opportunities for providers to unintentionally disclose confidential adolescent health information to parents during routine healthcare. For example, unintentional disclosure may happen if parents view EMR computer screens, problem lists, or medication lists during clinic visits; receive automatically printed AVS or discharge summaries that contain sensitive information; or have open access to adolescent patient portals with health information that should be controlled by the adolescent.

Processes to protect minor-controlled release of information from EMRs are complex, and have not been adequately addressed among current EMR vendors (Anosh iravani, Gaskin, Groshek, Kuelbs, & Longhurst, 2012; Blythe & Del Beccaro, 2012).

17.5   Special Populations

Confidential adolescent health services for several special populations of adolescents warrant further discussion because of their unique circumstances. These groups include youth in foster care and in juvenile justice settings, homeless youth, those at risk or infected with HIV, and those receiving care in military systems.

17.5.1 Youth in Foster Care

In 2011, an estimated total of 400,000 children and adolescents were in foster care in the United States (Administration for Children and Families, 2012). Of these, slightly more than an estimated 150,000 were ages 12–20. A significant number were in the older adolescent/young adult age group: 60,000 were age 16 or 17 and nearly 17,000 were ages 18–20. Slightly more than half of the total population was male. These youth are in a variety of placements including foster family homes (with relatives or unrelated families), pre-adoptive homes, group homes, institutions, and supervised independent living; the vast majority are in foster family homes. Youth in foster care are disproportionately from racial and ethnic minority groups, with 27 % of the total Black and 21 % Hispanic. The turnover in the foster care population is high, with approximately 250,000 entering care in 2011 and almost as many leaving in the same year.

Youth in and aging out of foster care experience physical and mental health problems at rates significantly higher than the general population (Childhood, 2012). About 30–40 % have mental health problems and more than one-third have a chronic illness or disability. Some of their health problems are directly related to factors leading to their placement in foster care, such as physical or sexual abuse, while others arise during placement. Adolescents in foster care often encounter significant problems gaining access to health care, and frequently lack access to health care providers experienced in caring for a population with their particular needs. While in foster care, most adolescents are eligible for Medicaid. Once they age out, however, the picture can change significantly, with studies finding that only about one half of foster youth had health insurance when they exited care. Beginning in 2014, as a result of the Affordable Care Act, all states will be required to provide Medicaid coverage for youth aging out of foster care until the age of 26, although outreach and enrollment challenges will remain for this vulnerable population (English & Park, 2012).

Many health concerns of youth in foster care are related to reproductive and sexual health, substance abuse, and mental health that give rise to the need for confidentiality protection. Maintaining confidentiality protection for youth in foster care entails significant challenges. As previously discussed, the relationship between consent and confidentiality is not straightforward, and for the foster care population is even more complex. State law determines who may or must consent for health care for a child or adolescent in foster care. Generally, unless parental rights have been terminated, consent may be given by the adolescent's parents, the court, or, if state law allows, the child welfare agency or caseworker. To the extent that state law authorizes an adolescent to consent for his or her own care, based on status or services being sought, an adolescent in foster care should also be able to do so.

Clarity is lacking, however, about the extent to which an adolescent in foster care who is consenting for his or her own care—such as for reproductive, substance abuse, or mental health care—can expect the care to be confidential. It is unclear when foster parents or the child welfare agency might have access to the information. Some child welfare agencies have policies stating that health care information about a foster child or adolescent should be available to them, and this policy is generally intended to facilitate appropriate health care for youth in foster care. When sensitive services are involved, however, such access can limit an adolescent's willingness to use care or the quality of the care they receive. The American Academy of Pediatrics has suggested that health care professionals taking care of adolescents in foster care should assume that minors with the capacity to consent have the right to confidentiality for issues related to family planning and reproduction, STIs, and substance abuse and that the information should not be shared with caseworkers, foster parents, or birth parents without the adolescent's consent (Task Force on Health Care for Children in Foster Care, 2005). Clinicians must be familiar with their state consent and confidentiality laws and any specific laws or policies related to the foster care population.

17.5.2   Youth in Juvenile Justice Settings

On a single date in 2008, a census indicated that approximately 80,000 juvenile offenders were held in public or private residential placements in the United States (Sickmund, 2010), although significantly higher numbers moved through such placements during a one-year period. These youth include both juvenile delinquents who have committed offenses that would be crimes for adults as well as status offenders who have committed offenses "for children only," such as school truancy or running away from home. The types of facilities in which they are placed include: secure and nonsecure; public (state or local), private, and tribal; and long-term and short-term holding facilities. Out-of-home placements include detention centers, juvenile halls, shelters, reception and diagnostic centers, group homes, wilderness camps, ranches, farms, youth development centers, residential treatment centers, training or reform schools, and juvenile correctional institutions.

The number of juveniles in residential placement is small in comparison to the 11 million juveniles who were arrested in 2008 (US Department of Justice, 2009), or to the more than 31 million youth who were under juvenile court jurisdiction in 2009, but not necessarily in residential placement (Puzzanchera, Adams, & Hockenberry, 2012). Racial and ethnic minority youth are disproportionately represented both among those who are arrested and those who are in custodial placements. Also in 2009, juvenile courts handled an estimated 1.5 million juvenile delinquency cases. More than 300,000 youth arrested for delinquency offenses were detained in 2009, while more than 130,000 of the adjudicated cases resulted in a disposition of out-of-home placement. More than one fourth of these cases (28 %) involved physical or sexual assaults or other violent offenses against persons, 33 % involved property offenses, and 9 % involved drug offenses.

Youth in juvenile justice settings experience significant health problems and encounter limitations in access to health care appropriate to address those problems. Youth in juvenile justice settings have health problems in the same broad categories as their counterparts in the community, but are at higher risk of mental health problems, suicide, substance abuse disorders, injuries associated with violence, and negative consequences of sexual behaviors (Adolescence, 2011). Youth placed in juvenile justice settings, both short-term detention and longer term correctional placements, receive health care of widely varying quality, even though the National Center on Correctional Health Care has detailed standards for the provision of health care in juvenile facilities (Care, 2011). These standards contain recommendations for screening, diagnosis, and treatment of sensitive health issues that trigger confidentiality concerns.

Health care for youth in juvenile justice settings raises complex issues related to confidentiality. The confidentiality concerns are important for several reasons: because so many of the health issues experienced by youth in these settings involve sensitive sexual behaviors, substance use, and mental health; because the settings vary so widely in terms of their structure, configuration, and management; and because there is a tension between the legitimate concerns of safety and privacy. Mental health professionals treating adolescents in juvenile justice settings need to be sensitive to confidentiality concerns and to the potential for role conflicts (Psychiatry, 2005). Taking care to avoid exploration of details of the youth's offense may be essential to avoiding conflicts over reporting and disclosure mandates. A youth who is receiving health care in a juvenile justice setting should not lose the consent and confidentiality protections available to them in the community according to their state's laws. Thus, a minor who is able to consent for confidential STI testing in the community should be able to do so in a juvenile justice setting. However, the policies and guidelines of specific agencies and institutions vary widely. It is essential for health care professionals providing care for youth in these settings to be familiar with both their state laws and local or institutional policies and guidelines.

17.5.3   Homeless Youth

The total number of adolescents who are homeless in the United States is difficult to estimate, and existing estimates vary widely. One estimate suggests that there are nearly 1.7 million homeless youth under age 18; approximately 380,000 of these remain homeless for more than one week and about 130,000 remain homeless for more than one month, with the remainder returning home quickly (Homelessness). Substantial variations exist among those who remain homeless for more than 1 week; some are "low-risk" and "transient" youth who retain relationships with their families while others are "high-risk" youth who have highly unstable or nonexistent family ties. The factors contributing to homelessness among adolescents include sexual orientation other than heterosexual, history of foster care placement, and school expulsion. The number of homeless young adults ages 18–24 is even more difficult to estimate and reliable estimates are not available, although these young people share many characteristics and health care needs with their younger counterparts.

Homeless youth have numerous health problems and extensive health care needs, which are insufficiently met (Pediatrics, 2013; Toro, Dworsky, & Fowler, 2007). The health problems they experience are similar to those affecting youth in foster care and juvenile justice settings. These problems are exacerbated by their living conditions, with limited sanitation and exposure to the elements. Also, homeless youth are at increased risk for being sexually exploited and trafficked, with the associated risk for physical injuries, substance abuse, mental health trauma, and sexual health problems.

Confidentiality issues for homeless youth vary in important ways from the confidentiality issues affecting youth in foster care or juvenile justice settings (Halley & English, 2009). This is because homeless youth are generally not in the custody or under the control of a child welfare or juvenile justice agency or institution, and are less likely than youth in the community to have parents insisting on access to information about health care they may have received for sensitive issues. Homeless youth who are age 18 or older are legally adults and are generally able to give consent for their own care on the same basis as other adults. They are also entitled to the same legal protections of confidentiality as other adults. However, homeless or unaccompanied youth who are under age 18 are legally minors. They may or may not be able to give their own consent for care, depending on specific provisions of state and federal law and the services they are seeking. Of particular importance for homeless youth, slightly less than one half of states have enacted statutes that enable minors who are living apart from their parents to consent for their own health care. Homeless youth under age 18 should be entitled to the same confidentiality protections as adolescent minors in the community, depending on their specific status and the services they are seeking. Health care professionals caring for homeless youth should be familiar with their state's consent and confidentiality laws.

17.5.4 Youth Living with and At-Risk for HIV/AIDS

Currently, there are approximately 1.2 million people in the United States living with HIV/AIDS and over 50,000 new infections occur each year (CDC, 2010b). Since the beginning of the epidemic nearly 40,000 adolescents have been diagnosed with HIV in the USA and an estimated 39 % of all new infections occur among young people ages 13–29, even though they represent only approximately 21 % of the total population (CDC, 2010b). According to recent Center for Disease Control and Prevention (CDC) estimates there are over 25,000 individuals 13–24 years of age living with HIV in the USA (CDC, 2010a).

The demographics of young people living with HIV/AIDS in the USA have changed during the last three decades. A combination of public health interventions has dramatically reduced the incidence of perinatal HIV infections. From 1998 to 2005, there have been less than 150 infected infants identified each year (CDC, 2007b). At the same time, with the advent of combination anti-retroviral therapy many youth with perinatally acquired HIV are now surviving into adulthood. Such longevity was never expected in the beginning of the epidemic and these perinatally infected teens now comprise almost one-third of adolescents living with HIV/AIDS (CDC, 2007a). This increase in the population of perinatally infected teenagers has been mirrored by an increasing incidence in behaviorally infected adolescents, primarily in those infected through sexual contact. At this time, the majority of newly infected adolescents are young men who have sex with men (YMSM), with Latino and particularly Black YMSM being disproportionately affected (CDC, 2010b). Male-to-female (MTF) transgender youth also have a particularly high incidence of HIV infection (Garofalo, Deleon, Osmer, Doll, & Harper, 2006). According to the most recent CDC data, among youth ages 13–19, the highest rates of new infection are in the South and Southeastern regions of the USA (CDC, 2010a). Finally, heterosexual transmission of HIV accounts for about 30 % of the cases in this age group with the overwhelming majority of patients being young Black and Hispanic/Latina women (CDC, 2010b; Garofalo et al., 2006). In addition to those living with HIV/AIDS, many young people are at risk for acquiring HIV infection, due to high rates of unprotected sex, presence of other STIs, substance abuse, and lack of awareness or education (CDC, 2007).

In general, youth living with and at-risk for HIV/AIDS have poor access to appropriate healthcare. According to the CDC, less than a quarter of all young people who reported being sexually active had ever been tested for HIV, despite recommendations for routine screening of sexually active adolescents and adults (Balaji et al., 2012; Branson et al., 2006). Additionally, it is estimated that approximately 60 % of youth living with HIV do not know their diagnosis (Centers for Disease Control and Prevention & Vital Signs, November 2012). Among people who have tested positive for HIV, data show that youth and particularly YMSM of color are less likely to engage in routine medical care than their adult counterparts.

Many people living with or at-risk for HIV/AIDS continue to experience stigma, both perceived and enacted, due to their HIV status and/or minority sexual orientation or gender identity (Dowshen, Binns, & Garofalo, 2009). It is within this context that confidentiality protections are particularly important. Many youth with HIV face isolation due to lack of community and family support if their infection status is known, and concerns about privacy are often cited as a barrier for not seeking healthcare. Furthermore, concerns about privacy can influence HIV testing. While adolescents can consent to care for STI testing and treatment in all 50 states, only 31 states explicitly include HIV testing and treatment, 18 states allow physicians to inform a minor's parents that he or she is receiving STI services, and 1 state requires parental notification of a minor's positive HIV test result (Guttmacher Institute, 2013). Additionally, state laws vary as to how HIV-related information must be treated and released to family members and other healthcare providers. Even when providers aim to protect confidentiality for adolescents and young adults regarding HIV testing or treatment, inadvertent disclosures often may occur due to insurance related issues including denial, acknowledgement, or payment of claims or EOBs to the primary beneficiary of the insurance plan (English et al., 2012). Such disclosures can have devastating consequences for youth living with and at-risk for HIV including violence or loss of stable housing. Of note, the recent success of preexposure prophylaxis (daily oral tenofivir/emtricitabine) as a promising biomedical HIV prevention strategy among YMSM and serodiscordant heterosexual couples has led to discussions of minor's right to consent and receive confidential care for this treatment (Culp & Caucci, 2013).

17.5.5   Military Adolescents and Young Adults

Adolescents and young adults associated with the US Armed Forces include two unique groups. The first group includes young military service members. The second group includes family members of military service members (e.g., children, spouses), also referred to as military dependents. During 2012, the total number of young people age 15–25, including both dependents and young military service members age 18–25, who were affiliated with the military medical system either through seeing military medical providers or having their healthcare paid for by Tricare (the organization responsible for funding healthcare for military personnel and their dependents), was approximately 1.63 million (*Evaluation of the TRICARE Program: Fiscal Year* 2012 *Report to Congress*, 2012). A separate report in 2011 showed there were approximately 642,000 young people between the ages of 12 and 23 who were dependents of military personnel, including both children and spouses (*2011 Demographics: Profile of the Military Community*, 2012). While many of these young people receive health care in military treatment facilities (MTFs), an increasing number are served in civilian practices around the USA; from 2008 to 2010 the percent of military dependents with a civilian primary care provider increased from 39 to 48 % (*Evaluation of the TRICARE Program: Fiscal Year* 2012 *Report to Congress*, 2012). While military personnel are primarily cared for at MTFs, they may be referred to civilian providers for specialty services and care that is not available at their MTF. Accordingly, it is imperative that healthcare providers, both military and civilian, have an understanding of some of the unique issues surrounding confidentiality for young people affiliated with the US military.

When we see images of soldiers, sailors, and marines, we rarely associate the word "adolescent" with them. However, when we recognize that 43.2 % (610,274) of all active duty military personnel and 33.5 % (286,797) of military reservists are under the age of 25, it is apparent that meeting the healthcare needs of this population of young adults is critical (*2011 Demographics: Profile of the Military Community*, 2012). The primary policy statement that guides issues related to confidentiality regarding their health information is Department of Defense (DoD) 6025.18-R (*Department of Defense Health Information Privacy Regulation*, 2003). In this statement, all of the rules related to the protection of military service members' health information are the same as their civilian counterparts, with a caveat. Under DoD 6025.18-R, and policy directives from the Army, Navy, and Air Force, military commands can request an individual service member's medical records without his or her consent in a select circumstance—ensuring the ability of the command to fulfill its mission (*Air Force Instruction 41-210*, 2000; *Department of*

Defense Health Information Privacy Regulation, 2003; Lenhart, Ling, Campbell, & Purcell, 2010; *MARADMIN 308/11*, 2011). To do this requires that the commanding officer determine the service member's health information is required for assessing and maintaining the health and readiness of the military command for carrying out its mission, or determining whether the particular military service member is fit for his or her duty or assignment. In this situation, the commanding officer must request the medical records in writing, with a specification of the information required and a justification for requiring it. Whether this information is requested from an MTF or civilian institution, the health care provider is to supply the minimum amount of information required to meet the specified needs of the command. A military service member has the right to request an accounting of what information was requested and given, and why this was done (Rushenberg, 2007). For assistance with these and other issues that arise with confidentiality concerns, military service members should be referred to the legal office of their commands or the privacy office at their MTFs.

The adolescent children of military parents and the civilian spouses of young service members are much more likely to see a civilian health care provider than military service members. As noted above, 48 % of military dependents have a civilian primary care provider, while this is true of less than 4 % of military service members (*Evaluation of the TRICARE Program: Fiscal Year* 2012 *Report to Congress*, 2012). For adolescents and young adults cared for by civilian providers in civilian institutions, the regulations and policies surrounding their confidentiality are the same as for any other adolescent or young adult in that practice. For the military dependents cared for in MTFs, the regulations of HIPAA and state laws regarding confidentiality are also in full effect, and some of the military services (like the Army) explicitly state in their regulations that 15–17-year-old dependents should have private medical records (*Air Force Instruction 33-332 Communications and Information Air Force Privacy Program*, 2011; English, Ford, & Santelli, 2009; *Manual of the Medical Department of the Navy, NAVMED P-117*, 2013). However, similar to the civilian sector, the practical application of these regulations and directives is more complicated. Because of the transient nature of this population, who frequently moving from military base to military base, and from the USA to overseas and back, the risk of losing paper records in transfer from one treatment center to another is a real concern. In the past, to help circumvent this problem, military service members could request the records of his or her dependents allowing the service members to hand carry these records between duty stations to facilitate the transition and prevent the loss of records. The ability to have records available upon arrival at a new location is vitally important in many situations, particularly for young people who have ongoing healthcare needs. However, this often meant that adolescent and young adults have no foolproof means of guaranteeing their records are completely confidential, even when MTFs are directed to provide this confidentiality. To ameliorate some of these concerns, TRICARE along with the medical departments of the branches of the US Military has updated their policies regarding dependents medical records, now requiring signed release of information documentation prior to the release or transfer of medical records for adult dependents

(*Evaluation of the TRICARE Program: Fiscal Year* 2012 *Report to Congress*, 2012; "TRICARE Management Activity," 2013). Similar to many sectors of the civilian medical system, it remains relatively easy for a service member to access his or her dependents' medical records. However, TRICARE in coordination with MTFs is actively working on improving ways to maintain confidentiality and facilitate record transfer through the use of nationally integrated EMR systems with increased protections around sensitive topics (*Evaluation of the TRICARE Program: Fiscal Year* 2012 *Report to Congress*, 2012).

17.6 Conclusion

Adolescents should have access to developmentally appropriate high quality confidential health care within professional, ethical, and legal guidelines. Clinicians and health care systems who provide this care have a higher likelihood of being able to effectively address the types of sensitive health issues linked to major causes of morbidity and mortality in this age group. Strategies to facilitate the ability to provide confidential adolescent healthcare include explaining its importance to parents and adolescents, routinely spending part of each adolescent visit alone with the patient, discussing confidentiality, and addressing issues that increase risk of unintentional disclosure of protected information related to billing, EOBs, release of health records, and EMRs. Clinicians need to become familiar with federal and state laws that influence practice and policies in their specific setting, and how to provide health care within this context to adolescent patients during routine and acute care.

NOTE: The opinions expressed in this chapter are those of the individual authors, and do not necessarily reflect the opinion or policy of the US Department of Defense.

References

Administration for Children and Families, Administration on Children, Youth and Families, Children's Bureau. (2012). *Preliminary estimates for 2011 as of July 2012* (Vol. 19, AFCARS Report No. 19). Washington: U.S. Department of Health and Human Services.

Adolescence, AAP Committee on Adolescence. (2011). Health care for youth in the juvenile justice system. *Pediatrics, 128*, 1219–1235.

Air Force Instruction 33-332 Communications and Information Air Force Privacy Program. (2011). Washington, DC.

Air Force Instruction 41-210. (2000). Retrieved from http://afpubs.hq.af.mil

Anoshiravani, A., Gaskin, G. L., Groshek, M. R., Kuelbs, C., & Longhurst, C. A. (2012). Special requirements for electronic medical records in adolescent medicine. *Journal of Adolescent Health, 51*(5), 409–414. doi: 10.1016/j.jadohealth.2012.08.003, S1054-139X(12)00335-7 [pii].

Balaji, A. B., Eaton, D. K., Voetsch, A. C., Wiegand, R. E., Miller, K. S., & Doshi, S. R. (2012). Association between HIV-related risk behaviors and HIV testing among high school students in the United States, 2009 [Comparative Study Multicenter Study]. *Archives of Pediatrics & Adolescent Medicine, 166*(4), 331–336. doi:10.1001/archpediatrics.2011.1131.

Beauchamp, T., & Childress, J. (1994). *Principles of biomedical ethics* (4th ed.). New York: Oxford University Press.

Blythe, M. J., & Del Beccaro, M. A. (2012). Standards for health information technology to ensure adolescent privacy. *Pediatrics, 130*(5), 987–990. doi:10.1542/peds.2012-2580, peds.2012-2580 [pii].

Boekeloo, B., Schamus, L., Cheng, T., & Simmens, S. (1996). Young adolescents' comfort with discussions about sexual problems with their physician. *Archives of Pediatrics and Adolescent Medicine, 150*, 1146–1152.

Branson, B. M., Handsfield, H. H., Lampe, M. A., Janssen, R. S., Taylor, A. W., Lyss, S. B., & Clark, J. E. (2006). Revised recommendations for HIV testing of adults, adolescents, and pregnant women in health-care settings [Practice Guideline]. MMWR. Recommendations and reports: Morbidity and mortality weekly report. Recommendations and reports/Centers for Disease Control, vol. 55(RR-14), pp. 1–17; quiz CE11-14.

Care, National Commission on Correctional Health Care. (2011). Standards for Health Services in Juvenile Detention and Confinement Facilities. Chicago, IL: National Commission on Correctional Health Care.

CDC. (2007a). CDC HIV/AIDS fact sheet: HIV/AIDS among youth.

CDC. (2007b). CDC HIV/AIDS fact sheet: Mother-to-child HIV transmission and prevention.

CDC. (2010a). HIV surveillance in adolescents and young adults. Divisions of HIV/AIDS Prevention. National Center for HIV/AIDS, Viral Hepatitis, STD, and TB Prevention.

CDC. (2010b). *HIV/AIDS surveillance report* (Vol. 20).

Centers for Disease Control and Prevention. (2007). *CDC HIV/AIDS fact sheet: HIV/AIDS among youth*. Retrieved 2013, from http://www.cdc.gov/hiv/resources/factsheets/PDF/youth.pdf

Centers for Disease Control and Prevention, & Vital Signs. (2012, November). *HIV among youth in the US*. Retrieved 2013, from http://www.cdc.gov/vitalsigns/hivamongyouth/

Cheng, T., Savageau, J., Sattler, A., & DeWitt, T. (1993). Confidentiality in health care: A survey of knowledge, perceptions, and attitudes among high school students. *JAMA, 269*(11), 1404–1407.

Childhood, AAP Council on Foster Care Adoption and Kinship Care and Committee on Early Childhood. (2012). Policy statement: Health care of youth aging out of foster care. *Pediatrics, 130*, 1170–1174.

Council, Institute of Medicine National Research Council. (2009). *Adolescent health services: Missing opportunities*. Washington, DC: The National Academies Press.

Culp, L., & Caucci, L. (2013). State adolescent consent laws and implications for HIV pre-exposure prophylaxis. [Research Support, U.S. Gov't, P.H.S. Review]. *American Journal of Preventive Medicine, 44*(1 Suppl 2), S119–S124. doi:10.1016/j.amepre.2012.09.044.

2011 Demographics: Profile of the Military Community. (2012). Washington, DC. Retrieved from http://www.militaryonesource.mil/12038/MOS/Reports/2011_Demographics_Report.pdf

Department of Defense Health Information Privacy Regulation. (2003). Washington, DC. Retrieved from http://www.dtic.mil/whs/directives/corres/pdf/602518r.pdf

Dowshen, N., Binns, H. J., & Garofalo, R. (2009). Experiences of HIV-related stigma among young men who have sex with men [Research Support, N.I.H., Extramural]. *AIDS Patient Care and STDs, 23*(5), 371–376. doi:10.1089/apc.2008.0256.

Edman, J. C., Adams, S. H., Park, M. J., & Irwin, C. E., Jr. (2010). Who gets confidential care? Disparities in a national sample of adolescents. *Journal of Adolescent Health, 46*(4), 393–395. doi:10.1016/j.jadohealth.2009.09.003, S1054-139X(09)00364-4 [pii].

English, A. (1990). Treating adolescents: Legal and ethical considerations. In J. Farrow (Ed.), *The medical clinics of North America* (pp. 1097–1112). Philadelphia: WB Saunders Company.

English, A. (2000). Reproductive health services for adolescents: Critical legal issues. *Obstetrics and Gynecology Clinics of North America, 27*(1), 195–211.

English, A., Bass, L., Boyle, A. D., & Eshragh, F. (2010). *State minor consent laws: A summary* (3rd ed.). Chapel Hill, NC: Center for Adolescent Health and the Law.

English, A., & Ford, C. A. (2004). The HIPAA Privacy Rule and adolescents: Legal questions and clinical challenges. *Perspectives on Sexual and Reproductive Health, 36*(2), 80–86.

English, A., Ford, C. A., & Santelli, J. S. (2009). Clinical preventive services for adolescents: Position paper of the Society for Adolescent Medicine. *American Journal of Law and Medicine, 35*(2–3), 351–364.

English, A., Gold, R. B., Nash, E., & Levine, J. (2012). *Confidentiality for individuals insured as dependents: A review of state laws and policies.* Retrieved from http://www.guttmacher.org/pubs/confidentiality-review.pdf

English, A., & Morreale, M. (2001). A legal and policy framework for adolescent health care: Past, present, and future. *Houston Journal of Health Law and Policy, 1*(1), 63–108.

English, A., & Park, M. (2012). The Supreme Court ACA decision: What happens now for adolescents and young adults. Chapel Hill, NC: Center for Adolescent Health & the Law and National Adolescent and Young Adult Health Information Center.

Evaluation of the TRICARE Program: Fiscal Year 2012 Report to Congress. (2012). Falls Church, VA. Retrieved from http://tricare.mil/tma/dhcape/program/evaluation.aspx

Force, U.S. Preventive Services Task Force. (2013). *Child and adolescent recommendations.* U.S. Preventive Services Task Force. Retrieved from http://www.uspreventiveservicestaskforce.org/tfchildcat.htm

Ford, C. A. (2010). Which adolescents have opportunities to talk to doctors alone? *Journal of Adolescent Health, 46*(4), 307–308.

Ford, C. A., Bearman, P. S., & Moody, J. (1999). Foregone health care among adolescents. *JAMA, 282*(23), 2227–2234. joc90755 [pii].

Ford, C., Best, D., & Miller, W. (2001). Confidentiality and adolescents' willingness to consent to STD testing. *Archives of Pediatrics and Adolescent Medicine, 155*(9), 1072–1073.

Ford, C., English, A., & Sigman, G. (2004). Confidential health care for adolescents: Position paper of the society for adolescent medicine. *Journal of Adolescent Health, 35*(1), 160–167.

Ford, C., Millstein, S., Halpern-Felsher, B., & Irwin, C. (1997). Influence of physician confidentiality assurances on adolescents' willingness to disclose information and seek future health care. *JAMA, 278*(12), 1029–1034.

Ford, C., Thomsen, S. L., & Compton, B. (2001). Adolescents' interpretations of conditional confidentiality assurances. *Journal of Adolescent Health, 29*(3), 156–159.

Gans, J. (1993). *Policy compendium on confidential health services for adolescents.* Chicago: American Medical Association.

Garofalo, R., Deleon, J., Osmer, E., Doll, M., & Harper, G. W. (2006). Overlooked, misunderstood and at-risk: Exploring the lives and HIV risk of ethnic minority male-to-female transgender youth. *Journal of Adolescent Health, 38*(3), 230–236. doi:10.1016/j.jadohealth.2005.03.023. S1054-139X(05)00204-1 [pii].

Ginsburg, K., Slap, G., Cnaan, A., Forke, C., Balsley, C., & Rouselle, D. (1995). Adolescents' perceptions of factors affecting their decisions to seek health care. *JAMA, 273*(24), 1913–1918.

Guttmacher Institute. (2013, July 1). *State policies in brief: Minors' access to STI services.* Retrieved 2013 from http://www.guttmacher.org/statecenter/spibs/spib_MASS.pdf

Hagan, J., Shaw, J., & Duncan, P. (2008). *Bright futures: Guidelines for health supervision of infants, children, and adolescents* (3rd ed.). Elk Grove Ill: American Academy of Pediatrics.

Halley, M., & English, A. (2009). *Health care for homeless youth: Policy options for improving access.* Retrieved from http://nahic.ucsf.edu/download/health-care-for-homeless-youth-policy-options-for-improving-access/

Holder, A. (1985). *Legal issues in the health care of children and adolescents* (2nd ed.). New Haven: Yale University Press.

Homelessness, National Alliance to End Homelessness. *An emerging framework to end unaccompanied youth homelessness.* Retrieved from http://b.3cdn.net/naeh/1c46153d87d15eaaff9zm6i2af5.pdf

Jackson, S., & Hafemeister, T. L. (2001). Impact of parental consent and notification policies on the decisions of adolescents to be tested for HIV. *Journal of Adolescent Health, 29*(2), 81–93.

Jones, R. K., Purcell, A., Singh, S., & Finer, L. B. (2005). Adolescents' reports of parental knowledge of adolescents' use of sexual health services and their reactions to mandated parental notification for prescription contraception. *Journal of the American Medical Association, 293*(3), 340–348.

Klein, J., Wilson, K., McNulty, M., Kapphahn, C., & Collins, K. (1999). Access to medical care for adolescents: Results from the 1997 Commonwealth Fund Survey of the Health of Adolescent Girls. *Journal of Adolescent Health, 25*(2), 120–130.

Law, National Center for Youth Law. (2010). *HIPAA or FERPA? A primer on school health information sharing in California.* Oakland, CA: National Center for Youth Law.

Lenhart, A., Ling, R., Campbell, S., & Purcell, K. (2010). *Teens and mobile phones.* Washington, DC: Pew Internet & American Life Project, Pew Research Center.

Levenberg, P., & Elster, A. (1995). *Guidelines for Adolescent Preventive Services (GAPS)—Implementation and resource manual.* Chicago, IL: American Medical Association.

Manual of the Medical Department of the Navy, NAVMED P-117. (2013). Washington, DC. Retrieved from http://www.med.navy.mil/directives/Pages/NAVMEDP-MANMED.aspx

MARADMIN 308/11. Department of the Navy. (2011). Washington, DC. Retrieved from http://www.doncio.navy.mil/uploads/0601CZD27871.pdf

Marks, A., Malizio, J., Hoch, J., Brody, R., & Fisher, M. (1983). Assessment of health needs and willingness to utilize health care resources of adolescents in a suburban population. *Journal of Pediatrics, 102*(3), 456–460.

Meehan, T. M., Hansen, H., & Klein, W. C. (1997). The impact of parental consent on the HIV testing of minors. *American Journal of Public Health, 97*(8), 1338–1341.

Nowell, D., & Spruill, J. (1993). If it's not absolutely confidential, will information be disclosed? *Professional Psychology: Research and Practice, 24*(3), 367–369.

Pediatrics, AAP Council on Community Pediatrics. (2013). Providing care for children and adolescents facing homelessness and housing insecurity. *Pediatrics, 131*, 1206–1210.

Psychiatry, American Academy of Child and Adolescent Psychiatry. (2005). Official action: Practice parameter for the assessment and treatment of youth in juvenile detention and correctional facilities. *Journal of the American Academy of Child and Adolescent Psychiatry, 44*(10), 1085–1098.

Puzzanchera, C., Adams, B., & Hockenberry, S. (2012). *Juvenile Court Statistics 2009.* Pittsburgh, PA: National Center for Juvenile Justice.

Reddy, D. M., Fleming, R., & Swain, C. (2002). Effect of mandatory parental notification on adolescent girls' use of sexual health care services. *JAMA, 288*(6), 710–714.

Rushenberg, T. J. (2007, October/November). HIPAA: A military perspective. *GPSolo, 24*.

Sickmund, M. (2010, February). Juveniles in residential placement: 1997–2008 (Vol. February). Washington, DC: Office of Juvenile Justice and Delinquency Prevention, Office of Justice Programs, U.S. Department of Justice.

Sigman, G., & O'Conner, C. (1991). Exploration for physicians of the mature minor doctrine. *Journal of Pediatrics, 199*, 520–525.

Silber, T. (1989). Justified paternalism in adolescent health care. *Journal of Adolescent Health Care, 10*, 449–453.

Sugerman, S., Halfon, N., Fink, A., Anerson, M., Valle, L., & Brook, R. (2000). Family planning clinic clients: Their usual health care providers, insurance status, and implications for managed care. *Journal of Adolescent Health, 27*(1), 25–33.

Task Force on Health Care for Children in Foster Care, AAP., District II, New York State. (2005). *Fostering health: Health care for children and adolescents in foster care* (2nd ed.). American Academy of Pediatrics.

Teare, C., & English, A. (2002). Nursing practice and statutory rape. Effects of reporting and enforcement on access to care for adolescents. *Nursing Clinics of North America, 37*(3), 393–404.

Thrall, J., McCloskey, L., Ettner, S., Rothman, E., Tighe, J., & Emans, S. (2000). Confidentiality and adolescents' use of providers for health information and for pelvic exams. *Archives of Pediatrics and Adolescent Medicine, 154*(9), 885–892.

Toro, P., Dworsky, A., & Fowler, P. (2007). *Homeless youth in the United States: Recent research findings and intervention approaches.* Retrieved from http://www.huduser.org/publications/pdf/p6.pdf

TRICARE Management Activity. (2013). Retrieved June 22, 2013, from www.tricare.mil

US Department of Justice, Office of Juvenile Justice and Delinquency Prevention. (2009). *Juvenile Arrests 2008.* Washington, DC: Office of Juvenile Justice and Delinquency Prevention.

Weiss, C. (2003). *Protecting minors' health information under the Federal Medical Privacy Regulations.* Retrieved July 9, 2013, from http://www.aclu.org/FilesPDFs/med_privacy_guide.pdf

Zabin, L., Stark, H., & Emerson, M. (1991). Reasons for delay in contraceptive clinic utilization: Adolescent clinic and nonclinic populations compared. *Journal of Adolescent Health, 12,* 225–232.

Chapter 18
Wellbeing of Children in the Foster Care System

Lindsey M. Weiler, Edward F. Garrido, and Heather N. Taussig

18.1 Foster Care Overview

The Adoption and Safe Families Act (ASFA), passed by Congress in 1997, identified *child well-being* as a major goal of the child welfare system. Since the recognition that safety and permanency are necessary but not sufficient for well-being, there has been a renewed focus on health promotion for youth in foster care. An Information Memorandum (ACYF-CB-IM-12-04; April 2012) issued by the U.S. Department of Health and Human Services, Administration on Children, Youth, and Families highlighted its focus on promoting well-being as follows: "To focus on social and emotional well-being is to attend to children's behavior, emotional, and social functioning—those skills, capacities, and characteristics that enable young people to understand and navigate their world in healthy, positive ways" (p. 1).

The term, *foster care*, will be used throughout this chapter as an umbrella term to refer to any type of court-ordered out-of-home placement including *nonrelative foster care and group homes* (i.e., children cared for in private homes by nonrelatives

L.M. Weiler, Ph.D. (✉)
University of Minnesota, 1985 Buford Ave, 290 McNeal Hall, St. Paul, MN 55108, USA
e-mail: lmweiler@umn.edu

E.F. Garrido, Ph.D.
Kempe Center for the Prevention and Treatment of Child Abuse and Neglect,
University of Colorado School of Medicine, 13123 E 16th Ave, B390, Aurora, CO 80045,
USA
e-mail: edward.garrido@childrenscolorado.org

H.N. Taussig, Ph.D.
Graduate School of Social Work, University of Denver; Kempe Center for the Prevention
and Treatment of Child Abuse and Neglect, University of Colorado School of Medicine,
2148 S. High Street, Denver, CO 80208, USA
e-mail: heather.taussig@du.edu

© Springer Science+Business Media New York 2016
M.R. Korin (ed.), *Health Promotion for Children and Adolescents*,
DOI 10.1007/978-1-4899-7711-3_18

who are licensed and supervised by child welfare agencies), *kinship care* (i.e., children cared for in private homes by relatives who are approved and supervised by child welfare agencies), *residential treatment* (i.e., children cared for by nonrelative professional staff in milieu settings typically designed for the treatment of emotional and behavioral difficulties), and temporary placements, such as emergency shelters, crisis centers, and psychiatric hospitals.

18.1.1   Prevalence and Characteristics of Children and Adolescents in Foster Care

The Adoption and Foster Care Analysis and Reporting System (AFCARS) of the U.S. Department of Health and Human Services, Children's Bureau Administration on Children, Youth, and Families collects annual data from all 50 states on children placed in foster care. The most recent statistics revealed that over 400,000 children and adolescents were in foster care on the last day of the 2013 fiscal year (US DHHS, 2014). Forty-three percent were 4 years old or less, 32 % were 5–12 years old, 25 % were 13–18 years old, and less than 1 % were 19–20 years old. The median age of children entering foster care was 6.4 years, and the median age of children exiting foster care was 8.1 years. A little over half of the children in foster care were male, with 42 % identified as White, 24 % as African-American, 22 % as Hispanic (of any race), 6 % as two or more races, and less than 3 % as American Indian/ Alaskan Native or Asian.

Statistics on the reasons children enter foster care come from the National Survey of Child and Adolescent Well-Being (NSCAW), which is a nationally representative longitudinal study of over 6200 children who had contact with the child welfare system (2007). Caseworkers reported that neglect was the primary cause for placement for over half of the youth, followed by physical abuse, sexual abuse, and other forms of abuse or neglect (e.g., abandonment, emotional abuse). Less than one-tenth of children were placed due to reasons other than maltreatment. These percentages represent the most serious form of maltreatment reported, but of note is that 41 % of youth in foster care experience more than one type of maltreatment (NSCAW).

18.1.2   Foster Care Placement Types and Length of Stay

According to the 2013 AFCARS report, nearly half of children were living in non-relative foster care, more than a quarter were living in kinship care, 15 % were living in an institution or group home, and 5 % or fewer were in a pre-adoptive home, supervised independent living program, or trial home visit. One percent was categorized in the report as having runaway. The average length of stay in foster care has declined from over 30 months in 2002 to about 22 months in 2012. These declines were evident among all racial/ethnic groups over this period (US DHHS, 2013).

While in care, many children experience multiple placements. Data from Chapin Hall's Center for State Child Welfare Data indicate that of school-aged youth who entered foster care in 2005–2009, nearly 60% had experienced two or more placements by the end of 2011, including 10% who had experienced six or more placements (National Working Group on Foster Care and Education, 2014). About half of the children who exited foster care in 2012 were reunited with their biological families (US DHHS, 2013).

18.1.3   Service Costs and Utilization

The United States spends close to $30 billion in federal, state, and local funds annually on child welfare services (DeVooght, Fletcher, Vaughn, & Cooper, 2012), while an estimated $9 billion is spent on providing placement and support services to children in foster care (Bess, Andrews, Jantz, Russell, & Geen, 2002). Due to the overrepresentation of foster youth in other service systems, substantial additional costs are incurred. For example, among children on Medicaid, young children in foster care had twice as many outpatient medical visits as children who were not in foster care, while older children (ages 6–11) in foster care spent, on average, 15 more days in inpatient settings than children who were not in foster care (SAMHSA, 2013). Similarly, in regard to inpatient mental health services, adolescents in foster care had an average length of stay that was 30 days longer than it was for adolescents who were not in foster care; for substance abuse stays, it was 60 days longer (SAMHSA, 2013).

Despite the high rates of service utilization, many children are left in need of physical or mental health services or receive services that are not beneficial. Although caseworkers report that more than half of youth in foster care would benefit from mental health services, only a quarter receive them (Bellamy et al., 2010). Furthermore, a study using NSCAW data found that foster children who received traditional mental health services did not evidence better outcomes; in fact, they demonstrated more mental health problems than foster children who did not receive such services (McCrae, Barth, & Guo, 2010). Bellamy and colleagues concluded after finding no benefit of treatments for children in long-term foster care that youth were receiving "untested treatments with questionable effectiveness" (2010, p. 474). As such, a major focus of later sections of this chapter is to review the challenge and promise of interventions for foster youth.

18.2   Functioning of Children and Adolescents in Foster Care

Children and adolescents placed in foster care have high rates of physical, emotional, and behavioral problems, likely due to many risk factors including adverse prenatal conditions, abuse and neglect, disrupted attachments, exposure to substance use and violence in their homes and communities, disruptions in living situations, and school and community transitions (Felitti et al., 1998; Garland, Hough, McCabe, Yeh, Wood, & Aarons, 2001, Garrido, Culhane, Petrenko, & Taussig, 2011a, 2011b; Garrido, Culhane, Raviv, & Taussig, 2010; Jouriles, Garrido, Rosenfield, & McDonald, 2009). Such disruptions may increase children's vulnerability to deleterious cascading problems. Without access to appropriate resources (internal and external), children are less likely to successfully cope with the many stressors associated with placement in foster care and the likelihood of negative physical, emotional, educational, and behavioral consequences increases.

18.2.1   Physical Health Problems

Few children enter foster care having regularly seen a medical doctor or dentist, and many present with co-occurring problems. Between 45 and 87 % of children placed in foster care have one or more chronic illness (Woods, Farineau, & McWey, 2012). High rates of untreated acute conditions, poor nutrition, and inadequate immunization coverage are also observed (Hansen, Mawjee, Barton, Metcalf, & Joye, 2004; Kools & Kennedy, 2003; Simms, Dubowitz, & Szilagyi, 2000). For example, the National Survey of Child and Adolescent Well-Being II study (NSCAW II), which is a nationally representative longitudinal study of over 5800 children ranging from birth to 17.5 years old, found that foster children had higher rates of asthma as compared to national norms (Casanueva, Ringeisen, Wilson, Smith, & Dolan, 2011). According to Medicaid claims, young children in foster care have a much higher prevalence of disorders of the teeth and jaw, whereas eye and dental problems are overrepresented among adolescents in foster care (SAMHSA, 2013).

18.2.2   Developmental, Cognitive, and Academic Problems

Foster children experience deficits in developmental and neurocognitive functioning, including poorer visuospatial processing, poorer memory skills, lower scores on intelligence tests, and less developed language capacities in comparison to children reared in biological, non-maltreating families (Leslie et al., 2005; Pears & Fisher, 2005). Early cognitive development was assessed as part of the battery of assessments within the NSCAW II study. Over half of toddlers were designated high risk for developmental delays and neurological impairments, especially in regard to poor reasoning skills and perception. Assessments of language development for children less than 5 years old indicated that 26 % scored two or more standard deviations below the normative mean for total language, 25 % for expression communication, and 18 % for auditory comprehension (Casanueva et al., 2011).

Once children reach school age, many struggle to achieve academically, which may be a result of high absenteeism prior to placement, multiple changes in schools, and/or cognitive and learning problems. An estimated 56–75% of children change schools when first entering foster care and over one-third experience five or more school changes (National Working Group on Foster Care and Education, 2014). This instability may diminish youths' abilities to succeed. Approximately 20–40% of foster youth are in special education classes (Scherr, 2007), 10–24% have repeated a grade (NCSAW, 2007), and only 50% complete high school (Wertheimer, 2002; Wolanin, 2005). Despite high rates of educational service utilization, 84% of preadolescent foster children who received recommendations for educational services had not received them 1 year later (Petrenko, Culhane, Garrido, & Taussig, 2011). Older youth in foster care are also twice as likely to receive an out-of-school suspension and three times more likely to be expelled than other students (National Working Group on Foster Care and Education, 2014).

18.2.3   Emotional and Behavioral Health Problems

Children entering foster care are significantly more likely to evidence emotional and behavioral problems than children who are not in foster care. Among children on Medicaid, nearly half of children in foster care were diagnosed with a mental health disorder, compared with 11% of children not in foster care; mood, anxiety, and adjustment disorders were 2–3 times higher for foster youth than non-foster youth (SAMHSA, 2013). In comparison to national norms, older adolescents and young adults in foster care report significantly higher scores on self-report mental health inventories (including those that measure symptoms of Conduct Disorder, Major Depressive Disorder, Attention Deficit and Hyperactivity Disorder, and Posttraumatic Stress Disorder), and half report receiving mental health services within the past year (Courtney, Piliavin, Grogan-Kaylor, & Nesmith, 2001; McMillen et al., 2005; Shin, 2005).

In addition to mental health problems, adolescents in foster care demonstrate high engagement in health-risking behaviors. A study of 17- and 18-year-olds in foster care found that 71% had committed a delinquent act (Courtney et al., 2001), while another study found that 2% of foster youth run away from placements each year, placing them at an increased risk for delinquent behavior, substance use, victimization, and long-term homelessness (Lin, 2012). Estimates of the degree to which youth are using substances indicate that nearly one in ten foster youth meets diagnostic criteria for drug dependence (Pilowsky & Wu, 2006). Several studies have also indicated high rates of risky sexual behavior and associated problems, including low contraceptive use and high pregnancy rates (Carpenter, Clyman, Davidson, & Steiner, 2001; Oshima, Narendorf, & McMillen, 2013; Risley-Curtiss, 1997). Finally, children in foster care have high rates of self-destructive behaviors and suicidal ideation and attempts (Anderson, 2011; Katz et al., 2011; Pilowsky & Wu, 2006). In fact, a recent study found that the prevalence of suicidality among children (ages 9–11) was 26 % (Taussig, Harpin, & Maguire, 2014).

18.3 Emancipated Young Adults

Approximately 23,000 adolescents "age out" or emancipate from foster care each year (US DHHS, 2013). Emancipated young adults experience high rates of physical, social, emotional, and behavior problems (Ahrens et al., 2010, Courtney & Dworsky, 2006; Courtney & Heuring, 2005; Garland et al., 2001; Taussig & Culhane, 2005). In addition to higher rates of psychosocial dysfunction, these young adults are at high risk for unemployment, homelessness, receipt of public assistance, incarceration, substance dependence, early childbearing, and significant mental health problems (Courtney et al., 2011). Despite the fact that 84 % of older youth in foster care have an interest in going to college, only 2–9 % attain a Bachelor's degree (National Working Group on Foster Care and Education, 2014). Without intervention, many young adults formerly in foster care will struggle to live stable, successful lives.

18.4 Protective Factors for Children and Adolescents in Foster Care

Despite the recent focus on promoting child well-being within the child welfare system, much of the research and practice in this area is concentrated on reducing vulnerability and risk. An exception to this is a recent report by the Administration for Children, Youth, and Families which examined protective factors for a number of children and adolescent populations, including youth in, or transitioning out of, foster care (Development Services Group, Inc., 2013). The report states, "ACYF's decision to examine protective factors for children and youth considered to be in-risk is an important step in understanding and promoting the well-being in young people" (p. 3). Although there is significant literature citing the importance of identifying protective factors for *at-risk* groups (e.g., Botvin & Griffin, 2004; Catalano, 2007; Hawkins, 2006), far less is known about protective factors for *in-risk* children (i.e., those already exposed to adversity;Development Services Group, Inc., 2013).

One way to conceptualize protective factors is through the lens of positive youth development (PYD). PYD is relatively new approach to health promotion that rejects deficit models focused on reducing undesirable behaviors and focuses instead on promotion of health across multiple domains (physical, intellectual, social, and emotional). Programs developed within this framework are designed to foster the development of skills and competencies within multiple contexts (individual, family, school, and community) in order to help youth chart a future that will make them healthy, productive citizens (Birkhead, Riser, Mesler, Tallon, & Klein,

2006; Gavin, Catalano, & Markham, 2010). It is hypothesized that the promotion of positive development will naturally lead to reductions in problem behaviors and may also buffer high-risk youth from the impact of prior adversities, such as maltreatment, exposure to violence, and chronic instability (Bernat & Resnick, 2006; Lerner, Almerigi, Theokas, & Lerner, 2005).

Because PYD programs are more likely to be efficacious when they are based on well-specified models (Catalano et al., 2002; Durlak, Weissberg, & Pachan, 2010), it is critical to know which protective factors are most salient among the unique population of youth in, and transitioning out of, foster care. The 2013 ACFY report reviewed evidence from the extant literature, including cross-sectional, longitudinal, and intervention studies, to identify protective factors for children in foster care at the individual, relationship, and community levels. Similar to the individual developmental assets identified by many general PYD programs, the report revealed evidence for the protective role of emotional and behavioral self-regulation, relational skills (e.g., ability to interact with foster parents, teachers, and positive peers), and academic skills in promoting positive outcomes. At the relationship level, living with kin, having relationships with caring adults, and living with competent caregivers (i.e., caregivers who use positive parenting practices) were identified as important protective factors. Finally, community-level factors including a positive school environment, a stable living situation, and support for the development of independent living skills were highlighted.

18.5 Interventions for Children and Adolescents in Foster Care

The remainder of the chapter focuses on prevention and intervention efforts for children and adolescents in foster care. Prior to reviewing programs with some evidence of efficacy or effectiveness within this population, we highlight some common challenges to receiving adequate care that partially explain the dearth of evidence-based programs for this population.

18.5.1 Barriers to Receiving Adequate Physical and Mental Health Care

1. **Consent and confidentiality issues**. Because foster youth can change placements and custody frequently, it can be difficult for providers to know who has the legal authority to consent to services. States also differ on the age of consent and who can receive results of testing or procedures. Additionally, services are typically provided in the context of an open child welfare case in which permanency determinations are being made. This may, in turn, impact youths' and families' willingness to disclose candid information.

2. **Incomplete or inaccurate health histories**. Demographic and other identifying information (e.g., names) may be incorrect or may change due to adoption. It may also be difficult to identify previous providers due to placement changes and inadequate documentation. Furthermore, medical and immunization records are often incomplete or missing. If medications are not tracked from placement to placement, youth may inappropriately discontinue or skip medication.

3. **Screening challenges**. Determining who, and when, to screen can be challenging. Should all children entering foster care be screened? Only those exhibiting behavioral problems? Those with documented physical concerns? Should screenings be done when the child first enters care? After each placement? Furthermore, due to a history of trauma, youth in foster care may be especially sensitive to painful or invasive screening procedures such as blood draws or pelvic examinations.

4. **Diagnostic challenges**. Because youth in foster care have often experienced early, chronic trauma, there is an increased risk that they will develop a profile called "complex trauma." This profile is characterized by a constellation of difficulties including significant problems in the formation and maintenance of attachments and relationships with adults and peers, dysregulation of emotions and behaviors, poor self-concept, and cognitive difficulties (Cook et al., 2005). In the absence of a diagnosis that encompasses all these areas of impairment, children often receive multiple other diagnoses (e.g., Attention Deficit Hyperactivity Disorder, Oppositional Defiant Disorder, Major Depressive Disorder), making it difficult to find appropriate services.

5. **Multiple system issues**. Coordinating services for youth involved in multiple systems (i.e., child welfare, juvenile justice, school) can be challenging. Providers and services may change abruptly due to placement changes or for legal reasons. The fragmentation of these systems may result in children receiving no, inappropriate, or duplicate services.

6. **Challenges for substitute caregivers**. The demands on substitute caregivers (i.e., foster parents and kinship providers) are often great, as they typically care for multiple children and are responsible for providing transportation and managing schedules for various activities (e.g., visitation with biological parents, therapy appointments, medical visits). Some caregivers may also be resistant to services focused on their parenting practices. Thus, it is particularly important for these interventions to establish the importance of parenting skills for child well-being, even in the context of adoption or reunification.

7. **Sociodemographic, maltreatment, and placement characteristics**. The lack of contextual and cultural sensitivity in service settings may pose an additional barrier. Receipt of mental health services for children in foster care (after controlling for need for services) differs by sociodemographic, maltreatment, and placement characteristics. Studies have found that ethnic minority children and children in kinship care are less likely to receive services. Some studies have shown that sexually and physically abused youth are more likely to receive services than children who have experienced neglect but not abuse (Burns et al., 2004; Garland et al., 1996, 2001; Leslie, Landsverk, Ezzet-Lofstrom, Tschann, Slymen, & Garland, 2000).

18.5.2   Psychosocial Interventions for Youth in Foster Care

Successful interventions must be grounded in theory and research, be effective in recruiting and retaining youth and families, and be contextually sensitive. Because concerning evidence has emerged of the ineffectiveness of mental health services "as usual" for children within foster care (Bellamy et al., 2010), it is imperative that children are screened and referred to programs specifically designed or adapted for youth in foster care. Below, we briefly review interventions above and beyond placement in foster care that promote healthy development. This is not meant to be an exhaustive list, and our focus is on those that have been rigorously tested.

18.5.2.1   Early Childhood

Most early childhood interventions are designed to encourage the formation of secure, positive relationships with caregivers and emotional and behavioral regulation skills, two important developmental tasks for infants and young children in foster care. One example of an intervention designed specifically for children in foster care is the *Attachment and Biobehavioral Catch-up* (ABC) program—a 10-session, manualized in-home intervention designed to help foster caregivers provide sensitive care to maltreated infants and toddlers (aged 0–3) in order to promote children's attachment and self-regulation skills. The intervention focuses on helping caregivers provide nurturing care, learn to follow the child's lead, appreciate the value of affectionate touch, and create conditions that encourage emotional expression and teach emotion recognition to their children. Results of two randomized controlled trials demonstrated significant improvements in children's cortisol regulation, indicating decreases of this stress hormone from pre- to post-intervention (Dozier et al., 2006; Dozier, Peloso, Lewis, Laurenceau, & Levine, 2008). An independent randomized controlled trial found decreases in children's internalizing and externalizing problems and parent's negative parenting attitudes and stress (Sprang, 2009). Another study found that children in the intervention demonstrated more cognitive flexibility and theory of mind skills approximately 2 years post-intervention, relative to foster children in the control condition (Lewis-Morrarty, Dozier, Bernard, Terracciano, & Moore, 2012).

The *Multidimensional Treatment Foster Care for Preschoolers* (MTFC-P) program incorporates several components of the *Multidimensional Treatment Foster Care for Adolescents* (MTFC-A) program initially designed for youth with chronic delinquency who were referred for foster care due to their behavioral difficulties. MTFC-A core components include placing children in specialized foster homes with caregivers who are trained to provide intense supervision and monitoring, as well as consistent limit setting within a well-defined behavior management program. Caregivers also receive daily phone calls that provide supervision and support and also allow for ongoing data collection (Chamberlain & Reid, 1998; Leve, Chamberlain, & Reid, 2005). The MTFC-P program includes these parent training and support components, but adds a weekly playgroup session for the children. This strength-based intervention has demonstrated better attachment outcomes among treatment group participants, and has improved children's ability to respond to stress, as measured by diurnal cortisol (Fisher, Burraston, & Pears, 2005; Fisher & Kim, 2007; Fisher, Stoolmiller, Gunnar, & Burraston, 2007).

Although not originally designed for children in foster care, *Parent–child Interaction Therapy* (PCIT) has undergone testing with foster families. PCIT was developed for children ages 2–7 with externalizing behavior problems, and includes a phase focused on enhancing the parent–child interactions and a second phase focused on improving child functioning (Eyberg & Robinson, 1982; Hembree-Kigin & McNeil, 1995). Parents are coached by therapists through an observation room to practice specific skills of communication and behavior management with their child. In a study seeking to determine its effectiveness for foster parents and their foster children as compared to a group of non-abusive biological families, strong treatment effects were found on measures of parent and child functioning for both groups, suggesting that PCIT had beneficial effects for foster families (Timmer, Urquiza, & Zebell, 2006).

Another effective intervention that has been adapted for children in foster care is the *Incredible Years* (IY) program, a parent training intervention designed to promote emotional and social competence and to prevent, reduce, and treat aggression and emotional problems in young children 0–12 years old. IY has demonstrated positive impacts on strengthening parental behavior management skills and reducing children's behavior problems in non-maltreated youth (Webster-Stratton, 1984) and has also shown positive results when implemented with maltreating parents whose children were not placed in foster care (Letarte et al., 2010). An adaptation of the IY intervention was conducted to meet the needs of a foster care population (Linares, Montalto, Li, & Oza, 2006). The first component involves 4–7 foster parents and biological parents pairs participated together in a small group. The second component involves a newly created co-parenting curriculum aimed at individual families comprising the child, foster parent, and biological parent. The randomized trial of the IY adaptation indicated improved positive parenting practices and collaborative co-parenting among foster and biological parents in the intervention group, but no differences in child internalizing or externalizing behavior problems between groups. IY has also been implemented and tested in Wales as part of initial training for foster caregivers. Results of the small-scale study showed a significant reduction in child behavior problems and improvement in caregivers' depression levels for intervention families at follow-up, compared with control (Bywater et al., 2011).

18.5.2.2 Middle Childhood and Adolescence

Several interventions for foster children and families have been identified as having some evidence of effectiveness or efficacy related to child well-being (Goldman et al., 2013; Leve et al., 2012). Two of the interventions were developed by researchers at the Oregon Social Learning Center and are similar to, or have been adapted from, MTFC-A. First, *Keeping Foster Parents Trained and Supported* (KEEP), an intervention for foster caregivers who had a new child placed in their care, was tested in a randomized controlled trial. Similar to MTFC-A, the chief components of the intervention include parent training in behavior management and ongoing parent support. The intervention demonstrated a reduction in child behavior problems (Chamberlain et al., 2008; Price, Chamberlain, Landsverk, Reid, Leve, & Laurent, 2008). The most recent adaptation of MTFC-A for children in foster care due to maltreatment is *Middle School Success* (MSS) for girls entering 6th grade. As part of MSS, parents receive group-based training in behavior management techniques, while youth participate in group sessions prior to the start of middle school and then individual coaching sessions throughout the school year. Intervention participants evidenced fewer mental health and behavior problems, less substance use, and greater prosocial behaviors up to 3 years post-baseline (Kim & Leve, 2011; Smith et al., 2011).

The *Fostering Healthy Futures* program is a preventive intervention for maltreated youth, ages 9–11, who entered foster care over the prior year. The intervention provides one-on-one mentoring and skills groups to children over a 30-week period. Mentoring is provided by graduate students in social work and psychology, who spend 3–4 h per week with each child, advocate for services to ameliorate challenges, and connect them with resources and activities to build on their strengths. Children attend a 1.5-h manualized weekly skills group that consists of sessions on social skills, healthy coping strategies, and resisting peer pressure for risky behaviors. Mentors work with children to generalize these skills in real-world settings. A randomized controlled trial has demonstrated positive outcomes, including: (1) an improvement in quality of life immediately post-intervention, (2) a reduction in mental health symptoms (including trauma symptoms) according to youth, their caregivers, and teachers 6-months post-intervention, (3) a reduction in mental health service utilization 6-months post-intervention, and (4) fewer placements changes, fewer placements in residential treatment centers, and increased permanency (Taussig et al., 2007, 2012; Taussig & Culhane, 2010).

Another intervention designed specifically for children in foster care is the *Fostering Individualized Assistance Program*, an intervention designed to improve permanency, placement stability, and behavioral and emotional adjustment of 7- to 15-year-old children. The intervention includes: (1) a comprehensive strengths-based assessment conducted by a family specialist; (2) life-domain planning conducted by a team of adults in the child's life who met regularly to create and evaluate plans to address the child's needs; (3) clinical case management that included short-term home-based counseling and advocacy; and (4) linkage to follow-along supports and services. Results of a randomized controlled trial demonstrated improvements in caregiver-reported behavior problems, attention problems, and symptoms of withdrawal in the short term, and improvements in externalizing and delinquent behaviors for males, less runaway behavior and fewer days on the run or incarcerated for older youth, as well as greater permanency, an average of 3.5 years post-study entry (Clark et al., 1994, 1998).

Finally, *Trauma-Focused Cognitive Behavioral Therapy* (TF-CBT) is an evidence-based intervention for children exposed to trauma designed to address behavior problems and trauma-related symptoms (Cohen, Mannarino, & Staron, 2006). TF-CBT includes 12–24 individual sessions with non-offending caregivers and children and conjoint child-caregiver sessions focused on psychoeducation, skill building, exposure, and cognitions. Several studies have evaluated and supported its efficacy for children in the general population (Cohen, Deblinger, Mannarino, & Steer, 2004; Cohen, Mannarino, & Knudsen, 2005; Cohen, Mannarino, & Murray, 2011), while a recent open trial examining TF-CBT with children in foster care found that treatment completion was linked to foster parent involvement (Weiner, Schneider, & Lyons, 2009). Only those families who participated in 11 or more sessions demonstrated significant reductions in posttraumatic stress symptoms. Given the importance of engaging foster families in the program, a recent randomized controlled trial tested the efficacy of TF-CBT plus evidence-based engagement strategies with 47 foster families (Dorsey, Pullmann, Berliner, Koschmann, McKay, & Deblinger, 2014). Families who participated in TF-CBT plus evidence-based engagement strategies were less likely to drop out of treatment, as compared to families who participated in TF-CBT, but clinical outcomes did not differ by study condition.

Although mental health is the domain most frequently discussed and researched within the realm of well-being for youth in foster care, educational interventions are sorely needed. Children in foster care have high rates of academic failure, grade retention, and dropout. Despite the need for intervention, a recent systematic review of the literature on promoting success in school among foster children found no study robust enough to provide evidence of effectiveness (Liabo, Gray, & Mulcahy, 2013). One quasi-experimental study was conducted in which an educational liaison was used, but the results were equivocal (Zetlin, Weinberg, & Kimm, 2004).]

18.5.3 *Physical Health Assessments and Interventions*

The American Academy of Pediatrics (AAP, 2005) and the Child Welfare League of America (CWLA, 2007) have published guidelines regarding the need for comprehensive physical health assessments, appropriate referrals, and case management. Unlike the psychosocial interventions reviewed above, however, there have not been rigorous trials of physical health interventions for children in foster care, likely due to ethical concerns. One quasi-experimental study found that young adults who had received "enhanced" foster care (consisting of better-trained caseworkers) when they were adolescents had fewer mental disorders, ulcers, and cardiometabolic disorders (but more respiratory disorders) than did young adults in traditional foster care (Kessler et al., 2008). Currently "best practice" for addressing physical health concerns among youth in foster care includes recognition of their special health care needs and following the published guidelines from AAP and CWLA regarding the assessment and treatment of children in foster care. There is also a growing focus on the health care needs, especially continuity of care, of young adults emancipating from care. Beginning in 2014, the Affordable Care Act requires all states to provide Medicaid coverage for youth who emancipate from foster care at age 18 or older. This coverage lasts until the age of 26, but experts have concerns about young adults navigating the enrollment procedures (English, Scott, & Park, 2014).

18.6   Conclusion

As evidenced by the research, children and adolescents in foster care experience high rates of physical, emotional, behavioral, and educational difficulties. Although some efficacious interventions exist, significant gaps exist when examining the array of effective programming available for this special-needs population. First, trials of interventions to promote positive educational and physical health outcomes are nonexistent. Most of the interventions reviewed in this chapter target only a narrow age range, and their efficacy for other ages is unknown. In addition, few interventions have demonstrated long-term outcomes. The few successful interventions that do promote well-being in foster youth do not represent a menu of options for child welfare workers that would be near comprehensive enough to cover the great demand for evidence-based programming for their heterogeneous clients. As such, the promotion of health among children and adolescents in foster care is reliant on the field's continued development, testing, and implementation of theoretically grounded and contextually sensitive interventions.

References

Administration on Children, Youth and Families [ACYF], U.S. Department of Health and Human Services. (2012). *Information Memorandum: Promoting social and emotional well-being for children and youth receiving Child Welfare services* (ACYF-CB-IM-12-04). Washington, DC.

Ahrens, K. R., Richardson, L. P., Courtney, M. E., McCarty, C., Simoni, J., & Katon, W. (2010). Laboratory-diagnosed sexually transmitted infections in former foster youth compared with peers. *Pediatrics, 126*(1), e97–e103.

American Academy of Pediatrics, Task Force on Health Care for Children in Foster Care. (2005). *Fostering health: Health care for children and adolescents in foster care* (2nd ed.). Retrieved from http://www.aap.org/en-us/advocacy-and-policy/aap-health-initiatives/healthy-foster-care-america/Pages/Fostering-Health.aspx

Anderson, H. D. (2011). Suicide ideation, depressive symptoms, and out-of-home placement among youth in the U.S. child welfare system. *Journal of Clinical Child & Adolescent Psychology, 40*, 790–796.

Bellamy, J. L., Gopalan, G., & Traube, D. E. (2010). A national study of the impact of outpatient mental health services for children in long-term foster care. *Clinical Child Psychology and Psychiatry, 15*(4), 467–479.

Bernat, D. H., & Resnick, M. D. (2006). Healthy youth development: Science and strategies. *Journal of Public Health Management and Practice, 12*, S10–S16.

Bess, R., Andrews, C., Jantz, A., Russell, V., & Geen, R. (2002). *The cost of protecting vulnerable children III: What factors affect states' fiscal decisions?* Washington, DC: The Urban Institute.

Birkhead, G. S., Riser, M. H., Mesler, K., Tallon, T. C., & Klein, S. J. (2006). Youth development is a public health approach. *Journal of Public Health Management and Practice, 12*, S1–S3.

Botvin, G. J., & Griffin, K. W. (2004). Life skills training: Empirical findings and future directions. *The Journal of Primary Prevention, 25*(2), 211–232.

Burns, B. J., Phillips, S. D., Wagner, H. R., Barth, R. P., Kolko, D. J., Campbell, Y., & Landsverk, J. (2004). Mental health need and access to mental health services by youths involved with child welfare: A national survey. *Journal of the American Academy of Child and Adolescent Psychiatry, 43*(8), 960–970.

Bywater, T. T., Hutchings, J. J., Linck, P. P., Whitaker, C. C., Daley, D. D., Yeo, S. T., & Edwards, R. T. (2011). Incredible Years parent training support for foster carers in Wales: A multi-centre feasibility study. *Child Care, Health and Development, 37*, 233–243.

Carpenter, S. C., Clyman, R. B., Davidson, A. J., & Steiner, J. F. (2001). The association of foster care or kinship care with adolescent sexual behavior and first pregnancy. *Pediatrics, 108*(3), e46–e46.

Casanueva, C., Ringeisen, H., Wilson, E., Smith, K., & Dolan, M. (2011). *NSCAW II baseline report: Child well-being* (OPRE Report #2011-27b). Washington, DC: Office of Planning, Research and Evaluation, Administration for Children and Families, U.S. Department of Health and Human Services.

Catalano, R. F., Berglund, M. L., Ryan, J. A., Lonczak, H. S., & Hawkins, J. D. (2002). Positive youth development in the United States: Research findings on evaluations of positive youth development programs. *Prevention & Treatment, 5*(1), 15a.

Catalano, R. F. (2007). Prevention is a sound public and private investment. *Criminology and Public Policy, 6*(3), 377–397.

Substance Abuse and Mental Health Services Administration [SAMHSA]. (2013). *Diagnoses and health care utilization of children who are in foster care and covered by Medicaid.* HHS Publication No. (SMA) 13-4804. Rockville, MD: Center for Mental Health Services and Center for Substance Abuse Treatment.

Chamberlain, P., Price, J., Leve, L. D., Laurent, H., Landsverk, J. A., & Reid, J. B. (2008). Prevention of behavior problems for children in foster care: Outcomes and mediation effects. *Prevention Science, 9*(1), 17–27.

Chamberlain, P., & Reid, J. B. (1998). Comparison of two community alternatives to incarceration for chronic juvenile offenders. *Journal of Consulting and Clinical Psychology, 66*(4), 624–633.

Clark, H. B., Prange, M. E., Lee, B., Boyd, L. A., McDonald, B. A., & Stewart, E. S. (1994). Improving adjustment outcomes for foster children with emotional and behavioral disorders: Early findings from a controlled study on individualized services. *Journal of Emotional and Behavioral Disorders, 2*(4), 207–218.

Clark, H. B., Prange, M. E., Lee, B., Stewart, E. S., McDonald, B. B., & Boyd, L. A. (1998). An individualized wraparound process for children in foster care with emotional/behavioral disturbances: Follow-up findings and implications from a controlled study. In M. H. Epstein, K. Kutash, & A. Duchnowski (Eds.), *Outcomes for children and youth with emotional and behavioral disorders and their families: Programs and evaluation best practices* (pp. 513–542). Austin, TX: Pro-ED, Inc.

Cohen, J. A., Deblinger, E., Mannarino, A. P., & Steer, R. A. (2004). A multisite, randomized controlled trial for children with sexual abuse-related PTSD symptoms. *Journal of the American Academy of Child and Adolescent Psychiatry, 43*(4), 393–402.

Cohen, J. A., Mannarino, A. P., & Knudsen, K. (2005). Treating sexually abused children: 1 year follow-up of a randomized controlled trial. *Child Abuse & Neglect, 29*(2), 135–145.

Cohen, J. A., Mannarino, A. P., & Murray, L. K. (2011). Trauma-focused CBT for youth who experience ongoing traumas. *Child Abuse & Neglect, 35*(8), 637–646.

Cohen, J. A., Mannarino, A. P., & Staron, V. R. (2006). A pilot study of modified cognitive-behavioral therapy for childhood traumatic grief (CBT-CTG). *Journal of the American Academy of Child & Adolescent Psychiatry, 45*(12), 1465–1473.

Cook, A., Spinazzola, J., Ford, J., Lanktree, C., Blaustein, M., Cloitre, M., … van der Kolk, B. (2005). Complex trauma in children and adolescents. *Psychiatric Annals, 35*(5), 390–398.

Courtney, M. E., & Dworsky, A. (2006). Early outcomes for young adults transitioning from out-of-home care in the USA. *Child & Family Social Work, 11*(3), 209–219.

Courtney, M. E., Dworsky, A., Brown, A., Cary, C., Love, K., & Vorhies, V. (2011). *Midwest evaluation of the adult functioning of former foster youth: Outcomes at age 26*. Chicago, IL: Chapin Hall at the University of Chicago.

Courtney, M. E., & Heuring, D. (2005). The transition to adulthood for youth 'aging out' of the foster care system. In D. Osgood, E. Foster, C. Flanagan, & G. R. Ruth (Eds.), *On your own without a net: The transition to adulthood for vulnerable populations* (pp. 27–67). Chicago, IL: University of Chicago Press.

Courtney, M. E., Piliavin, I., Grogan-Kaylor, A., & Nesmith, A. (2001). Foster youth transitions to adulthood: A longitudinal view of youth leaving care. *Child Welfare, 80*(6), 685–717.

Development Services Group. (2013). Protective factors for populations served by the Administration on Children, Youth, and Families: A Literature review and theoretical framework. Administration on Children, Youth, and Families Research Report.

DeVooght, K., Fletcher, M., Vaughn, B., & Cooper, H. (2012). *Federal, state, and local spending to address child abuse and neglect in SFYs 2008 and 2010*. Baltimore, MD: Annie E. Casey Foundation.

Dorsey, S., Pullmann, M. D., Berliner, L., Koschmann, E., McKay, M., & Deblinger, E. (2014). Engaging foster parents in treatment: A randomized trial of supplementing Trauma-focused Cognitive Behavioral Therapy with evidence-based engagement strategies. *Child Abuse & Neglect, 38*, 1508–1520. doi:10.1016/j.chiabu.2014.03.020.

Dozier, M., Peloso, E., Lewis, E., Laurenceau, J. P., & Levine, S. (2008). Effects of an attachment-based intervention on the cortisol production of infants and toddlers in foster care. *Development and Psychopathology, 20*(03), 845–859.

Dozier, M., Peloso, E., Lindhiem, O., Gordon, M. K., Manni, M., Sepulveda, S., … Levine, S. (2006). Developing evidence-based interventions for foster children: An example of a randomized clinical trial with infants and toddlers. *Journal of Social Issues, 62*, 767–785.

Durlak, J. A., Weissberg, R. P., & Pachan, M. (2010). A meta-analysis of after-school programs that seek to promote personal and social skills in children and adolescents. *American Journal of Community Psychology, 45*(3–4), 294–309.

English, A., Scott, J., & Park, M. J. (2014). *Fact Sheet: Impact of the ACA on vulnerable youth*. Chapel Hill, NC: Center for Adolescent Health & The Law; San Francisco, CA: National Adolescent and Young Adult Health Information Center.

Eyberg, S., & Robinson, E. A. (1982). Parent-child interaction training: Effects on family functioning. *Journal of the Clinical Child & Adolescent Psychology, 39*, 1356–1364.

Felitti, V. J., Anda, R. F., Nordenberg, D., Williamson, D. F., Spitz, A. M., Edwards, V., … Marks, J. S. (1998). Relationship of childhood abuse and household dysfunction to many of the leading causes of death in adults: The Adverse Childhood Experiences (ACE) Study. *American Journal of Preventive Medicine, 14*(4), 245–258.

Fisher, P. A., Burraston, B., & Pears, K. (2005). The early intervention foster care program: Permanent placement outcomes from a randomized trial. *Child Maltreatment, 10*, 61–71.

Fisher, P. A., & Kim, H. K. (2007). Intervention effects on foster preschoolers' attachment-related behaviors from a randomized trial. *Prevention Science, 8*(2), 161–170.

Fisher, P. A., Stoolmiller, M., Gunnar, M. R., & Burraston, B. O. (2007). Effects of a therapeutic intervention for foster preschoolers on diurnal cortisol activity. *Psychoneuroendocrinology, 32*(8), 892–905.

Garland, A. F., Hough, R. L., McCabe, K. M., Yeh, M. A. Y., Wood, P. A., & Aarons, G. A. (2001). Prevalence of psychiatric disorders in youths across five sectors of care. *Journal of the American Academy of Child & Adolescent Psychiatry, 40*(4), 409–418.

Garland, A. F., Landsverk, J. L., Hough, R. L., & Ellis-MacLeod, E. (1996). Type of maltreatment as a predictor of mental health service use for children in foster care. *Child Abuse & Neglect, 20*(8), 675–688.

Garrido, E. F., Culhane, S. E., Petrenko, C. L., & Taussig, H. N. (2011a). Psychosocial consequences of intimate partner violence (IPV) exposure in maltreated adolescents: Assessing more than IPV occurrence. *Journal of Family Violence, 26*(7), 511–518.

Garrido, E. F., Culhane, S. E., Petrenko, C. L., & Taussig, H. N. (2011b). Psychosocial consequences of caregiver transitions for maltreated youth entering foster care: The moderating impact of community violence exposure. *American Journal of Orthopsychiatry, 81*(3), 382–389.

Garrido, E. F., Culhane, S. E., Raviv, T., & Taussig, H. N. (2010). Does community violence exposure predict trauma symptoms in a sample of maltreated youth in foster care? *Violence and Victims, 25*(6), 755–769.

Gavin, L. E., Catalano, R. F., & Markham, C. M. (2010). Positive youth development as a strategy to promote adolescent sexual and reproductive health. *Journal of Adolescent Health, 46*(3), S1–S6.

Goldman Fraser, J., Lloyd, S. W., Murphy, R. A., Crowson, M. M., Casanueva, C., Zolotor, A., … Viswanath, M. (2013). *Child exposure to trauma: Comparative effectiveness of interventions addressing maltreatment.* Comparative Effectiveness Review No. 89. (Prepared by the RTI-UNC Evidenced-based Practice Center under Contract No. 290-2007-10056-I). AHRQ Publication No. 13-EHC002-EF. Rockville, MD: Agency for Healthcare Research and Quality. Retrieved from www.effectivehealthcare.ahrq.gov/reports/final.cfm

Child Welfare League of America [CWLA]. (2007). *Standards of excellence: CWLA standards of excellence for health care services for children in out-of-home care.* Washington, DC: Child Welfare League of America.

Hawkins, J. D. (2006). Science, social work, prevention: Finding the intersections. *Social Work Research, 30*(3), 137–152.

Hansen, R. L., Mawjee, F. L., Barton, K., Metcalf, M. B., & Joye, N. R. (2004). Comparing the health status of low-income children in and out of foster care. *Child Welfare, 83*(4), 367–380.

Hembree-Kigin, T., & McNeil, C. (1995). *Parent-child interaction therapy.* New York: Plenum.

Jouriles, E. N., Garrido, E., Rosenfield, D., & McDonald, R. (2009). Experiences of psychological and physical aggression in adolescent romantic relationships: Links to psychological distress. *Child Abuse & Neglect, 33*(7), 451–460.

Katz, L. Y., Au, W., Singal, D., Brownell, M., Roos, N., Martens, P. J., … Sareen, J. (2011). Suicide and suicide attempts in children and adolescents in the child welfare system. *Canadian Medical Association Journal, 183,* 1977–1981.

Kim, H. K., & Leve, L. D. (2011). Substance use and delinquency among middle school girls in foster care: A three-year follow-up of a randomized controlled trial. *Journal of Consulting and Clinical Psychology, 79*(6), 740–750.

Kools, S., & Kennedy, C. (2003). Foster child health and development: Implications for primary care. *Pediatric Nursing, 29*(1), 39–41.

Lerner, R. M., Almerigi, J. B., Theokas, C., & Lerner, J. V. (2005). Positive youth development: A view of the issues. *The Journal of Early Adolescence, 25*(1), 10–16.

Leslie, L. K., Gordon, J. N., Lambros, K., Premji, K., Peoples, J., & Gist, K. (2005). Addressing the developmental and mental health needs of children in foster care. *Journal of Developmental and Behavioral Pediatrics, 26*(2), 140–151.

Leslie, L. K., Landsverk, J., Ezzet-Lofstrom, R., Tschann, J. M., Slymen, D. J., & Garland, A. F. (2000). Children in foster care: Factors influencing outpatient mental health service use. *Child Abuse & Neglect, 24*(4), 465–476.

Letarte, M., Normandeau, S., & Allard, J. (2010). Effectiveness of a parent training program "Incredible Years" in a child protection service. *Child Abuse & Neglect, 34,* 253–261.

Leve, L. D., Chamberlain, P., & Reid, J. B. (2005). Intervention outcomes for girls referred from juvenile justice: Effects on delinquency. *Journal of Consulting and Clinical Psychology, 73*(6), 1181.

Leve, L. D., Harold, G. T., Chamberlain, P., Landsverk, J. A., Fisher, P. A., & Vostanis, P. (2012). Practitioner review: Children in foster care—Vulnerabilities and evidence-based interventions that promote resilience processes. *Journal of Child Psychology and Psychiatry, 53*(12), 1197–1211.

Lewis-Morrarty, E., Dozier, M., Bernard, K., Terracciano, S., & Moore, S. (2012). Cognitive flexibility and theory of mind outcomes among foster children: Preschool follow-up results of a randomized clinical trial. *Journal of Adolescent Health, 51,* S17–S22.

Liabo, K., Gray, K., & Mulcahy, D. (2013). A systematic review of interventions to support looked-after children in school. *Child & Family Social Work, 18*(3), 341–353.

Lin, C. H. (2012). Children who run away from foster care: Who are the children and what are the risk factors? *Children and Youth Services Review, 34*(4), 807–813.

Linares, L. O., Montalto, D., Li, M., & Oza, V. S. (2006). A promising parenting intervention in foster care. *Journal of Consulting and Clinical Psychology, 74*(1), 32–41.

McCrae, J. S., Barth, R. P., & Guo, S. (2010). Changes in maltreated children's emotional–behavioral problems following typically provided mental health services. *American Journal of Orthopsychiatry, 80*(3), 350–361.

McMillen, J. C., Zima, B. T., Scott, L. D., Jr., Auslander, W. F., Munson, M. R., Ollie, M. T., & Spitznagel, E. L. (2005). Prevalence of psychiatric disorders among older youths in the foster care system. *Journal of the American Academy of Child & Adolescent Psychiatry, 44*(1), 88–95.

National Survey of Child and Adolescent Well-Being [NSCAW]. (2007). *Who are the children in foster care? Research brief, findings from the NSCAW study* (NSCAW No. 1). Retrieved from http://www.acf.hhs.gov/sites/default/files/opre/children_fostercare.pdf

National Working Group on Foster Care and Education. (2014). *Fostering success in education: National factsheet on the educational outcomes of children in foster care.* Retrieved from http://www.cacollegepathways.org/sites/default/files/datasheet_jan_2014_update.pdf

Oshima, K. M., Narendorf, S. C., & McMillen, J. C. (2013). Pregnancy risk among older youth transitioning out of foster care. *Children and Youth Services Review, 35*(10), 1760–1765.

Pears, K., & Fisher, P. A. (2005). Developmental, cognitive, and neuropsychological functioning in preschool-aged foster children: Associations with prior maltreatment and placement history. *Journal of Developmental & Behavioral Pediatrics, 26*(2), 112–122.

Petrenko, C. L. M., Culhane, S. E., Garrido, E., F., & Taussig, H. N. (2011). Do youth in out-of-home care receive recommended mental health and educational services following screening evaluations?. *Children and Youth Services Review, 33*(10), 1911–1918.

Pilowsky, D. J., & Wu, L. T. (2006). Psychiatric symptoms and substance use disorders in a nationally representative sample of American adolescents involved with foster care. *Journal of Adolescent Health, 38*(4), 351–358.

Price, J. M., Chamberlain, P., Landsverk, J., Reid, J. B., Leve, L. D., & Laurent, H. (2008). Effects of a foster parent training intervention on placement changes of children in foster care. *Child Maltreatment, 13*(1), 64–75.

Risley-Curtiss, C. (1997). Sexual activity and contraceptive use among children entering out-of-home care. *Child Welfare, 76*(4), 475–499.

Scherr, T. (2007). Educational experiences of children in foster care: Meta-analyses of special education, retention and discipline rates. *School Psychology International, 28*, 419–436.

Shin, S. H. (2005). Need for and actual use of mental health service by adolescents in the child welfare system. *Children and Youth Services Review, 27*(10), 1071–1083.

Simms, M. D., Dubowitz, H., & Szilagyi, M. A. (2000). Health care needs of children in the foster care system. *Pediatrics, 106*(Supple 3), 909–918.

Smith, D. K., Leve, L. D., & Chamberlain, P. (2011). Preventing internalizing and externalizing problems in girls in foster care as they enter middle school: Impact of an intervention. *Prevention Science, 12*(3), 269–277.

Sprang, G. (2009). The efficacy of a relational treatment for maltreated children and their families. *Child and Adolescent Mental Health, 14*(2), 81–88.

Taussig, H. N., & Culhane, S. E. (2005). Foster care as an intervention for abused and neglected children. In *Child victimization: Maltreatment, bulling and dating violence, prevention and intervention* (pp. 1–20).

Taussig, H. N., & Culhane, S. E. (2010). Impact of a mentoring and skills group program on mental health outcomes for maltreated children in foster care. *Archives of Pediatrics & Adolescent Medicine, 164*(8), 739–746.

Taussig, H. N., Culhane, S. E., Garrido, E., & Knudtson, M. D. (2012). RCT of a mentoring and skills group program: Placement and permanency outcomes for foster youth. *Pediatrics, 130*(1), e33–e39.

Taussig, H. N., Culhane, S. E., & Hettleman, D. (2007). Fostering healthy futures: An innovative preventive intervention for preadolescent youth in out-of-home care. *Child Welfare, 86*(5), 113.

Taussig, H. N., Harpin, S. B., & Maguire, S. A. (2014). Suicidality among preadolescent maltreated children in foster care. *Child Maltreatment, 19*(1), 17–26.

Timmer, S. G., Urquiza, A. J., & Zebell, N. (2006). Challenging foster caregiver–maltreated child relationships: The effectiveness of parent–child interaction therapy. *Children and Youth Services Review, 28*(1), 1–19.

United States Department of Health and Human Services [US DHHS], Administration for Children and Families. (2014, July). *The AFCARS report: Preliminary FY 2013 estimates*. Retrieved from http://www.acf.hhs.gov/sites/default/files/cb/afcarsreport21.pdf

Webster-Stratton, C. (1984). Randomized trial of two parent-training programs for families with conduct-disordered children. *Journal of Consulting & Clinical Psychology, 52*, 666–678.

Weiner, D. A., Schneider, A., & Lyons, J. S. (2009). Evidence-based treatments for trauma among culturally diverse foster care youth: Treatment retention and outcomes. *Children and Youth Services Review, 31*, 1199–1205.

Woods, S. B., Farineau, H. M., & McWey, L. M. (2012). Physical health, mental health, and behavior problems among early adolescents in foster care. *Child: Care, Health and Development, 30*, 220–227.

Zetlin, A., Weinberg, L., & Kimm, C. (2004). Improving education outcomes for children in foster care: Intervention by an education liaison. *Journal of Education for Students Placed at Risk, 9*(4), 421–429.

Index

A
Aban Aya Youth Project, 174–175
ABC program. *See Attachment and Biobehavioral Catch-up* (ABC) program
ACE. *See* Adverse childhood experience (ACE)
Adolescent health
  cognitive behavioral therapy, 330
  treatment planning, 331
Adolescents, health promotion, 6–7
Adolescents, substance misuse. *See* Substance misuse prevention
Adoption and Foster Care Analysis and Reporting System (AFCARS), 372
Adoption and Safe Families Act (ASFA), 371
Adverse childhood experience (ACE), 86–88, 244
AFCARS. *See* Adoption and Foster Care Analysis and Reporting System (AFCARS)
Alcohol
  consumption, 222
  effects, 223
  use and abuse, 223
Alcohol-intervention research, 290
American Academy of Pediatrics (AAP), 266
American Community Survey (ACS), 31
American Medical Association (AMA), 277
Anorexia nervosa (AN), 285
Attachment and Biobehavioral Catch-up (ABC) program, 379
Attention-deficit/hyperactivity disorder (ADHD)
  adaptive/maladaptive outcomes, 147
  behavioral/pharmacological interventions, 147
  counseling/psychological and social services, 154
  CSH and MTSS, 153
  developmental psychopathology, 147
  disruptive behaviors, 161
  EBIs, 152
  health consequences and correlates, 148–152
  health risk behaviors, 152
  healthy eating, 156–157
  individual/environmental level, 147
  injury prevention, prosocial relationships and violence, 157–158
  integration, 152
  middle school and adolescence, 149–152
  minimal brain damage, 146
  moral imbecility, 146
  neurodevelopmental disorder, 145
  ODD and CD, 145
  preschool and elementary years, 148–149
  race/ethnicity, 146
  SAMHSA, 154
  school- and clinic-based professionals, 146
  SEL, 156
  self-injury and suicide, 160
  social exclusion, 147
  substance use and sexual risk taking, 158–159
  vertical integration, 153, 154, 161
Attitude–behavior discrepancies, 219

© Springer Science+Business Media New York 2016
M.R. Korin (ed.), *Health Promotion for Children and Adolescents*,
DOI 10.1007/978-1-4899-7711-3

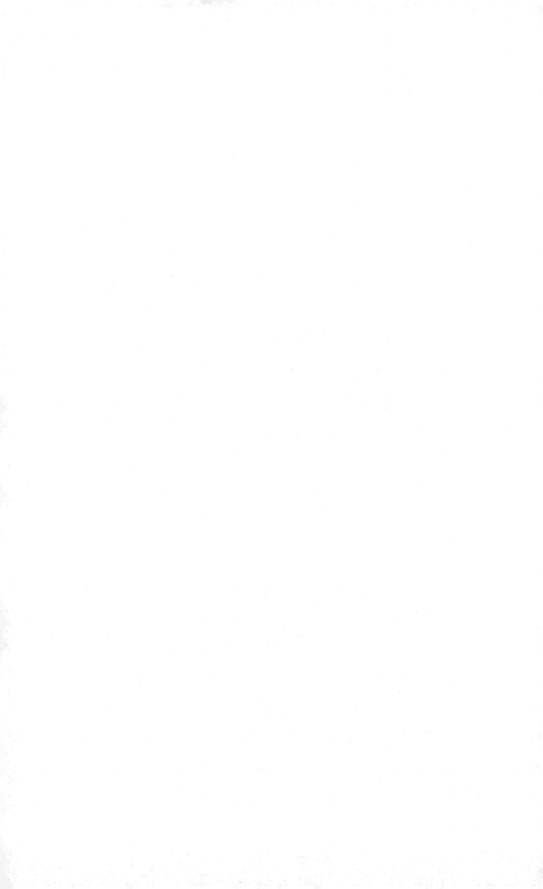

Made in the USA
Monee, IL
05 January 2021

56655666R00227